Noninvasive Mechanical Ventilation

JOHN R. BACH, MD
Professor and Vice Chairman
Department of Physical Medicine and Rehabilitation
Professor of Neurosciences
University of Medicine and Dentistry of New Jersey
New Jersey Medical School

Director of Research and Associate Medical Director
Department of Physical Medicine and Rehabilitation
Medical Director, Center for Ventilator Management
    Alternatives and Pulmonary Rehabilitation
Co-director, UMDNJ-New Jersey Medical School's Jerry
    Lewis Muscular Dystrophy Association Clinic
University Hospital
Newark, New Jersey

HANLEY & BELFUS, INC. / Philadelphia

Publisher: HANLEY & BELFUS, INC.
Medical Publishers
210 South 13th Street
Philadelphia, PA 19107
(215) 546-7293; 800-962-1892
FAX (215) 790-9330
Web site: http://www.hanleyandbelfus.com

All Mahler quotes from de la Grange H: *Gustav Mahler*. Paris, Fayard, 1979.

Back Cover Photograph

Makoto (*left*) and Kazu (*right*) performing in the Japanese jazz-rock group DMD—that is, Dream Music Directory. The five musicians who comprise DMD have muscular dystrophy, and four are ventilator users with Duchenne muscular dystrophy. Three of the performers require around-the-clock noninvasive ventilation and, as seen here, use mouthpiece ventilation for daytime ventilatory support and for the deep insufflations needed when singing. The members of DMD write, sing, and, with the assistance of computers, perform their own music and have recorded two compact disks.

Library of Congress Control Number: 2002106244

Noninvasive Mechanical Ventilation   ISBN 1-56053-549-0

Last digit is the print number: 9   8   7   6   5   4   3   2   1

——— **Dedication**

Arete, *an ancient Greek word meaning "the striving for intellectual, physical, and moral excellence"*

Arete, you whom the mortal race wins by much toil, the fairest prey in life.

—Aristole

This book is dedicated to the memory of Mr. John Haven (Jack) Emerson. During World War II, Mr. Emerson developed high-altitude demand-flow valves that provided tactical advantages for American fighter pilots by increasing altitude tolerance. Mr. Emerson's contributions to pulmonary and critical care medicine, home mechanical ventilation, and noninvasive mechanical ventilation include the development and production of Iron Lungs, wrap ventilators such as the Red Poncho and Pneumosuit, the Rocking Bed Ventilator, Pneumobelt Ventilator, positive-pressure and negative-pressure ventilators, jet ventilation and airway oscillators, hyperbaric oxygen treatment tanks, and mechanical forced exsufflation devices. In 1979, the American Thoracic Society honored Mr. Emerson with its Chadwick Medal for advancements in respiratory medicine.

Mr. Emerson's work continues to make it possible for people with ventilatory impairment to remain healthy and free of hospitalizations and tracheostomy tubes. In the late 1980s and early 1990s, accompanied by patients who had been using Cof-flators (mechanical forced exsufflation devices) since the 1950s and others who desperately needed these devices, I implored numerous ventilator manufacturers to remanufacture these machines. It was only Jack Emerson who had the wisdom to listen and the energy to do so. Ultimately his In-exsufflator™ came onto the market in February of 1993.[1] I remember Mr. Emerson fondly for his energy, wit, and gracious personality, as well as for his stories about Upper West Side life in Manhattan during the teens and Roaring Twenties.

Arete is typified by Mr. Emerson as it is by so many of the patients who have benefited from Mr. Emerson's innovations. These include Mr. Ira Holland, President of Disability Options, Inc., New York City, Mr. Roger Duell, Mr. Jeffrey Gray, the Piazza and Schepis families, the late Mr. James Starita, and so many others who, with great effort and perseverance, taught me that noninvasive alternatives to tracheotomy were usually better.

I also dedicate this book to all who struggle for *arete* but who are not graced with the time to achieve it. This fate has been shared by many people with neuromuscular disease, prematurely deceased because of inadequacies in their care, as well as by my late wife, Muguette, whose creative endeavors were prematurely ended by cancer.

—JRB

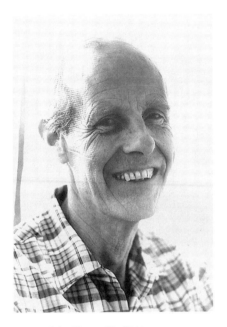

John Haven (Jack) Emerson.

REFERENCE

1. Round Table Conference on Poliomyelitis Equipment. Sponsored by the National Foundation for Infantile Paralysis, Inc. New York City, May 28–29, 1953.

There is just one point I would like to mention, which has just come along which, I think, makes it (noninvasive positive pressure ventilation) even more feasible. It is so simple that why it wasn't thought of long ago I don't know. Actually, some of our physical therapists, in struggling with the patients, noticed that they could simply take the positive pressure attachment, apply a small plastic mouthpiece..., and allow that to hang in the patient's mouth. You can take him to the Hubbard tank by such means and you can do any nursing procedure, if the patient is on the rocking bed and has a zero vital capacity, if you want to stop the bed for any reason, or if you want to change him from the tank respirator to the bed, or put the cuirass respirator on, or anything to stop the equipment, you can simply attach this, hang it by the patient, he grips it by his lips, and thus it allows for the excess to blow off which he doesn't want.

It works very well. We even had one patient who has no breathing ability who has fallen asleep and been adequately ventilated by this procedure, so that it appears to work very well, and I think does away with a lot of complications of difficulty of using positive pressure. You just hang it by the patients and they grip it with their lips, when they want it, and when they don't want it, they let go of it.

It is just too simple.

Dr. John Affeldt
Round Table Conference on Poliomyelitis Equipment
New York City
May, 1953

Men will have to work a long time at cracking the nuts that I'm shaking down from the tree for them.

—Gustav Mahler, *Briefe*

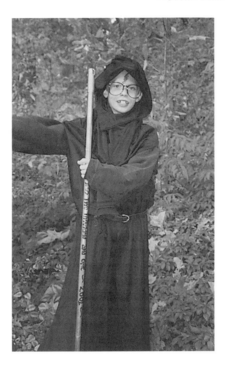

Noninvasive mechanical ventilation: it's not wizardry!

Contents

─── Contributors

John R. Bach, M.D.
Professor and Vice Chairman, Department of Physical Medicine and Rehabilitation; Professor of Neurosciences, University of Medicine and Dentistry of New Jersey, New Jersey Medical School; Director of Research and Associate Medical Director, Department of Physical Medicine and Rehabilitation; Medical Director, Center for Ventilator Management Alternatives and Pulmonary Rehabilitation; Co-director, UMDNJ-New Jersey Medical School's Jerry Lewis Muscular Dystrophy Association Clinic, University Hospital, Newark, New Jersey

Mark W. Elliott, M.D., FRCP
Consultant Respiratory Physician and Senior Clinical Lecturer in Medicine, Department of Respiratory Medicine, University of Leeds; St James's University Hospital, Leeds, England

Jill Gaydos, M.S.
Department of Nutrition, University Hospital, University of Medicine and Dentistry of New Jersey, New Jersey Medical School, Newark, New Jersey

Irving I. Habcr, D.O.
Clinical Assistant Professor, Department of Physical Medicine and Rehabilitation, Indiana University School of Medicine, Indianapolis, Indiana; Therapy Alternatives, Terre Haute, Indiana

Nicholas S. Hill, M.D.
Professor of Medicine, Division of Pulmonary, Critical Care, and Sleep Medicine, Department of Medicine, Tufts University School of Medicine; New England Medical Center, Boston, Massachusetts

John R. Hotchkiss, M.D.
Assistant Professor, Department of Pulmonary and Critical Care Medicine, University of Minnesota Medical School, Minneapolis, Minnesota; Regions Hospital, St. Paul, Minnesota

John J. Marini, M.D.
Department of Pulmonary and Critical Care Medicine, University of Minnesota Medical School, Minneapolis, Minnesota; Regions Hospital, St. Paul, Minnesota

Vis Niranjan, M.D.
Assistant Professor, Department of Pediatrics, University of Medicine and Dentistry of New Jersey, New Jersey Medical School; University Hospital, Newark, New Jersey

Barbara Rogers, B.A.
President, Respiratory Resources, Inc.; Director, Breethezy, New York, New York

Bruce K. Rubin, M.D., MEngr, FCCP, FRCPC
Professor and Vice-Chair for Research, Department of Pediatrics; Professor of Medicine, Medical Engineering, Physiology, and Pharmacology; Acting Section Chief, Pediatric Pulmonary Medicine, Wake Forest University School of Medicine, Winston-Salem, North Carolina

Cees P. van der Schans, Ph.D., P.T.
Department of Rehabilitation, University Hospital, Groningen, The Netherlands

About the Editor

After completing studies in science and engineering at Stevens Institute for Technology in Hoboken, NJ, John R. Bach received his medical degree from the UMDNJ–New Jersey Medical School in 1976. He completed postgraduate studies in pediatrics and in physical medicine and rehabilitation at New York University in 1980. In 1979, as a house physician on the Howard Rusk Ventilator Unit at Goldwater Memorial Hospital, he reported the long-term use of noninvasive positive-pressure ventilation by patients with Duchenne muscular dystrophy. He managed the ventilator unit from 1980 to 1981. He then became the technical advisor to Professor Yves Rideau, working to develop a service for noninvasive ventilation for the University of Poitiers, France, from 1981 to 1983. It was during the winter of 1981–82 that he, along with Drs. Rideau and Delaubier, first used nasal ventilation. He joined the faculty of the UMDNJ–New Jersey Medical School in June 1983.

Dr. Bach is a fellow of the American Academy of Physical Medicine and Rehabilitation, the American College of Chest Physicians, the Association of Academic Physiatrists, the American Paraplegia Society, the New Jersey Association of Electromyography and Electrodiagnosis, l'Association Française d'Actions et de Recherches sur les Dystrophies Musculaires, Sigma Xi, Alpha Omega Alpha National Honor Society, the American Spinal Injury Association, and the Institut Duchenne pour la Recherche dans les Maladies Neuromusculaires. He is a Professor of Physical Medicine and Rehabilitation, Department of Physical Medicine and Rehabilitation; Professor of Neurosciences, Department of Neurosciences; Vice Chairman of the Department of Physical Medicine and Rehabilitation, UMDNJ–New Jersey Medical School; Director of Research and Associate Medical Director of the Department of Physical Medicine and Rehabilitation at University Hospital, Newark, NJ; Co-director of the UMDNJ–New Jersey Medical School's Jerry Lewis Muscular Dystrophy Association Clinic; and Medical Director of the Center for Ventilator Management Alternatives and Pulmonary Rehabilitation, University Hospital, Newark, NJ. He has over 200 peer-reviewed scientific articles and book chapters and eight books on neuromuscular and pulmonary medicine and has lectured on these topics in over 30 countries around the globe.

Dr. Bach has received numerous awards including:

- *American Journal of Physical Medicine and Rehabilitation:* Award for Excellence in Research Writing (1990)
- *American Journal of Physical Medicine and Rehabilitation:* Award for Excellence in Research Writing (1994)
- William H. McLean UPTAM Alumni Honor Award, Stevens Institute of Technology (1994)
- American Academy of Physical Medicine and Rehabilitation: Award for the Best Research Paper Published by a Physiatrist (1994)
- University of Medicine and Dentistry of New Jersey: University Excellence Award for Patient Care (1994)
- University of Medicine and Dentistry of New Jersey, New Jersey Medical School: Special Faculty Achievement Award presented by the Faculty Organization (1996)

- American Academy of Physical Medicine and Rehabilitation: Education and Research Fund Best Scientific Research Paper (1997)
- Newark Beth Israel Health Care Foundation Humanism in Medicine Award (1998)
- The American Paraplegia Society: A. Estin Colmarr Memorial Award for Clinical Service (1999)
- New Jersey Society for Respiratory Care/American Association of Respiratory Care: A. Gerald Shapiro, M.D., Award for Outstanding Leadership in the Field of Respiratory Care (2000)

Dr. Bach is an internationally recognized pioneer in the rehabilitation of patients with neuromuscular conditions and in the use of physical medicine interventions as noninvasive alternatives to intubation and tracheostomy for these patients. He brought the Rideau protocol for early, essentially prophylactic lower extremity musculotendinous release surgery to the United States. This permits a prolongation of brace-free ambulation for children with muscular dystrophy. He was part of the group that defined indications for spinal instrumentation to treat scoliosis for patients with Duchenne muscular dystrophy. He was the first to describe the use of robot arms to facilitate activities of daily living for people with neuromuscular disease. In 1981 he first tried nasal ventilation and was the first to use it for patients with no autonomous breathing ability in 1984. He was also the first to report the nocturnal use of intermittent positive-pressure ventilation (IPPV) via a mouthpiece for a large population of ventilator users with no autonomous breathing ability. He defined criteria for extubation and tracheostomy tube decannulation and described normalization of ventilatory drive and blood carbon dioxide levels by conversion of patients from tracheostomy to noninvasive ventilatory support methods. He is responsible for the reintroduction of mechanical insufflation-exsufflation. He described possible mechanisms whereby open, noninvasive systems of ventilatory support can be successful for patients with no autonomous breathing ability. Along with Dr. Ishikawa, he first reported the effective medical management of cardiomyopathy in patients with neuromuscular cardiomyopathy. He developed the protocol that spares people with respiratory muscle weakness from respiratory complications, hospitalizations, intubations, and tracheostomies. He has treated celebrities and statesmen including a former Prime Minister of Greece. He also published key studies on cost-effectiveness issues concerning mechanical ventilation and rehabilitation for lung disease and neuromuscular disease patients.

——— Preface

An estimated 16 million Americans have chronic obstructive pulmonary disease (COPD).[1] In addition, 500,000 people in the United States have neuromuscular diseases,[2] more than 500,000 have spinal cord injury or post-polio respiratory impairment, and 3–5% of the population have thoracic wall restrictive lung disease, sleep-disordered breathing, or obesity hypoventilation. In this era of cost containment, medical interventions are expected to be both efficacious and cost-effective. Both survival and quality of life are considered in equations designed to justify the cost-benefit for prospective interventions. Interestingly, noninvasive respiratory interventions are consistently preferred by patients over invasive alternatives. Use of these interventions has been shown to prolong survival while decreasing the risk of pulmonary complications, need for hospitalizations and intensive care, and cost. Likewise, the use of respiratory muscle aids can optimize function, quality of life, and life satisfaction. Despite these facts, physician surveys indicate that only a small minority of patients who could benefit from these methods are ever offered them. This book is unique in presenting the various inspiratory and expiratory muscle aids and the outcomes of their use in patients with respiratory muscle dysfunction.

John R. Bach, M.D.

REFERENCES

1. Beers MH, Berkow R: Chronic obstructive airway disorders. In Beers MH, Berkow R (eds): The Merck Manual of Diagnosis and Therapy, 17th ed. Whitehouse Station, NJ, Merck & Co., 1999, pp 568–582.
2. Devereaux K: Bridging the information gap. In RRTCNMD Program Overview 1998–2003. Davis, CA, NIDRR Rehabilitation Research and Training Center in Neuromuscular Diseases at University of California, Davis. Available at www.rehabinfo.net/Clearinghouse/Virtual_Library/Index.html.

The Center for Noninvasive Mechanical Ventilation Alternatives and Pulmonary Rehabilitation, UMDNJ-NJMS at University Hospital, Newark, New Jersey

This book reflects the efforts of the Center for Noninvasive Mechanical Ventilation Alternatives and Pulmonary Rehabilitation of the University of Medicine and Dentistry of New Jersey, New Jersey Medical School (UMDNJ-NJMS), at University Hospital in Newark, New Jersey. The Center, founded in 1992, consists of health care professionals dedicated to the holistic and comprehensive care of people with respiratory impairment from any cause. The staff at the Center work to prevent or allay respiratory morbidity and mortality. With the use of inspiratory and expiratory muscle aids developed by the Center, surgery can be performed on patients who have little or no respiratory muscle function with minimal risk of respiratory complications and no need to resort to tracheotomy. The center has removed over 100 tracheostomy tubes from ventilator users with little or no functioning respiratory muscles or ability to breathe and has taught alternative methods of breathing without ventilators.

Staff:

John R. Bach, MD, Medical Director; Professor of Physical Medicine and Rehabilitation and Vice Chairman, Department of Physical Medicine and Rehabilitation; Professor of Neurosciences

Lou Saporito, BS, RRT, Technical Director

Kathy Opromollo, BS, Administrative Director; Associate, Department of Physical Medicine and Rehabilitation

Scott Baird, MD, Assistant Professor of Pediatrics; Director of Pediatric Intensive Care Services

Soly Baredes, MD, Associate Professor of Surgery; Chief of the Division of Otopharyngology

Colin Bethel, MD, Assistant Professor of Surgery; Assistant Professor of Pediatrics; Chief of Pediatric Surgery

Melissa Davidson, MD, Associate Professor of Anesthesiology

Jill Gaydos, MS, Department of Nutrition

Ann Guylas, MA, SLP, Division of Speech and Language Therapy, Department of Physical Medicine and Rehabilitation

John Katz, MD, Associate Professor of Anesthesiology

Jose Navado, MD, Assistant Professor of Pediatrics

Sanjeev Sabharwal, MD, Assistant Professor of Orthopedics; Assistant Professor of Pediatrics; Chief of Pediatric Orthopedics

Kenneth Swan, MD, Professor of General and Trauma Surgery

Brian Weaver, BS, RRT, RPFT, Technical Advisor for Pediatrics

List of Abbreviations

AHI	Apnea/hypopnea index
ALS/MND	Amyotrophic lateral sclerosis/motor neuron disease
BMD	Becker muscular dystrophy
CHF	Congestive heart failure
CNEP	Continuous negative expiratory pressure
CNS	Central nervous system
CPAP	Continuous positive airway pressure
DAG	Dystrophin-associated glycoprotein
DMD	Duchenne muscular dystrophy
$dSpO_2$	Oxyhemoglobin desaturation
EDMD	Emery-Dreifuss muscular dystrophy
EPAP	Expiratory positive airway pressure
EPP	Equal pressure point
EPR	Electrophrenic respiration
$EtCO_2$	End-tidal carbon dioxide
FEV_1	Forced expiratory volume in 1 second
FRC	Functional residual capacity
FSH	Facioscapulohumeral muscular dystrophy
GPB	Glossopharyngeal breathing
IAPV	Intermittent abdominal pressure ventilator
ICU	Intensive care unit
I/E	Inspiratory/expiratory (ratio)
IPAP	Inspiratory positive airway pressures
IPPB	Intermittent positive-pressure breathing
IPPV	Intermittent positive-pressure ventilation
LGMD	Limb-girdle muscular dystrophy
MAC	Mechanically assisted coughing
MELAS	Mitochondrial myopathy, encephalopathy, lactic acidosis, and stroke-like episodes
MERRF	Mitochondrial myopathy with myoclonic epilepsy and ragged red fibers

MIC	Maximum insufflation capacity
MI-E	Mechanical insufflation-exsufflation
NMD	Neuromuscular disease
NPBV	Negative pressure body ventilator
OSAS	Obstructive sleep apnea syndrome
PCF	Peak cough flows
PEEP	Positive end-expiratory pressure
PEF	Peak expiratory flow
PEP	Positive expiratory pressure
PIP + PEEP	Positive inspiratory pressure plus positive end-expiratory pressure
REE	Resting energy expenditure
REM	Rapid eye movement
ROM	Range of motion
SCI	Spinal cord injury/injured
SIMV	Synchronized intermittent mandatory ventilation
SMA	Spinal muscular atrophy
SONI	Strapless oral nasal interface
SpO_2	Oxyhemoglobin saturation
VC	Vital capacity

1 —— Disease Profiles of Noninvasive Ventilation Users

JOHN R. BACH, M.D.

Comment donc parvient-on à connaitre les hommes, qui sont bien plus profonds et plus complexes que leurs oeuvres? Il faut observer avec attention et tendresse.
(How then can one come to know men, who are indeed more profound and more complex than their works? It is necessary to observe them with attention and affection.)

Gustav Mahler

Most patients with lung disease are referred to and managed by pulmonologists long before ventilator use becomes an issue. Chest physicians are well schooled in the primary pathologic processes of lung diseases and in their evaluation and treatment. Pulmonary journals are devoted largely to lung disease. Because of the great variety of lung pathology, this chapter reviews only the most common lung diseases of patients using respiratory muscle aids.

Patients with neuromuscular respiratory dysfunction who can benefit from the use of noninvasive respiratory muscle aids, on the other hand, are most often diagnosed by physicians who have little experience in preventing the respiratory complications of neuromuscular disease (NMD). The clinicians to whom these patients are likely to be referred are equally unlikely to teach and equip them with the respiratory muscle aids needed to prevent respiratory failure. Indeed, most patients with NMD or respiratory muscle impairment from any cause are evaluated and treated as though they have primarily lung disease rather than ventilatory impairment. As a result, acute respiratory failure is inevitable. Most clinicians other than neurologists have little understanding of the NMD processes that cause muscle dysfunction and rarely feel qualified to manage the nonrespiratory aspects of these conditions.

This chapter surveys the diagnoses for which respiratory muscle aids are useful and considers options for respiratory and nonrespiratory management.

CANDIDATES FOR PHYSICAL MEDICINE RESPIRATORY INTERVENTIONS

Patients who can most benefit from respiratory muscle aids, as well as from general habilitation and rehabilitation interventions, must be able to learn and must have adequate

1

bulbar muscle function to use specific respiratory techniques and equipment Most patients with the diagnoses considered in Table 1 retain adequate bulbar muscle and cognitive function to be candidates for the use of physical medicine alternatives to tracheal intubation for invasive ventilatory support and secretion management. Some patients with severe lung or airways disease or severe bulbar muscle weakness that precludes effective use of noninvasive inspiratory aids may still benefit from manually and mechanically assisted coughing

TABLE 1. Conditions with Functional Bulbar Musculature That Can Result in Chronic Alveolar Hypoventilation

Myopathies
  Muscular dystrophies[5,113,114]
    Dystrophinopathies—Duchenne and Becker dystrophies
    Other muscular dystrophies—limb-girdle, Emery-Dreifuss, facioscapulohumeral, congenital, childhood autosomal recessive, and myotonic dystrophy[5,115,116]
  Non-Duchenne myopathies[5,114]
    Congenital and metabolic myopathies such as acid maltase deficiency,[116] acid alpha glucosidase deficiency,[117] mucopolysaccharidoses,[118] mitochondrial myopathies[119–121]
    Inflammatory myopathies such as polymyositis[122]
    Diseases of the myoneural junction such as myasthenia gravis,[123] congenital myasthenic syndromes,[124] mixed connective tissue disease[122]
    Myopathies of systemic disease such as carcinomatous myopathy, cachexia/anorexia nervosa,[125] medication-associated myopathy

Neurologic disorders
  Spinal muscular atrophies[126]
  Motor neuron diseases[5,114]
  Poliomyelitis[5,114]
  Neuropathies
    Hereditary sensory motor neuropathies,[127,128] including familial hypertrophic interstitial polyneuropathy, phrenic neuropathies[64]—associated with cardiac hypothermia,[91] surgical or other trauma,[129] radiation, phrenic electrostimulation, familial, paraneoplastic or infectious etiology, and lupus erythematosus[122]
    Guillain-Barré syndrome
  Multiple sclerosis[5–8]
  Disorders of supraspinal tone such as Friedreich's ataxia
  Myelopathies of rheumatoid, infectious, spondylitic, vascular, traumatic,[3,4,130,131] or idiopathic etiology[100,132]
  Tetraplegia associated with pancuronium bromide,[133] botulism
  Static encephalopathies associated with Arnold-Chiari malformation and syringomyelia,[134] myelomeningocele,[135,136] encephalitis[137]

Sleep-disordered breathing, including obesity hypoventilation,[5,114,138] central and congenital hypoventilation syndromes,[139–142] retrognathism,[143] and hypoventilation associated with diabetic microangiopathy,[144] familial dysautonomia, or Prader-Willi syndrome[145]

Kyphoscoliosis, idiopathic[5,114,146] or from osteogenesis imperfecta, rigid spine syndrome,[113] spondyloepiphyseal dysplasia congenita,[147] tuberculosis[104,114,148]

Restrictive lung disease associated with lung resection,[5,149] tuberculosis,[150] Milroy's disease,[151] congenital diaphragmatic hernia[152]

Vocal cord paralysis,[153] laryngotracheal reconstruction[154]

Endocrine abnormalities, as with hypothyroidism, acromegaly[155]

Mixed ventilatory–respiratory impairment

Chronic obstructive pulmonary disease,[5,155] cystic fibrosis[156–158]

Pneumonia[159–161]

Trauma[162]

Postoperative cancer,[163] lung transplantation[164]

Hematopoietic progenitor transplantation[165]

(MAC). Likewise, some patients unable to maintain a patent airway when trying to use expiratory aids may benefit from inspiratory aids. In addition, virtually any patient with adequate cognition and at least one reliable volitional movement, such as eye blink, can use robotics and computers to communicate, operate sophisticated environmental control systems, and function in society.

Patients with chronic lung or airways disease often have intermittent exacerbations associated with hypercapnic respiratory failure. These episodes are often triggered by exacerbations of respiratory muscle dysfunction and inability to clear the secretions of hyperproductive and hypercollapsible airways. Others may have sudden onset of respiratory muscle failure, as occurs with acute poliomyelitis,[1,2] acute traumatic high level spinal cord injury (SCI),[3,4] and airway mucus plugging during chest colds. Still others can have insidiously progressive respiratory muscle dysfunction that eventually results in hypercapnic ventilatory failure. The clinical course of the latter patients is often punctuated by episodes of acute respiratory failure during periods of increased airway secretion production (e.g., upper respiratory tract infections or chest infections).

In addition to patients with primarily lung disease, skeletal disease, or NMDs, patients with certain degenerative central nervous system (CNS) conditions such as multiple sclerosis and Friedreich's ataxia also can develop chronic ventilatory insufficiency and episodes of respiratory failure.[5–8] Debilitated patients with any CNS disorder that results in severe dysphagia and aspiration of upper airway secretions or food also can develop pneumonias and episodes of hypercapnic respiratory failure. Likewise, there can be an element of central hypoventilation, as in familial dysautonomia and congenital hypoventilation syndromes. Patients with obesity-hypoventilation syndrome and others with sleep-disordered breathing complicated by inspiratory muscle dysfunction also may require the nocturnal use of inspiratory muscle aids. A discussion of key clinical aspects of the least familiar pertinent diagnoses follows. The reader is referred to other sources for additional information.[9–14]

MYOPATHIES

The term *myopathy* applies to disorders attributed to pathologic, biochemical, or electrical changes in muscle fibers or in the interstitial tissues of the skeletal musculature in the absence of nervous system dysfunction.[15] In 1891 Erb described the histopathology of "muscular dystrophy."[16] Walton suggested that this term be reserved for cases of progressive, genetically determined, primary, degenerative myopathy in which active muscle degeneration and regeneration are observed in muscle biopsy specimens.[15] Thus, myopathies traditionally have been recognized and differentiated by characteristic histopathologic findings, electromyography (EMG), and increased titers of serum muscle enzymes. Now, however, many myopathies are diagnosed by identification of specific DNA defects. As of this writing, over 250 specific genetic defects have been identified for various NMDs.

Dystrophin-deficient Muscular Dystrophies

Duchenne muscular dystrophy (DMD), the most common severe myopathy, and Becker muscular dystrophy (BMD) are caused by a defect in the 21 region on the short arm (p) of the X-chromosome (Xp21 defect).[17] The nature and precise position of the defect or deletion affect the quantity and quality of the encoded dystrophin and, thereby, phenotypic expression.[18] DMD, in which no dystrophin is seen in biopsy specimens, has an incidence of 1 per 3500 male births.[19,20] BMD, with reduced quantity or abnormal dystrophin, has an incidence of 1 per 25,000 male births.

Children with DMD may be somewhat hypotonic at birth, but weakness is often not formally evaluated by the pediatrician before 3 years of age. Such children have pseudohypertrophic calves and a relentless, progressive, fairly symmetrical and predictable pattern of

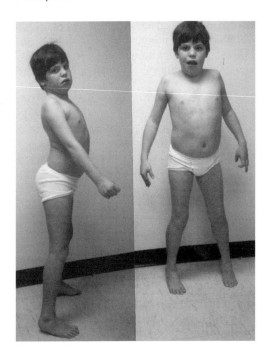

FIGURE 1. Seven-year-old boy with Duchenne muscular dystrophy. Hip extensor weakness leads to anterior pelvic tilt, hip flexor contractures, and increased lumbar lordosis. The patient must keep his weight line behind the hips to avoid jack-knifing at the hips. Tensor fascia lata and iliotibial band contractures lead to a wide-based gait. With increasing quadriceps weakness the patient must stabilize the knee by keeping the weight line anterior to the knee (as well as behind the hips). The stronger plantarflexors encourage toe-walking and lead to ankle equinus, which in the early stages may help to stabilize the knee. Iliotibial tract tightness increases torque on the femur to flex the knee and eventually prevents adequate hyperextension of the hip and lumbar spine. Once knee flexion contractures develop, it becomes impossible to keep the center of gravity both behind the hip and in front of the knee. Imbalance of foot evertor strength with the stronger tibialis posterior destabilizing the subtalar joint leads to falls at first on uneven and eventually on all surfaces.

muscle weakness and contractures. The child may be slow in attaining the motor "milestones," but no correlation has been found between late walking and rapid progression (Fig. 1).[21] The average age at wheelchair dependence ranges from 8.6 to 9.5 years,[22–24] although it can be delayed by about 1.5 years for children who tolerate prednisone therapy or who undergo judicious lower extremity surgery. Nevertheless, children with DMD generally do not walk unassisted beyond 13 years of age. They have an average intelligence quotient of 90 but tend to have specific deficits in verbal working-memory skills, including deficits in measures of story recall, digit span, and auditory comprehension as well as in reading, writing, and mathematics.[25] Most patients with BMD have a much milder course with later onset and slower progression and may not be diagnosed until after 25 years of age. The genetics, evaluation, and management principles are basically the same as for DMD.

Medical and surgical strategies for treating DMD date back to 1845.[26] Most attempts at medical treatment have been unsuccessful,[27–29] but corticosteroid therapy temporarily increases strength and slows muscle deterioration in DMD.[30–32] Optimal dosage schedule for prednisone is unclear, but a daily dose of 0.75 mg/kg for at least 6 months between ages 4 and 8 years appears to be highly beneficial. When tolerated, treatment can be begun by age 3 and extended indefinitely. Intermittent or "pulsed" prednisone therapy for several weeks six or more times per year from age 3 to 17 years also has been reported to be beneficial. Blood pressure, growth, and urinary/blood glucose must be monitored. Patients also must be evaluated for possible cushingoid appearance, acne, behavioral changes (e.g., hyperactivity, irritability, insomnia, euphoria, depression), easy bruising, increased appetite, nausea, stomach discomfort, hypertrichosis, and intercurrent infections. Diets low in sodium and sugar are prudent, and supplemental calcium carbonate is recommended with each meal.[33] Glucocorticoids may increase surgical and anesthetic risks; they have not been shown to change significantly serum creatine kinase concentrations[31,33,34] or to prolong life.[35] Deflazacort, a relatively new corticosteroid, is equally as effective and may have fewer side effects than prednisone but has not been approved by the Food and Drug Administration.[36]

Myoblast transfer therapy has been a failure. However, in extensive, ongoing work, gene therapy—the introduction of the dystrophin gene into muscle tissues using viral vectors, liposomes, or other carriers—appears promising. In addition, attempts are being made to promote continued production of utrophin. Utrophin is the smaller dystrophin-like membrane protein that is present in the fetus but gradually disappears and is replaced by dystrophin during early childhood. It is believed that, if utrophin can be maintained, the subsequent development of muscle weakness may be less severe.

Without optimal treatment, severe spinal deformity occurs in at least 90% of patients with DM.[37,38] Scoliosis can be prevented or minimized only by surgery.[39]

Up to 90%[40–44] of conventionally managed patients with DMD die from the pulmonary complications associated with untreated respiratory muscle dysfunction between 16 and 19 years of age (Fig. 2).[19,43] Respiratory complications unnecessarily remain the most common cause of death for patients with DMD.[19]

Cardiomyopathy is also a common complication of many myopathies, especially the muscular dystrophies.[45] Most myopathic patients who die before developing chronic hypercapnia, who die suddenly despite effective use of noninvasive respiratory muscle aids, or who die without profuse airway secretion die from complications of cardiomyopathy.[40]

Children with DMD have delayed gastric emptying (up to 3 times longer than normal).[46] Gastrointestinal motility is decreased in association with smooth muscle dystrophin deficiency.[20] Degeneration of the outer, longitudinal, smooth-muscle layer of the stomach has been observed at autopsy.[47] Constipation results from decreased intestinal motility and loss of effective Valsalva maneuver due to abdominal muscle weakness in all patients with NMDs.

Patients with DMD and some patients with NMDs have a high incidence of dysphagia and choking associated with bulbar muscle dysfunction.[48] Although 15–20% of patients with DMD eventually require gastrostomy tubes for nutritional supplementation, bulbar muscle weakness of sufficient severity to necessitate tracheostomy virtually never occurs in DMD, even after 25 years or more of continuous ventilatory support by noninvasive means.[49]

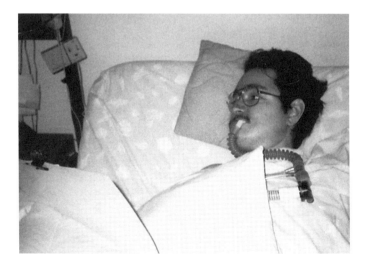

FIGURE 2. Thirty-four-year-old patient with Duchenne muscular dystrophy who has used 24-hour mouthpiece/lipseal IPPV since the age of 12 years. He has had little or no breathing tolerance for the past 20 years but has had no respiratory complications or hospitalizations.

Other Muscular Dystrophies

Emery-Dreifuss muscular dystrophy is an X-linked recessive (distal long arm at Xq27-28)[50] condition caused by emerin deficiency. Autosomal dominant inheritance also has been described.[51] Possibly as a result of connective tissue as well as muscle involvement, prominent flexion contractures develop at the elbows and heel cords before muscle weakness becomes prominent. The cervical spine is hyperextended, and flexion of the entire spine is limited. The two typical patterns of weakness are (1) elbow flexion and extension and peroneal muscle weakness (humeroperoneal dystrophy) and (2) elbow and pelvic muscle weakness (humeropelvic dystrophy). Most patients are able to walk until the third decade.[24] Cardiac arrhythmias are common and often life-threatening when not adequately treated.

The predominantly autosomal recessive muscular dystrophies include limb-girdle muscular dystrophy (LGMD) and the congenital muscular dystrophies. Thus far, defects have been found at 13 loci on various chromosomes in patients with LGMD. At least three of the chromosomal defects associated with LGMD result in autosomal dominant inheritance. When no genetic correlate is found, the diagnoses of these conditions are necessarily made on the basis of muscle biopsy histopathology and phenotypic expression of muscle weakness. These conditions are equally expressed in both sexes.

Onset of LGMD is between 5 and 30 years of age. The shoulder and pelvic girdle muscles are involved initially, and the rate of progression is highly variable. Calf hypertrophy may occur. Severe disability, muscular contractures, skeletal deformities, cardiomyopathy, and chronic alveolar hypoventilation are common (Fig. 3).

Pediatric-onset autosomal recessive muscular dystrophy can be confused with DMD, and its course can be almost as severe.[52] However, muscle dystrophin is normal, and there is no Xp21 defect. History of parental consanguinity may help to establish the diagnosis. Wheelchair dependence occurs at the mean age of 18 years[53] but can occur from age 10 to 45 years. If untreated, scoliosis can become severe, and ventilatory impairment can begin as early as age 20, although it more commonly appears after age 25.

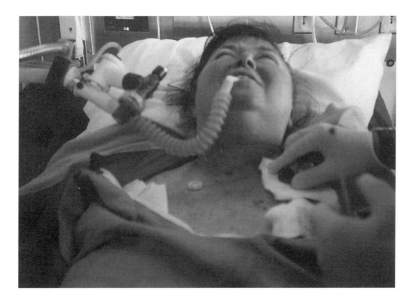

FIGURE 3. Woman with limb-girdle muscular dystrophy (onset at age 5 years, diagnosed at age 10 years). The patient became wheelchair-dependent at age 22 years and was tracheostomized for continuous ventilatory support at age 37 years. After 6 years of 24-hour tracheostomy IPPV, she was converted to 24-hour noninvasive IPPV (see Case Study 12 in Chapter 15 for details).

Congenital muscular dystrophy without CNS involvement usually presents as hypotonia at birth or soon thereafter.[54] Static to rapidly progressive forms have been described.[55–57] Except for some static, relatively mild forms, such as the stick-man type, patients develop predominantly proximal muscle weakness, joint contractures, and occasionally facial muscle weakness, but other cranial musculature is generally spared. About 50% remain severely disabled and never achieve the ability to walk. Scoliosis and chronic alveolar hypoventilation may become early and severe problems.

The most common predominantly autosomal dominant forms of muscular dystrophy include facioscapulohumeral muscular dystrophy (FSH) and myotonic dystrophy, although autosomal recessive forms also have been described for FSH.[52] FSH can present in adult, juvenile, or infantile forms.[58] It varies greatly in severity, but each form leads to the development of life-threatening lung hypoventilation. The pattern of weakness is distinct. Facial muscles are usually markedly weakened, and scapular winging becomes prominent. Limb weakness usually begins in the upper arms but typically spares the biceps. Weakness in the legs may be more prominent in distal musculature. Patients can lose the ability to close their eyes; speech can become indistinct and smiling and whistling impossible. Cardiomyopathy can be severe.

Myotonic dystrophy is common, with an incidence of 13 per 100,000 population (Fig. 4).[59] The defective gene, a triplet repeat sequence of DNA abnormally expanded many times, has been located on chromosome 19.[60] Clinical severity increases with the number of triplet repeats. The size of the expansion increases in succeeding generations, particularly when the affected parent is the mother. With few exceptions, the most severe form, congenital myotonic dystrophy, is inherited from the mother.[61]

Myotonic dystrophy can present from birth until 50 years of age with some combination of myotonia, hand weakness, gait difficulties, temporal muscle atrophy, frontal baldness (in men), and complaints of poor vision, ptosis, weight loss, impotence, and hypertrichosis. Patients have a predilection for neck flexor and distal limb muscle weakness. Ankle and occasionally other musculotendinous contractures can develop, along with weakness and wasting of the limbs. Systemic manifestations may include cataracts, gonadal atrophy and other endocrine anomalies, cardiomyopathy, bony changes, abnormalities of serum immunoglobulins, chronic alveolar hypoventilation, and hypersomnia with or without sleep-disordered breathing.[62] Hypersomnolence may be associated with disturbed function of the

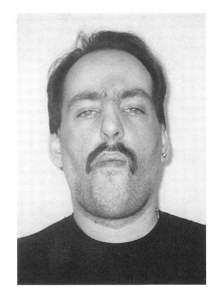

FIGURE 4.   40-year-old man with myotonic dystrophy demonstrating typical dolicocephalic facies, temporal atrophy, and frontal balding. He also has cataracts, cardiomyopathy, and chronic alveolar hypoventilation, for which he uses nocturnal nasal IPPV.

TABLE 2. Neuromuscular Diseases of Floppy Infants In Order of Incidence

Spinal muscular atrophy
Congenital myopathies
Congenital muscular dystrophies
Congenital myotonic dystrophy
Congenital myasthenic syndrome
Acid maltase deficiency (Pompe's disease)
Debranching enzyme deficiency (type 3 glycogen storage disease)
Branching enzyme deficiency (type 4 glycogen storage disease)
Carnitine deficiency
Mitochondrial myopathies
Congenital peripheral neuropathies

hypothalamic-pituitary axis.[63] Mental retardation may be present and is especially pronounced in patients with congenital myotonic dystrophy. Dysarthria is a common problem. Creatine kinase is usually normal.

Nondystrophic Myopathies

The term *congenital myopathy* relates to conditions defined by specific morphologic abnormalities observed in muscle biopsy specimens. Patients with onset of congenital myopathy in childhood are often floppy neonates (Table 2). The best characterized congenital myopathies include central core disease, centronuclear myopathies, and nemaline myopathies. Central core disease usually presents as hypotonia at birth and is usually autosomal dominant; it is generally mild and nonprogressive. Centronuclear and nemaline myopathies can have mildly to rapidly progressive courses, leading to severe disability and chronic alveolar hypoventilation.[54,64,65] Nemaline myopathy has a rapidly progressive adult-onset form.[66] Spheroid body myopathy also can be rapidly progressive and lead to ventilatory failure.[67] Dilated cardiomyopathy (DCM) often occurs in these conditions. Most other congenital myopathies are less well characterized and have mild or nonprogressive courses (Fig. 5). It is possible that some severe myopathies thought to be congenital are actually of viral etiology.[68]

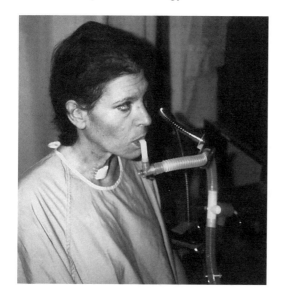

FIGURE 5. Woman with a congenital myopathy who was able to walk until age 16 years and remained stable until age 49 years, at which point respiratory failure led to a tracheostomy for ventilatory support. After 5 months of unsuccessful ventilator weaning attempts, she was converted to noninvasive IPPV (see Case Study 16 in Chapter 15 for details).

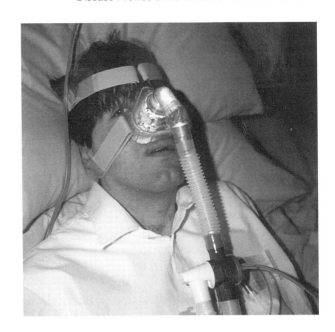

FIGURE 6. Man with acid maltase deficiency who was a successful high school athlete. Onset of weakness was noted at age 24 years, diagnosis was made at age 28, and severe dyspnea and chronic global alveolar hypoventilation led to use of a rocking bed ventilator for nocturnal ventilatory assistance at ages 30–35 years. At age 35 years, the rocking bed was minimally effective, and the patient required periods of daytime ventilatory assistance. He was switched to daytime mouthpiece IPPV and nocturnal nasal IPPV, which he has used for 9 years.

Except for certain mitochondrial myopathies, metabolic myopathies are autosomal recessive disorders for which defects in muscle metabolism have been identified—or are suspected. The defects can be in lipid, glycogen, or purine metabolism. Patients with most metabolic myopathies present with fatigue, muscle cramps, and exercise intolerance and ultimately have only mild muscle weakness. The diagnoses are suspected by elevated creatine kinase levels and myoglobinuria and are confirmed by muscle biopsy. However, progressive generalized muscular weakness resembling LGMD is characteristic of acid maltase deficiency and both branching and debranching enzyme deficiencies, which are disorders of glycolysis, and carnitine deficiency. For these disorders, generalized, predominantly proximal, often painless muscle weakness and possibly severe cardiomyopathy may be key findings. Acid maltase deficiency, which leads to accumulation of glycogen in lysosomes, not uncommonly presents with hypercapnia and cor pulmonale due to respiratory muscle involvement, particularly in the adult-onset form (Fig. 6). There is no medical treatment for acid maltase deficiency; the use of small frequent meals is recommended for patients with debranching enzyme deficiency; and liver transplantation has been highly effective in treating branching enzyme deficiency.[69] Some patients with carnitine deficiency respond well to restrictions in dietary fat and treatment with oral L-carnitine.[70]

Mitochondrial myopathies are metabolic disorders in which abnormalities in mitochondria are suspected and often can be detected by electronmicroscopy. The most common indication of mitochondrial NMD is progressive external ophthalmoplegia (PEO) and possibly ptosis.[71] Nonmuscular manifestations may include lipomas, ichthyosis, cataracts, retinitis pigmentosa, cardiac arrhythmias, cardiomyopathy, intestinal pseudo-obstruction, short stature, diabetes, goiter, primary ovarian failure, deafness, ataxia, neuropathy, seizures, and strokes. In Kearns-Sayre syndrome, a defect in mitochondrial DNA, PEO is accompanied by a myriad of other symptoms and signs,[71] including pigmentary degeneration of the retina, heart block, and depressed ventilatory drive (Fig. 7).[72] Familial PEO syndromes have been separated into a maternally inherited mitochondrial abnormality and an autosomal dominant disorder.[71] Maternally inherited PEO does not have multisystem involvement like Kearns-Sayre syndrome or autosomal dominant PEO, in which tremor, ataxia, sensorimotor peripheral neuropathy, and hearing loss may be present.

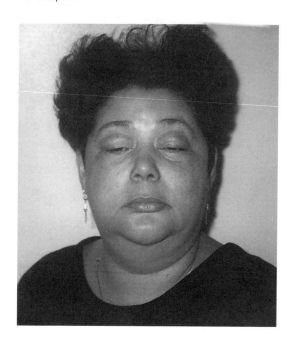

FIGURE 7. External ophthalmoplegia (PEO) and ptosis due to Kearns-Sayre syndrome. The patient had both depressed ventilatory drive and respiratory muscle weakness, which led to severe chronic alveolar hypoventilation and four episodes of respiratory failure before institution of respiratory muscle aids.

Other than some suggestion that coenzyme-Q administration may be helpful,[73] there are no medical treatments for the mitochondrial myopathies. For patients with mitochondrial myopathies—such as myoclonic epilepsy and ragged red fibers (MERRF) and mitochondrial myopathy with encephalopathy, lactic acidosis, and stroke-like episodes (MELAS)—severe systemic involvement and intellectual deterioration preclude the use of noninvasive respiratory muscle aids.

Polymyositis is an inflammatory myopathy that does not affect more than one member of a family. Presentation before age 20 years is uncommon, but childhood and infantile cases have been reported (Fig. 8).[74] Progression can be rapid or insidious, with symmetric, predominantly proximal and neck muscle weakness. Dysphagia is common; pseudohypertrophy is rare; muscular atrophy is often not severe; and deep tendon reflexes are relatively spared. Creatine kinase can be markedly elevated during disease activity but otherwise may be normal. Skin changes (dermatomyositis) or other manifestations of systemic disease may be present. Inflammation is not always seen in the muscle biopsies of inflammatory myopathies. Such conditions can imitate progressive myopathies with limb-girdle weakness.[75] When diagnosed and treated in a timely manner with corticosteroids or other immunosuppressives, an excellent response can be achieved. Such patients are susceptible to both acute[76] and late-onset ventilatory failure.

Myasthenia gravis is characterized by fatigue and intermittent exacerbations of muscle weakness after repetitive muscle activation. Patients experience at least partial recovery after a period of inactivity, especially with treatment. Bulbar and respiratory muscles can be markedly affected, particularly during acute exacerbations. Nonetheless, bulbar muscle function is usually adequate for effective physical medicine interventions.

Prevalence of myasthenia gravis is about 1 per 10,000 population, with females predominating. The modal age of onset is about 20 years[77]; however, incidences are highest in young women and middle-aged men. The onset is usually insidious but can be sudden. Diagnosis is based on the characteristic clinical picture, which often includes asymmetric ptosis and ophthalmoplegia, anti-acetylcholine receptor site antibodies, characteristic

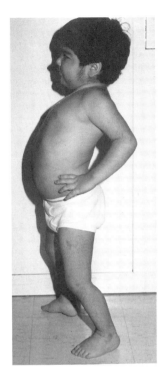

FIGURE 8.   Child with rapid onset of generalized weakness at age 2 years. His condition appeared to stabilize with gluco-corticoid therapy, and he remained stable without medications. However, he lost the ability to walk at age 7 years and had a severe restrictive pulmonary syndrome. He developed chronic alveolar hypoventilation in his early teens.

EMG findings (e.g., decremental evoked action potential amplitudes during repetitive supramaximal stimulation), and therapeutic response to anticholinesterases. Patients respond well to currently available treatments, including corticosteroid therapy, anticholinesterase administration, plasmapheresis, and thymectomy (Fig. 9).

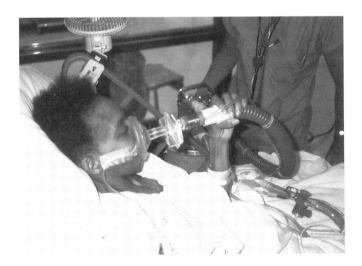

FIGURE 9.   Patient with myasthenia gravis who has relied heavily on auto-administration of mechanical insufflation-exsufflation, nocturnal nasal IPPV, and, during acute exacerbations, continuous noninvasive IPPV for 9 years. During this period she has been free of hospitalization despite intermittent exacerbations. Before this time she was hospitalized and underwent endotracheal intubation on numerous occasions during exacerbation-associated episodes of respiratory failure.

Many systemic diseases lead to some combination of muscle weakness and myopathic changes in muscle. Usually treating the primary medical disorder prevents the degree of respiratory muscle deterioration that otherwise would necessitate the use of respiratory muscle aids. On some occasions, however, conditions such as cancer, collagen disease, or endocrine disease can be complicated by one or more of the following risk factors: advanced age,[78] obesity, cardiopulmonary disease, malnutrition, ongoing glucocorticoid therapy, or use of certain chemotherapeutic agents or agents (e.g., penicillamine, cimetidine) that can produce an inflammatory myopathy. For many such patients the risk of pulmonary complications and even overt ventilatory failure can be prevented or managed strictly by noninvasive respiratory muscle aids.

DISEASE AFFECTING THE MOTOR NEURONS

Motor neurons are affected in the spinal muscular atrophies (SMAs), poliomyelitis, and amyotrophic lateral sclerosis/motor neuron disease (ALS/MND). The SMAs are inherited in an autosomal recessive fashion with the genetic defect at chromosome 5q exons 7 and 8. Gene deletions are detectable in 98% of patients. The incidence is about 1 per 5,000 population.[79] Severity, which is inversely proportional to the amount of survival motor neurons (SMNs), ranges from severe generalized paralysis and need for ventilatory support from birth[80] to relatively mild, static conditions presenting in young adults. SMAs have been arbitrarily separated into five types based largely on severity. In infantile SMA type 1 (Werdnig-Hoffmann disease), the infant never attains the ability to sit. Acute respiratory failure occurs during chest infections in the first 2 years of life (Fig. 10). With rare

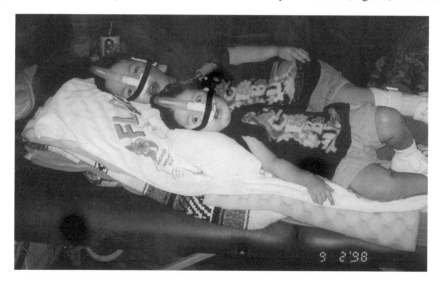

FIGURE 10. Brothers (6 years 7 months and 4 year 2 months old) with spinal muscular atrophy type 1. The older brother developed respiratory failure at 5 months of age and required continuous noninvasive ventilation before weaning to nocturnal-only high-span positive inspiratory pressure plus positive end-expiratory pressure (PIP + PEEP). After a second episode of respiratory failure at 11 months of age, he required PIP + PEEP continuously. He has a vital capacity of 90 ml and has received all nutrition via nasogastric tube since 5 months of age. His brother has been continuously dependent on PIP + PEEP and nutrition via nasogastric tube since 4 months of age and has never been hospitalized. He has up to 5 minutes of breathing tolerance in the supine position and a vital capacity of 70 ml. Both brothers use PIP + PEEP at an IPAP of 20 and an EPAP of 3 cmH$_2$O. Both are averbal but communicate via computer voice synthesizer. They are happy children with their own personalities and do extremely well with school work. Neither has any sign of pectus excavatum.

exception, patients die by 2 years of age (median: around 7 months); about 80% of affected children die by 12 months of age.[80] See below and Chapter 10 for a discussion of the diagnosis and treatment of SMA type 1.

Children with SMA type 2 at least temporarily attain the ability to sit independently. Children with SMA type 3 (Kugelberg-Welander disease) temporarily attain the ability to walk. For type 2 and type 3 patients, oropharyngeal musculature usually remains adequate for speaking and taking at least some nutrition by mouth throughout life. Muscle strength and function (motor milestones) can improve during childhood, and strength remains constant during adolescence. For some children, however, strength and function can decrease before adolescence. This decrease may result from metabolic factors or muscle wasting due to periods of undernutrition not directly related to the primary muscle pathology. Metabolic factors also may be responsible for strength and bulbar musculature weakening during chest infections and other periods of physiologic stress (see Chapter 14).[81] Musculotendinous contractures and scoliosis are inevitable in patients with infantile SMA.

Like SMA types 1–3, SMA type 4 is also an autosomal recessive condition, but it presents after adolescence. Most patients become wheelchair users in middle age and may require ventilator use 20–40 years after onset. Kennedy's disease, now considered type 5 SMA, is a sex-linked recessive motor neuron disease that affects predominantly males. It also presents after adolescence and often is associated with gynecomastia and other endocrine disturbances.

Although no medical treatments have been proved to be effective, a recent controlled study of thyrotropin-releasing hormone showed promising results for SMA types 2 and 3.[82] Folic acid, vitamin B_{12}, and creatinine have been shown to be beneficial in animal models of SMA. Sodium butyrate increases the amount of exon 7 SMN protein in SMA lymphoid cell lines by changing the alternative SMN splicing pattern of exon 7 in the SMN 2 gene. This process dramatically alters the course of SMA in mice. Nutritional modifications are also promising (see Chapter 14).

ALS is a disease of unknown etiology that affects both upper and lower motor neurons. Five to 10% of cases have an autosomal dominant pattern of transmission. ALS has an incidence of about 1 per 1800 population in the United States. ALS/MND usually presents between ages 25 and 74.[83] The mean age at onset is about 57 years.[84] Monomelic and juvenile forms may present before age 25. The first symptoms and signs are usually muscle cramps, weakness, and fasciculations; however, fatigue, dyspnea, slurred speech, dysphagia, and hypophonia also may be initial symptoms (Fig. 11). Flaccid paralysis and atrophy usually coexist with cramps, fasciculations, and spasticity. Pseudobulbar affect, or pathologic crying or laughing, can be quite troubling; it is not a mood disorder but an abnormal affective display that occurs in up to 50% of patients.[85] Amitriptyline and fluvoxamine have been reported to be helpful for treating pseudobulbar affect.[85]

The rate of disease progression is variable but most often linear. The rate of decline in pulmonary function most closely correlates with death for patients not managed with respiratory aids. For such patients, mean survival is 4 years.[84] It has been estimated that 15–20% of all patients have a slower form with survival for more than 5 years without ventilatory support.[17] Another study reported that only about 4% of mainly younger men had unusually long courses with milder paralysis, but such patients could not be identified early in the illness.[83] Patients with onset between 25 and 44 years survived 71.5 months; patients with onset between 45 and 54 years, 32.5 months; and patients with onset from 55 to 74 years, 32.5 months.[83] We and others have seen patients with typical ALS/MND who have had persistent improvement in vital capacity and strength of large muscle groups beginning 6-7 years after onset. In a sense, muscle function tends to plateau for most people with ALS/MND. We have had patients whose vital capacity stabilized at around 300 ml for years. Many retain some finger or arm function, and 67–90% retain the ability to blink the eyes.

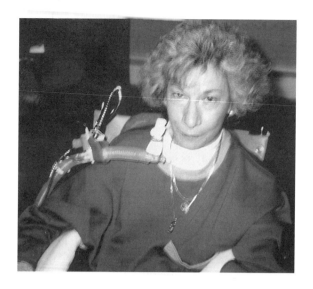

FIGURE 11. Woman with onset of amyotrophic lateral sclerosis at age 59 years. She was diagnosed 6 months later, developed hypophonia from alveolar hypoventilation 13 months after onset, and quickly became dependent on daytime mouthpiece and nocturnal nasal IPPV with no breathing tolerance. She lost bulbar function 6 months later and died after refusing tracheotomy.

It is possible that most survivors of the mid-century poliomyelitis pandemic are still alive. Over 500,000 people were afflicted in the United States (Fig. 12).[86] There also have been several hundred indigenous acute cases and many immigrants with postpolio sequelae.[87] In addition, non-polio virus anterior horn cell disease typical of poliomyelitis has been reported.

In one center, 10% of 500 patients who had required iron lungs remained ventilator-dependent, whereas 73% had become completely free of ventilators by 4–7 years after acute poliomyelitis.[88] The same center reported a 44% incidence of late-onset chronic ventilatory insufficiency.[89] Late complications of poliomyelitis present as a form of motor neuron disease with a constellation of symptoms that include fatigue, dysphagia, dyspnea, and increased functional difficulties.[90] The condition results from senescent loss of remaining anterior horn cells. Postpolio survivors are developing pulmonary complications associated

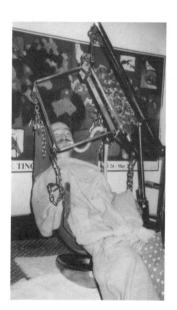

FIGURE 12. Patient with poliomyelitis who uses 24-hour mouthpiece (daytime) or lipseal (sleep) IPPV. He has had no measurable vital capacity and no volitional extremity movement since 1952 but has never been intubated or hospitalized for respiratory failure since having acute poliomyelitis. He uses a Hoyer lift to facilitate bowel movements. This approach has reduced the time needed to complete bowel movements from 3 hours to 15–20 minutes.

with respiratory muscle weakness and, occasionally, bulbar muscle weakness. Many patients who require ventilatory assistance are able to walk.

Neuropathies

The most common hereditary peripheral neuropathy is Charcot-Marie-Tooth disease. It is an autosomal dominant disorder with variable penetrance, symmetric distal greater than proximal weakness, and sensory involvement. EMG demonstrates severe nerve conduction slowing; however, an axonal form has been described in which conduction can be within normal limits while amplitudes are diminished. Although ankle deformities and distal extremity weakness and sensory loss are usually the only impairments, occasional patients (four in the author's experience) progress to severe generalized weakness and need for permanent ventilatory support.

Familial hypertrophic interstitial polyneuropathy (Dejerine-Sottas disease) is a rare disease of generalized weakness. It is diagnosed by peripheral nerve biopsy. Bulbar muscle involvement often precludes the optimal use of noninvasive inspiratory muscle aids because the lips are often too weak to grasp a mouthpiece and scoliosis can prevent the effective use of an intermittent abdominal pressure ventilator (IAPV). Expiratory muscle aids, however, can assist cough.

A multitude of conditions can cause phrenic nerve trauma and neuropathies (see Table 1). A common new cause is iatrogenic phrenic nerve damage during coronary artery bypass surgery.[91] Ventilatory failure occurs during the first few days after surgery. Because of bulbar and expiratory muscle sparing, patients require only inspiratory muscle aids, but they are conventionally managed by invasive means, often with dire consequences (see Case 21 in Chapter 15).

Acute postinfectious polyneuropathy (Guillain-Barré syndrome) is an acquired inflammatory, segmental, demyelinating neuropathy. Two-thirds of cases present with a history of preceding viral infection, immunization, surgery, or immunologic disorder.[92] Sensory loss is usually slight and is absent in one-third of patients.[92] Ascending weakness and paresthesias begin in the hands and feet and usually progress for 1–2 weeks. Partial to almost complete recovery usually takes 3–6 months. Protein concentration in cerebrospinal fluid is elevated at some time during the illness. The diagnosis is based on the history, clinical and laboratory picture, and observation of characteristically severe nerve conduction slowing. With recovery, residual weakness ranges from mild ankle dorsiflexion weakness to severe paralysis necessitating permanent ventilatory support (uncommon).

Other Neurologic Conditions

Multiple sclerosis is a disease of unknown etiology characterized by widespread patches of CNS demyelination followed by gliosis. Its incidence is 1–8 per 10,000 population.[93] The most common symptoms and signs include optic neuritis and nystagmus. Focal or generalized paralysis, incoordination, dysarthria, sensory abnormalities, bowel and bladder incontinence, vertigo, and mental symptoms are also common. The diagnosis is made by the characteristic appearance of high gammaglobulin levels in cerebrospinal fluid, occasional elevations of mononuclear cell levels, and the characteristic appearance of CNS plaques during nuclear magnetic resonance imaging. Remissions and relapses are characteristic and usually occur over many years. Acute relapses often respond well to administration of high doses of corticosteroids (Fig. 13).

Friedreich's ataxia, which is inherited in an autosomal recessive (rarely autosomal dominant) fashion, is a progressive condition that presents after 5 years of age. Symptoms include generalized CNS (especially spinal cord) degeneration and reactive gliosis. The anterior horn cells also may be involved.[94] About 50% of patients die from cardiomyopathy.[95] Chronic alveolar hypoventilation and severely impaired cough occur late in the disease.

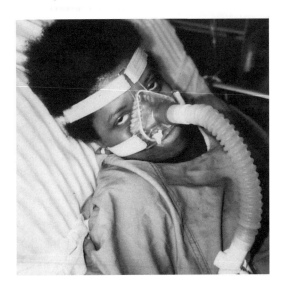

FIGURE 13. This 36-year-old woman with multiple sclerosis, blind from optic neuritis, presented with transverse myelitis and acute ventilatory failure. Her vital capacity decreased to as low as 100 ml. She received 24-hour nasal IPPV instead of intubation (see Case Study 1, Chapter 15).

Myelopathies

The most common cause of myelopathy is traumatic SCI, which most commonly results from motor vehicle accidents, diving accidents, and gunshot wounds. The incidence of acute SCI in the United States is 28–50 per million per year.[96] The number of tetraplegics slightly exceeds that of paraplegics.[97] The prevalence of people with SCI in the United States has been estimated at about 200,000[98] and is increasing yearly because of prolonged survival and longevity.[99] Untimely and inadequate treatment for impaired cough are the principal reasons that pneumonia is the leading cause of death both acutely and over the long term[100] (Fig. 14).

Myelitis, which refers to any condition that causes inflammation of the spinal cord, usually involves both gray and white matter and may involve any level of the spine. When limited to a few segments it is noted as transverse myelitis. It is most often due to neurotrophic viruses and is associated with small pox, measles, chicken pox, mononucleosis, herpes zoster, influenza, certain vaccinations, and tuberculosis.[15] An episode of apparent transverse myelitis may be a precursor to multiple sclerosis. Myelopathies also result from

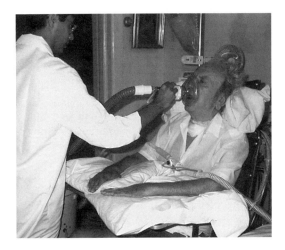

FIGURE 14. Seventy-two-year-old man who suffered a C2 fracture and complete C2 tetraplegia after falling from a tree. His tracheostomy tube, which was placed in the immediate postinjury period, was removed, and he relied on continuous noninvasive IPPV. Here he is using mechanical insufflation-exsufflation to eliminate food that he aspirated because of swallowing dysfunction.

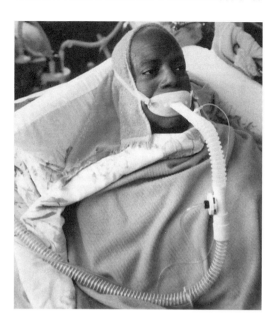

FIGURE 15. Man with idiopathic C2 transverse myelitis who developed complete tetraplegia over several months in 1967 and relied on continuous mouthpiece IPPV until his death from an unrelated cancer in 1997.

radiation exposure, tumors, vascular disease (especially of the anterior and posterior spinal arteries), fibrocartilaginous emboli to the spine,[101] cervical spondylosis, spondylitis associated with connective tissue diseases, and electric shock to the spine. Most often, however, the cause is unknown (Fig. 15). Myelopathies, which may be of sudden onset or develop over months or years, result in ventilatory failure. Bulbar musculature is most often spared.

Tetraplegia can result from administration of pancuronium bromide[102] or other curarization agents, which often are used to prevent self-extubation. Botulism, the generalized paralysis resulting from the toxin of intestinal *Clostridium botulinum* spores, also has been treated by noninvasive ventilatory support rather than endotracheal intubation.[103] Botulism immune globulin, which neutralizes the toxin in the intestine, may prove to be effective in limiting paralysis.

SKELETAL PATHOLOGY

Kyphoscoliosis invariably develops in children with progressive NMDs and is frequently seen in neurofibromatosis, osteogenesis imperfecta, tuberculosis of the spine,[104] rigid spine syndrome,[105] familial dysautonomia, and especially familial autosomal dominant idiopathic kyphoscoliosis (see Chapter 2). Table 3 lists reasons for attempting to prevent kyphoscoliosis whenever possible.

PULMONARY CANDIDATES FOR PHYSICAL MEDICINE RESPIRATORY INTERVENTIONS

In the United States more than 7.5 million people have chronic bronchitis, and 2.3 million have pulmonary emphysema. Over 70,000 deaths annually are due to chronic obstructive pulmonary disease (COPD). It is the 5th leading cause of death, directly causing 3% of all deaths.[106,107] Its incidence has more than doubled since 1970, and it is likely to become increasingly prevalent because of the prolonged survival of the general population. Fifty percent of patients have activity limitations, and 25% are bed-disabled.[108] COPD is the fourth largest cause of major activity limitation.

TABLE 3.   Reasons to Prevent Kyphoscoliosis

1. To permit intermittent abdominal pressure ventilator use as an option to treat alveolar hypoventilation
2. To prevent associated cardiopulmonary compromise
3. To prevent loss of ability to sit
4. To prevent loss of sitting balance and need for seating support systems
5. To prevent lumbar radiculopathies and lower limb radicular pain
6. To prevent ischial skin pressure pain and pressure ulcers

Chronic bronchitis, emphysema, asthmatic bronchitis, and cystic fibrosis are the most common causes of COPD. These conditions usually have significant elements of both airway obstruction and parenchymal lung disease. COPD often results from a combination of genetic predisposition and environmental factors in which allergic diatheses (e.g., asthma), respiratory infections (e.g., bronchopneumonitis), chemical inflammation (cigarette smoke, asbestoses), and possibly metabolic abnormalities (e.g., alpha1 antitrypsin deficiency) cause chronic inflammation and proliferation of mucus-producing cells, impair mucociliary clearance, and ultimately destroy the connective tissues that provide structure for the lungs. This process results in the collapsing airways and air trapping that are characteristic of COPD. Mucus hypersecretion and retention block airways and set the stage for recurrent infection, airway and alveolar damage, and irreversible lower airflow obstruction. Chronic bronchitis, which is characterized by mucus hypersecretion and air flow obstruction, also can develop from asthma.

One in 15 people who smoke one or more packs of cigarettes per day succumbs to lung cancer, and many others succumb from other cancers or the cardiovascular complications of cigarette smoking. On the average, a 30- to 35-year-old person who smokes 10–20 cigarettes per day will die 5 years sooner than a nonsmoker. A person of the same age who smokes 1–2 packs per day will die 6.5 years sooner.[109] Smoking is by far the most frequent cause of chronic bronchitis and emphysema. All smokers eventually develop emphysema if they survive long enough. Smokers are 3.5–25 times more likely (depending on the amount smoked) to die of COPD than nonsmokers.[110]

Pure emphysema is characterized by distention of air spaces distal to the terminal nonrespiratory bronchioles with destruction of alveolar walls. Pathologic changes include loss of lung recoil, excessive airway collapse on exhalation, and chronic airflow obstruction. Chronic bronchitis and cystic fibrosis are characterized by enlargement of tracheobronchial mucus glands, chronic mucus hypersecretion, and chest infections. Chronic bronchitis is defined by the daily presence of a productive cough (not caused by reflux) for 3 months or longer for at least 2 successive years. Mucus hypersecretion appears to be a nonspecific response to irritating airborne substances such as cigarette smoke. Some people have a chronic productive cough for many years without developing airway obstruction; they have simple bronchitis. In other cases, definite airway obstruction occurs. A bronchogram shows poor peripheral filling of terminal bronchi and distinct irregularities of the bronchial wall. Chronic bronchitis is distinguished from asthmatic bronchitis by its irreversibility, lack of bronchial hyperreactivity, lack of responsiveness to bronchodilators, and distinctive abnormalities in ventilation-perfusion.[111] It should not be forgotten, however, that the most common cause of a chronic productive cough in adults is not lung or airways disease but gastric reflux.

Chest-wall distortions occur in patients with COPD, and the resulting stretching of inspiratory and expiratory musculature alters normal length-contraction relationships. This process leads to respiratory muscle weakness and, along with airway mucus trapping, episodes of decompensation.

Cystic fibrosis is the most common life-threatening inherited disorder. About 30,000 Americans have cystic fibrosis. It develops in people who are homozygous for the defective gene on the long arm of chromosome 7. The gene codes for a protein called cystic fibrosis transmembrane conductance regulator. Chloride concentration is markedly elevated in the sweat. The presence of *Pseudomonas aeruginosa* in sputum is characteristic, and sinusitis is usually present. Males are usually azoospermic.

The basic defect is resistance to chloride permeability in epithelial cells, which prevents the reabsorption of chloride along the sweat duct tubules. Although there is no damage in utero, shortly after birth bacterial pathogens become impossible to eradicate from the lungs. Mucus-secreting glands hypertrophy, and thick secretions plug the airways. The structural integrity of the bronchi is disrupted, and cystic and cylindric bronchiectasis develops. Hemoptysis is common, and occasionally bronchial bleeding is fatal. Eventually hypoxemia, pulmonary hypertension, and cor pulmonale develop. These conditions are exacerbated late in the course of the disease when, as in patients with advanced emphysema or bronchitis, chronic hypercapnia develops. About one-half of such patients also exhibit reversible bronchospasm.

Noninvasive ventilation has been described as a bridge to lung transplantation for patients with cystic fibrosis.[112] Noninvasive facilitation of airway secretion elimination is also important as well as possible long-term antibiotic therapy, aerosolized bronchodilators for patients with reversible bronchospasm, aerosolized human recombinant DNAase, occasional glucocorticoid therapy, and transmembrane conductance regulator genes delivered by aerosolized adenovirus. See Chapter 2 for more information about pathophysiology.

In addition to chest hypoexpansion due to muscle weakness, restrictive pulmonary syndromes can result from lung resection, chest wall pathology, and morbid obesity. Patients with intrinsic lung diseases such as pulmonary fibrosis also may have restrictive pulmonary syndromes. Although restrictive syndromes associated with respiratory muscle dysfunction are characterized by low vital capacity, low total lung capacity, low minute ventilation, and decreased lung and chest wall compliance, in restrictive conditions caused by intrinsic lung disease minute ventilation is increased and $PaCO_2$ levels are low until late in the disease. Diffusion can be greatly reduced in such patients with pulmonary fibrosis or other infiltrative conditions.

✦

No tengas pena, amigo, porque yo har ahora el balsamo precioso, con el que sanaremos en un abrir y cerrar de ojos.
(Do not worry, friend, for I now have a precious balm with which we can cure you in the blink of un eye.)

Miguel de Cervantes, *Don Quijote de La Mancha*

✦

REFERENCES

1. Bach JR, Alba AS: Pulmonary dysfunction and sleep disordered breathing as post-polio sequelae: Evaluation and management. Orthopedics 14:1329–1337, 1991.
2. Fischer DA: Poliomyelitis: Late respiratory complications and management. Orthopedics 8:891–894, 1985.
3. Bach JR: Alternative methods of ventilatory support for the patient with ventilatory failure due to spinal cord injury. J Am Paraplegia Soc 14:158–174, 1991.
4. Bach JR: Inappropriate weaning and late onset ventilatory failure of individuals with traumatic quadriplegia. Paraplegia 31:430–438, 1993.
5. Bach JR, Alba AS, Saporito LR: Intermittent positive pressure ventilation via the mouth as an alternative to tracheostomy for 257 ventilator users. Chest 103:174–182, 1993.
6. Aisen M, Arlt G, Foster S: Diaphragmatic paralysis without bulbar or limb paralysis in multiple sclerosis. Chest 98:499–501, 1990.
7. Bach JR, Alba A, Mosher R, Delaubier A: Intermittent positive pressure ventilation via nasal access in the management of respiratory insufficiency. Chest 92:168–170, 1987.

8. Manon-Espaillat R, Gothe B, Ruff RL, Newman C: Sleep apnea in multiple sclerosis. J Neurol Rehabil 3:133–136, 1989.
9. Engel AG, Franzini-Armstrong C (eds): Myology: Basic and Clinical, vol 2. New York, McGraw-Hill, 1994.
10. Griggs RC, Mendell JR, Miller RG: Evaluation and treatment of myopathies. Philadelphia, F.A. Davis, 1995.
11. Roland LP, Laycer RB: The X-linked muscular dystrophies. In Vinken PJ, Bruyn GW (eds): Handbook of Clinical Neurology. New York, North Holland, 1979, pp 349–414.
12. Yang GF, Alba A, Lee M: Respiratory rehabilitation in severe restrictive lung disease secondary to tuberculosis. Arch Phys Med Rehabil 65:556–558, 1994.
13. Younger DS (ed): Paralysis. Part 1. Semin Neurol 13:241–315, 1991.
14. Younger DS (ed): Paralytic syndromes. Part II. Semin Neurol 13:319–379, 1991.
15. Walton JN: Brain's Diseases of the Nervous System, 8th ed. Oxford, Oxford University Press, 1977, pp 779–786.
16. Erb W: Dystrophia Muscularis Progressiva: Klinische und Pathologischanatomische Studien. Deutsch Z Nervenheilk 1:13–94, 173–261, 1891.
17. Mulder DW, Howard FM: Patient resistance and prognosis in amyotrophic lateral sclerosis. Mayo Clin Proc 51:537–541, 1976.
18. Liechti-Gallati S, Koenig M, Kunkel LM, et al: Molecular deletion patterns in Duchenne and Becker type muscular dystrophy. Hum Genet 81:343–348, 1989.
19. Emery AEH: Duchenne muscular dystrophy: Genetic aspects, carrier detection and antenatal diagnosis. Br Med Bull 36:117–122, 1980.
20. Miyatake M, Miike T, Zhao J, et al: Possible systemic smooth muscle layer dysfunction due to a deficiency of dystrophin in Duchenne muscular dystrophy. J Neurol Sci 93:11–17, 1989.
21. Hinge HF, Hein-Sorensen O, Reske-Nielsen E: X-linked Duchenne muscular dystrophy. Scand J Rehabil Med 21:27–31, 1989.
22. Demos J: Early diagnosis and treatment of rapidly developing Duchenne de Boulogne type myopathy. Am J Phys Med 50:271–284, 1971.
23. Gardner-Medwin D: Clinical features and classification of the muscular dystrophies. Br Med Bull 36:109–115, 1980.
24. Rowland LP, Fetell M, Olarte M, et al: Emery-Dreifuss muscular dystrophy. Ann Neurol 5:111–117, 1979.
25. Hinton VJ, DeVivo DC, Nereo NE, et al: Selective deficits in verbal working memory associated with a known genetic etiology: The neuropsychological profile of Duchenne muscular dystrophy. JINS 7:45–54, 2001.
26. Meryon E: On granular or fatty degeneration of the voluntary muscles. Medico-Chirurgical Trans 35:73–84, 1852.
27. Griggs RC, Moxley RT, Mendell JR, et al: Randomized, double-blind trial of mazindol in Duchenne dystrophy. Muscle Nerve 13:1169–1173, 1990.
28. Zatz J, Betti RTB: Benign Duchenne muscular dystrophy in a patient with growth hormone deficiency: A five year follow-up. Am J Med Genet 24:567–572, 1986.
29. Zatz J, Betti RTB, Frota-Pessoa O: Treatment of Duchenne muscular dystrophy with growth hormone inhibitors. Am J Med Genet 24:549–566, 1988.
30. DeSilva S, Drachman DB, Mellits D, Kunel RW: Prednisone treatment in Duchenne muscular dystrophy: Long-term benefit. Arch Neurol 44:818–822, 1987.
31. Drachman DB, Toyka RV, Myer E: Prednisone in Duchenne muscular dystrophy Lancet 2:1409–1412, 1974.
32. Backman E, Henriksson KG: Low dose prednisolone treatment in Duchenne and Becker muscular dystrophy. Neuromusc Disord 5:233–241, 1995.
33. Mendell JR, Moxley RC, Griggs RC, et al: Randomized, double-blind six-month trial of prednisone in Duchenne's muscular dystrophy. N Engl J Med 320:1592–1597, 1989.
34. Siegel IM, Miller JE, Ray RD: Failure of corticosteroid in the treatment of Duchenne (pseudo-hypertrophic) muscular dystrophy: Report of a clinically matched three year double-blind study. Illinois Med J 145:32–33, 1974.
35. Cohen L, Morgan J, Babbs Jr R, et al: Fast walking velocity in health and Duchenne muscular dystrophy: A statistical analysis. Arch Phys Med Rehabil 65:553–758, 1984.
36. Dubrovsky AL, Mesa L, Marco P, et al: Deflazacort treatment in Duchenne muscular dystrophy. Neurology 41(Suppl 1):136–141, 1991.
37. Heckmatt J, Rodillo E, Dubowitz V: Management of children: Pharmacological and physical. Br Med Bull 45:788–801, 1989.
38. Rideau Y, Glorion B, Delaubier A, et al: Treatment of scoliosis in Duchenne muscular dystrophy. Muscle Nerve 7:281–286, 1984.
39. Duport G, Gayet E, Pries P, et al: Spinal deformities and wheelchair seating in Duchenne muscular dystrophy: Twenty years of research and clinical experience. Semin Neurol 15:9–17, 1995.
40. Brooke MH, Fenichel GM, Griggs RC, et al: Duchenne muscular dystrophy: patterns of clinical progression and effects of supportive therapy. Neurol 39:475–480, 1989.
41. Mukoyama M, Kondo K, Hizawa K, and the DMDR Group: Life spans of Duchenne muscular dystrophy patients in the hospital care program in Japan. J Neurol Sci 81:155–158, 1987.

42. Inkley SR, Oldenberg FC, Vignos PJ: Pulmonary function in Duchenne muscular dystrophy related to stage of disease. Am J Med 56:297–306, 1974.
43. Rideau Y, Gatin G, Bach J, Gines G: Prolongation of life in Duchenne muscular dystrophy. Acta Neurol 5:118–124, 1983.
44. Vignos PJ. Respiratory function and pulmonary infection in Duchenne muscular dystrophy. Isr J Med Sci 13:207–214, 1977.
45. Tamura T, Shibuya N, Hashiba K, et al: Evaluation of myocardial damage in Duchenne's muscular dystrophy with thalium-201 myocardial SPECT. Jpn Heart J 34:51–61, 1993.
46. Barohn RJ, Levine EJ, Olson JO, Mendell JR: Gastric hypomotility in Duchenne's muscular dystrophy. N Engl J Med 319:15–18, 1988.
47. Leon SH, Schuffler MD, Kettler M, Rohrmann CA: Chronic intestinal pseudoobstruction as a complication of Duchenne's muscular dystrophy. Gastroenterology 90:455–459, 1986.
48. Jaffe KM, McDonald CM, Ingman E, Haas J: Symptoms of upper gastrointestinal dysfunction in Duchenne muscular dystrophy: Case-control study. Arch Phys Med Rehabil 71:742–744, 1990.
49. Bach JR, O'Brien J, Krotenberg R, Alba A: Management of end stage respiratory failure in Duchenne muscular dystrophy. Muscle Nerve 10:177–182, 1987.
50. Thomas NST, Williams H, Elsas LJ, et al: Localisation of the gene for Emery-Dreifuss muscular dystrophy to the distal long arm of the X chromosome. J Med Genet 23:596–598, 1986.
51. Miller RG, Layzer RB, Mellenthin MA, et al: Emery-Dreifuss muscular dystrophy with autosomal dominant transmission. Neurology 35:1230–1233, 1985.
52. Walton JN, Gardner-Medwin D: The muscular dystrophies. In Walton J (ed): Disorders of Voluntary Muscle, 5th ed. London, Churchill Livingstone, 1988, pp 519–568.
53. Rideau Y, Delaubier A, Foucault P, et al: Une forme meconnue de myopathie. II: Définition et caractères cliniques. Semin Hôp Paris 67:1343–1349, 1991.
54. McMenamin JB, Becker LE, Murphy EG: Congenital muscular dystrophy: A clinicopathologic report of 24 cases. J Pediatr 100:692–697, 1982.
55. O'Brien MD. An infantile muscular dystrophy· Report of a case with autopsy findings. Guys Hosp Rep 111:98–106, 1962.
56. Wharton BA: An unusual variety of muscular dystrophy. Lancet i:603–604, 1965.
57. Zellweger H, Afifi A, McCormick WF, Mergner W: Severe congenital muscular dystrophy. Am J Dis Child 114:591–602, 1967.
58. Bailey RO, Marzulo DC, Hans MB: Infantile fascioscapulohumeral muscular dystrophy: New observations. Acta Neurol Scand 74:51–58, 1986.
59. Brooke MH: A Clinician's View of Neuromuscular Diseases, 2nd ed. Baltimore, Williams & Wilkins, 1986, pp 194–212.
60. Aslanidis C, Jansen G, Amemiya C, et al: Cloning of the essential myotonic dystrophy region and mapping of the putative defect. Nature 355:548–551, 1992.
61. Rutherford MA, Heckmatt JZ, Dubowitz V: Congenital myotonic dystrophy: Respiratory function at birth determines survival. Arch Dis Childh 64:191–195, 1989.
62. Zucca MR, Martinetti C, Ottolini A, et al: Hypersomnia in dystrophia myotonica: a neurophysiological and immunogenetic study. Acta Neurol Scand 84:498–502, 1991.
63. Fernandez JM, Lara I, Gila L, et al. Disturbed hypothalamic-pituitary axis in idiopathic recurring hypersomnia syndrome. Acta Neurol Scand 82:361–363, 1990.
64. Chan CK, Loke J, Virgulto JA, et al: Bilateral diaphragmatic paralysis: Clinical spectrum, prognosis, and diagnostic approach. Arch Phys Med Rehabil 69:967–979, 1988.
65. Rimmer KP, Whitelaw WA: The respiratory muscles in multicore myopathy. Am Rev Respir Dis 148:227–231, 1993.
66. Brownell AKW, Gilbert JJ, Shaw DT, et al: Adult onset nemaline myopathy. Neurology 28:1306–1309, 1978.
67. Jerusalem F, Ludin H, Bischoff A, Hartmann G: Cytoplasmic body neuromyopathy presenting as respiratory failure and weight loss. J Neurol Sci 41:1–9, 1979.
68. Carpenter S, Karpati G, Holland P: New observations in reducing body myopathy. Neurology 35:818–827, 1985.
69. Selby R, Starzl TE, Yunis E, et al: Liver transplantation for type IV glycogen storage disease. N Engl J Med 324:39–42, 1991.
70. Stanley CA, DeLeeuw S, Coates PM, et al: Chronic cardiomyopathy and weakness or acute coma in children with a defect in carnitine uptake. Ann Neurol 30:709–716, 1991.
71. Griggs RC, Mendell JR, Miller RG: Evaluation and treatment of myopathies. Philadelphia, F.A. Davis, 1995, pp 294–313.
72. Barohn RJ, Clanton T, Sahenk Z, Mendell JR: Recurrent respiratory insufficiency and depressed ventilatory drive complicating mitochondrial myopathies. Neurology 40:103–106, 1990.
73. Bendahan D, Desnuelle C, Vanuxem D, et al: 31P NMR spectroscopy and ergometer exercise test as evidence for muscle oxidative performance improvement with coenzyme Q in mitochondrial myopathies. Neurology 42:1203–1208, 1992.
74. Thompson CE: Infantile myositis. Dev Med Child Neurol 24:307–313, 1982.

75. Fowler WM, Nayak NN: Slowly progressive proximal weakness: Limb-girdle syndromes. Arch Phys Med Rehabil 64:527–538, 1983.
76. Blumbergs PC, Byrne E, Kakulas BA: Polymyositis presenting with respiratory failure. J Neurol Sci 65:221–229, 1984.
77. Simpson JA: Myasthenia gravis and myasthenic syndromes. In Walton JN (ed): Disorders of Voluntary Muscle, 5th ed. London, Churchill Livingstone, 1988, pp 628–665.
78. Wang TG, Bach JR: Pulmonary dysfunction in residents of chronic care facilities. Taiwan J Rehabil 21:67–73, 1993.
79. Iannaccone ST: Spinal muscular atrophy. Semin Neurol 18:19–26, 1998.
80. Dubowitz V: Very severe spinal muscular atrophy (SMA type 0): An expanding clinical phenotype. Eur J Paediatr Neurol 3:49–51, 1999.
81 Mier-Jedrzejowicz A, Brophy C, Green M: Respiratory muscle weakness during upper respiratory tract infections. Am Rev Respir Dis 138:5–7, 1988.
82. Tzeng AC, Cheng JF, Fryczynski H, et al: Randomized double-blind prospective study of thyrotropin-releasing hormone for the treatment of spinal muscular atrophy: A preliminary report. Am J Phys Med Rehabil 79:435–440, 2000.
83. Norris F, Shepherd R, Denys E, et al: Onset, natural history and outcome in idiopathic adult motor neuron disease. J Neurol Sci 118:48–55, 1993.
84. Ringel SP, Murphy JR, Alderson MK, et al: The natural history of amyotrophic lateral sclerosis. Neurology 43:1316–1322, 1993.
85. Miller RG, Rosenberg JA, Gelinas DF, et al: Practice parameter: the care of the patient with amyotrophic lateral sclerosis: Report of the Quality Standards Subcommittee of the American Academy of Neurology ALS Practice Parameters Task Force. Neurology 52:1311–1323, 1999.
86. Historical Statistics of the United States: Colonial Times to 1970, Bicentennial Edition. Part 1. Washington, DC, U. S. Department of Commerce, Bureau of the Census, 1975, pp 8,77.
87. Statistical Abstracts of the United States, 110th ed. Washington, DC, U. S. Department of Commerce, Bureau of the Census, 1990, p 116.
88. Affeldt JE, Bower AG, Dail CW: The prognosis for respiratory recovery in severe poliomyelitis. Arch Phys Med Rehabil 38:383–388, 1957.
89. Baydur A, Layne E, Aral H, et al: Long term non-invasive ventilation in the community for patients with musculoskeletal disorders: 46 year experience and review. Thorax 55:4–11, 2000.
90. Halstead LS: Post-polio sequelae: Assessment and differential diagnosis for post-polio syndrome. Orthopedics 14:1209–1217, 1991.
91. Wilcox P, Baile EM, Hards J, et al: Phrenic nerve function and its relationship to atelectasis after coronary artery bypass surgery. Chest 93:693–698, 1988.
92. Lisak RP: The immunology of neuromuscular disease. In Walton JN (ed): Disorders of Voluntary Muscle, 5th ed. London, Churchill Livingstone, 1988, pp 345–371.
93. Walton JN: Brain's Diseases of the Nervous System, 8th ed. Oxford, Oxford University Press, 1977, pp 548–549.
94. Walton JN: Brain's Diseases of the Nervous System, 8th ed. Oxford, Oxford University Press, 1977, pp 672–674.
95. Hewer RL: Study of fatal cases of Friedreich's ataxia. Br Med J 3:649–652, 1968.
96. DeVivo MJ, Fine PR, Maetz HM, Stover SL: Prevalence of spinal cord injury: A re-estimation employing life table techniques. Arch Neurol 37:707–708, 1980.
97. Kennedy EJ (ed): Spinal Cord Injury: The Facts and Figures. Birmingham, AL, University of Alabama, 1986, p 27.
98. Kraus JF: Epidemiological aspects of acute spinal cord injury: A review of incidence, prevalence, causes, and outcome. In Becker DP, Povlishock JT (eds): Central Nervous System Trauma Status Report—1985. Bethesda, MD, National Institute of Neurological and Communicative Disorders and Stroke, National Institutes of Health, 1985, pp 313–322.
99. Kennedy EJ (ed): Spinal Cord Injury: The Facts and Figures. Birmingham, AL, University of Alabama, 1986, p 59.
100. DeVivo MJ, Black KJ, Stover SL: Causes of death during the first twelve years after spinal cord injury [abstract]. J Am Parapleg Soc 14:113, 1991.
101. Bockenek W, Bach JR: Fibrocartilaginous emboli to the spinal cord: A review of the literature. J Am Parapleg Soc 13:18–23, 1990.
102. Giostra E, Magistris MR, Pizzolato G, et al: Neuromuscular disorder in intensive care unit patients treated with pancuronium bromide: Occurrence in a cluster group of seven patients and two sporadic cases, with electrophysiologic and histologic examination. Chest 106:210–220, 1994.
103. Blackney DA: Negative pressure conquers infant botulism. In Lifecare's Alert Newsletter. Murrysville, PA, Respironics, Inc., Sept/Oct 1994.
104. Leger P, Robert D, Langevin B, Guez A: Indications of home mechanical ventilation in patients with chest wall deformities due to idiopathic kyphoscoliosis or sequelae of tuberculosis. Eur Respir Rev 2:362–368, 1992.

105. Efthmiou J, McLelland J, Round J, et al: Diaphragm paralysis causing ventilatory failure in an adult with rigid spine syndrome. Am Rev Respir Dis 136:1483–1485, 1987.
106. Higgins MW, Thom T: Incidence, prevalence, and mortality: Intra- and intercountry differences. In Hensley MJ, Saunders NA (eds): Clinical Epidemiology of Chronic Obstructive Pulmonary Disease. New York, Marcel Dekker, 1989, pp 23–39.
107. National Center for Health Statistics: Current estimates from the National Health Interview Survey, United States. Vital and Health Statistics, Series 10, No. 164. Washington, D.C., Department of Health and Human Services, Public Health Service, 1986, pp 897–1592.
108. Higgins ITT: Epidemiology of bronchitis and emphysema. In Fishman AP (ed): Pulmonary Diseases and Disorders, 2nd ed. New York, McGraw-Hill, 1988, pp 70–90.
109. Department of Health, Education, and Welfare: Smoking and Health: A Report of the Surgeon General. DHEW Publication No. (PHS) 79-50066. Washington, DC, 1979.
110. Fishman AP: The spectrum of chronic obstructive disease of the airways. In Fishman AP (ed): Pulmonary Diseases and Disorders. New York, McGraw-Hill, 1988, pp 1159–1171.
111. Tager I: Chronic bronchitis. In Fishman AP (ed): Pulmonary Diseases and Disorders. New York, McGraw-Hill, 1988, pp 1543–1551.
112. O'Brien G, Criner GJ: Mechanical ventilation as a bridge to lung transplantation. J Heart Lung Transplant 18:255–265, 1999.
113. Bach JR, Ishikawa Y, Kim H: Prevention of pulmonary morbidity for patients with Duchenne muscular dystrophy. Chest 112:1024–1028, 1997.
114. Bach JR, Alba AS: Management of chronic alveolar hypoventilation by nasal ventilation. Chest 97:52–57, 1990.
115. Estenne M, Borenstein S, De Troyer A: Respiratory muscle dysfunction in myotonia congenita. Am Rev Respir Dis 130:681–684, 1984.
116. Vercken JB, Raphael JC, DeLattre J, et al: Adult maltase acid deficiency myopathy: Treatment with long-term home mechanical ventilation. Biomed Pharmacother 42:343–349, 1988.
117. Tanaka C, Maegaki Y: Chronic respiratory failure in juvenile-onset acid alpha-glucosidase deficiency: Successful therapy with nasal intermittent positive pressure ventilation [in Japanese]. No To Hattatsu 1:51–54, 1997.
118. Sancho J, Servera E, Perez D, et al: Nocturnal noninvasive ventilation in a patient with mucopolysaccharidoses. Eighth Journees Internationales de Ventilation a Domicile, abstract 148, March 7, 2001, Hopital de la Croix-Rousse, Lyon, France.
119. Byrne E, Dennett X, Trounce I, Burdon J: Mitochondrial myoneuropathy with respiratory failure and myoclonic epilepsy: A case report with biochemical studies. J Neurol Sci 71:273–281, 1985.
120. Cros D, Palliyath S, DiMauro S, et al: Respiratory failure revealing mitochondrial myopathy in adults. Chest 101:824–828, 1992.
121. Bielen P, Sliwinski P, Kaminski D, Zielinski J: Respiratory failure in mitochondrial myopathy treated with noninvasive mechanical ventilation. Pneumonol Alergol Pol 66:555–559, 1998.
122. Martyn JB, Wong MJ, Huang SHK: Pulmonary and neuromuscular complications in mixed connective tissue disease: a report and review of the literature. J Rheumatol 15:703–705, 1988.
123. Quera-Salva MA, Guilleminault C, Chrevret S, et al: Breathing disorders during sleep in myasthenia gravis. Ann Neurol 31:86–92, 1992.
124. Iannaccone ST, Mills JK, Harris KM, et al: Congenital myasthenic syndrome with sleep hypoventilation. Muscle Nerve 23:1129–1132, 2000.
125. Ryan CF, Whittaker JS, Road JD: Ventilatory dysfunction in severe anorexia nervosa. Chest 102;1286–1288, 1992.
126. Bach JR, Wang TG: Noninvasive long-term ventilatory support for individuals with spinal muscular atrophy and functional bulbar musculature. Arch Phys Med Rehabil 76:213–217, 1995.
127. Dyck PJ, Litchy WJ, Minnerath S, et al: Hereditary motor and sensory neuropathy with diaphragm and vocal cord paresis. Ann Neurol 35:608–615, 1994.
128. LaRoche CM, Carroll N, Moxham J, et al: Diaphragm weakness in Charcot-Marie-Tooth disease. Thorax 43:478–479, 1988.
129. Maziak DE, Maurer JR, Kesten S: Diaphragmatic paralysis: A complication of lung transplantation. Ann Thorac Surg 61:170–173, 1996.
130. Bach JR: New approaches in the rehabilitation of the traumatic high level quadriplegic. Am J Phys Med Rehabil 70:13–20, 1991.
131. Bach JR, Alba AS: Noninvasive options for ventilatory support of the traumatic high level quadriplegic. Chest 98:613–619, 1990.
132. Bockenek W, Bach JR, Alba AS, Cravioto A: Cartilagenous emboli to the spinal cord: A case study. Arch Phys Med Rehabil 71:754–757, 1990.
133. Giostra E, Magistris MR, Pizzolato G, et al: Neuromuscular disorder in intensive care unit patients treated with pancuronium bromide: Occurrence in a cluster group of seven patients and two sporadic cases, with electrophysiologic and histologic examination. Chest 106:210–220, 1994.
134. Fanfulla F, Eleftheriou D, Patruno V, et al: Chronic respiratory failure in a patient with type 1 Arnold-Chiari malformation and syringomyelia. Monaldi Arch Chest Dis 53:138–141, 1998.

135. Ward SLD, Nickerson BG, van der Hal A, et al: Absent hypoxic and hypercapneic arousal responses in children with myelomeningocele and apnea. Pediatrics 78:44–50, 1986.
136. Kirk VG, Morielli A, Gozal D, et al: Treatment of sleep-disordered breathing in children with myelomeningocele. Pediatr Pulmonol 30:445–452, 2000.
137. Brouillette RT, Hunt CE, Gallemore GE: Respiratory dysrhythmia: A new cause of central alveolar hypoventilation. Am Rev Respir Dis 134:609–611, 1986.
138. Bott J, Baudouin SV, Moxham J: Nasal intermittent positive pressure ventilation in the treatment of respiratory failure in obstructive sleep apnea. Thorax 46:457–458, 1991.
139. Thommi G, Nugent K, Bell GM, Liu J: Termination of central sleep apnea episodes by upper airway stimulation using intermittent positive pressure ventilation. Chest 99:1527–1529, 1991.
140. Bullemer F, Heindl S, Karg O: "Ondine's curse" in adults [in German]. Pneumologie 53:S91–S92, 1999.
141. Paditz E, Dinger J, Reitemeier G, et al: Noninvasive ventilation of a 4-year-old boy with severe late onset hypoventilation syndrome. Med Klin 92(Suppl1):46–49, 1997.
142. Kerbl R, Litscher H, Grubbauer HM, et al: Congenital central hypoventilation syndrome (Ondine's curse) in two siblings: Delayed diagnosis and successful noninvasive treatment. Eur J Pediatr 11:977–980, 1996.
143. Banfi P, Bertoletti F, Piccioni L, et al: Hypercapnic respiratory failure in bird face syndrome: One case study. Eighth Journées Internationales de Ventilation à Domicile, abstract 151, March 7, 2001, Hôpital de la Croix-Rousse, Lyon, France.
144. Silverstein D, Michlin B, Sobel HJ, Lavietes MH: Right ventricular failure in a patient with diabetic neuropathy (myopathy) and central alveolar hypoventilation. Respiration 44:460–465, 1983.
145. Smith IE, King MA, Siklos PW, Shneerson JM: Treatment of ventilatory failure in the Prader-Willi syndrome. Eur Respir J 11:1150–1152, 1998.
146. Bach JR, Robert D, Leger P, Langevin B: Sleep fragmentation in kyphoscoliotic individuals with chronic alveolar hypoventilation treated by nasal IPPV. Chest 107:1552–1158, 1995.
147. Augenstein KB, Ward MJ, Nelson VS: Spondyloepiphyseal dysplasia congenita with ventilator dependence: Two case reports. Arch Phys Med Rehabil 77:1201–1204, 1996.
148. Smith IE, Laroche CM, Jamieson SA, Shneerson JM: Kyphosis secondary to tuberculosis osteomyelitis as a cause of ventilatory failure: Clinical features, mechanisms, and management. Chest 110:1105–1110, 1996.
149. Yang GF, Alba A, Lee M: Respiratory rehabilitation in severe restrictive lung disease secondary to tuberculosis. Arch Phys Med Rehabil 65:556–558, 1984.
150. Schulz MR, Herth FJ, Wiebel M, Schulz V: Intermittent positive pressure ventilation in post tuberculosis syndrome [in German]. Pneumologie 53:S116–S119, 1999.
151. Kirshblum SC, Bach JR: Walker modification for ventilator assisted individuals. Am J Phys Med Rehabil 71:304–306, 1992.
152. Shu SM, Hsieh WS, Lin JN, et al: Treatment and outcome of congenital diaphragmatic hernia. J Formos Med Assoc 99:844–847, 2000.
153. Chetty KG, McDonald RI, Berry RB, Mahutte CK: Chronic respiratory failure due to bilateral vocal cord paralysis managed with nocturnal nasal positive pressure ventilation. Chest 103:1270–1271, 1993.
154. Hertzog JH, Siegel LB, Hauser GJ, Dalton HJ: Noninvasive positive-pressure ventilation facilitates tracheal extubation after laryngotracheal reconstruction in children. Chest 116:260–263, 1999.
155. Seggev J, Shapiro MS, Levin S, Schey G: Alveolar hypoventilation and daytime hypersomnia in acromegaly. Eur J Respir Dis 68:381–383, 1986.
156. Piper AJ, Parker S, Torzillo PJ, et al: Nocturnal nasal IPPV stabilizes patients with cystic fibrosis and hypercapnic respiratory failure. Chest 102:846–850, 1992.
157. Fauroux B, Baculard A, Boule M, Tournier G: Noninvasive ventilation using nasal mask in mucoviscidosis. Rev Mal Respir 12:509–511, 1995.
158. Sprague K, Graff G, Tobias DJ: Noninvasive ventilation in respiratory failure due to cystic fibrosis. South Med J 93:954–961, 2000.
159. Keddissi HI, Metcalf JP: The use of noninvasive ventilation in acute respiratory failure associated with oral contrast aspiration pneumonitis. Respir Care 45:494–496, 2000.
160. Confalonieri M, Potena A, Carbone G, et al: Acute respiratory failure in patients with severe community-acquired pneumonia: A prospective randomized evaluation of noninvasive ventilation. Am J Respir Crit Care Med 160:1585–1591, 1999.
161. Marin D, Gonzalez-Barca E, Domingo E, et al: Noninvasive mechanical ventilation in a patient with respiratory failure after hematopoietic progenitor transplantation. Bone Marrow Transplant 22:1123–1124, 1998.
162. Beltrame F, Lucangelo U, Gregori D, Gregoretti C: Noninvasive positive pressure ventilation in trauma patients with acute respiratory failure. Monaldi Arch Chest Dis 54:109–114, 1999.
163. Varon J, Walsh GL, Fromm RE Jr: Feasibility of noninvasive mechanical ventilation in the treatment of acute respiratory failure in postoperative cancer patients. J Crit Care 13:55–57, 1998.
164. Kilger E, Briegel J, Haller M, et al: Noninvasive ventilation after lung transplantation. Med Klin 90(Suppl 1):26–28, 1995.
165. Marin D, Gonzalez-Barca E, Domingo E, et al: Noninvasive mechanical ventilation in a patient with respiratory failure failure after hematopoietic progenitor transplantation. Bone Marrow Transplant 22:1123–1124, 1998.

2 —— Physiology and Pathophysiology of Hypoventilation: Ventilatory vs. Oxygenation Impairment

JOHN R. BACH, M.D.

The Sphinx stares grimly, ominous with question,
Her stony, blank gray eyes tell nothing, nothing,
No single, saving sign, no ray of light:
And if I solve it not, my life is forfeit.

Gustav Mahler, sketch poem for
Des Knaben Wunderhorn, 1883

VENTILATION VS. OXYGENATION IMPAIRMENT

Most patients with impairment of pulmonary function can be placed into one of two categories: (1) those who suffer primarily from oxygenation impairment due mainly to intrinsic lung disease and (2) those with lung ventilation impairment due to respiratory muscle weakness. This distinction is important because, although many patients in the former category have been reported to benefit from noninvasive ventilation in the acute care setting, long-term use is controversial. Patients with primarily ventilatory impairment, on the other hand, can benefit from the use of both inspiratory and expiratory muscle aids. They often can avoid episodes of respiratory failure despite total respiratory muscle paralysis, do not require tracheostomy, and have excellent prognoses with long-term home mechanical ventilation.

It is useful to define terms that can distinguish between the natural courses of the two patient populations. Whereas patients with oxygenation impairment can develop respiratory insufficiency or respiratory failure, ventilatory impairment can be characterized as ventilatory insufficiency or ventilatory muscle failure. Ventilatory insufficiency is defined by hypercapnia in the presence of a normal arterial-alveolar (A-a) gradient. The hypercapnia is not caused by intrinsic lung disease or irreversible airway obstruction. The ventilatory insufficiency can be due to inspiratory muscle dysfunction or central hypoventilation. Patients with ventilatory insufficiency secondary to respiratory muscle dysfunction can have airway obstruction due to bronchial mucus plugging. This obstruction causes an elevated A-a gradient. However, because the mucus plugging is reversible with the use of respiratory muscle aids, these patients still belong in the category of primarily ventilation impairment. A typical example of ventilatory insufficiency is the hypercapnic patient with Duchenne muscular dystrophy (DMD) who has normal SpO_2 when awake and is asymptomatic or minimally symptomatic with little or no ventilator use. Patients with symptoms due to ventilatory insufficiency most often have dips in SpO_2 below 95%. Symptomatic hypercapnic patients benefit from the use of noninvasive ventilation for at least part of the day, most often overnight. With progressive ventilatory muscle weakness, withdrawal of daily or nightly aid eventually results in ventilatory failure.

Ventilatory muscle failure is defined by the inability of the inspiratory and expiratory muscles to sustain respiration without immediate resort to ventilator use. Patients with ventilatory muscle failure do not have unlimited breathing tolerance and require ventilatory support. Ventilatory insufficiency leading to respiratory failure can be nocturnal only and result from diaphragm failure (the patient is unable to breathe when supine); it also can result from a lack of central ventilatory drive, as in patients with congenital central hypoventilation, or severe generalized respiratory muscle dysfunction. This point deserves further elucidation. Many patients with ventilatory insufficiency survive for years without ventilator use at the cost of increasingly severe hypercapnia, its associated symptoms and dangers, and a compensatory metabolic alkalosis that depresses the hypoxic and hypercapnic central ventilatory drive. The alkalosis allows the brain to accommodate to hypercapnia without overt symptoms of acute ventilatory failure. When such patients are treated with noninvasive intermittent positive pressure ventilation (IPPV), blood gases normalize and the metabolic alkalosis resolves as the kidneys excrete excessive bicarbonate ions. Then, because of the need to take larger breaths to maintain normal $PaCO_2$ and blood pH levels, the ventilator user becomes intolerably short of breath when ventilator use is discontinued and, at least temporarily, loses any significant breathing tolerance. Breathing tolerance can be lost in supine, sitting, side-lying, or all positions. Without ventilator use, the untreated patient with severe ventilatory muscle dysfunction develops increasingly severe hypercapnia that eventually results in coma due to carbon dioxide narcosis or ventilatory (respiratory) arrest. Respiratory arrest occurs despite the absence of significant intrinsic lung disease. Thus, patients with ventilatory muscle dysfunction may require daily periodic (but often not continuous) ventilatory support. Some patients with ventilatory muscle failure and no measurable vital capacity with their breathing muscles use only nocturnal aid and rely on glossopharyngeal breathing (GPB) to ventilate their lungs during daytime hours.

Patients who suffer primarily from oxygenation impairment, on the other hand, have an increased A-a gradient with or without hypercapnia. The A-a gradient increases whenever there is decreased diffusion or increased blood flow. The increased blood flow that occurs with increased physical activity can exacerbate the A-a oxygen gradient and cause or exacerbate dyspnea. Arterial pO_2 decreases before there is an observed rise in $PaCO_2$ because of the greater rate of carbon dioxide diffusion. Thus, hypoxia in the presence of eucapnia or hypocapnia is characteristic of intrinsic lung diseases, such as emphysema, pulmonary fibrosis, and pneumonia, and may be associated with either respiratory insufficiency or respiratory failure. Unlike patients with ventilation impairment due to respiratory muscle dysfunction, hypercapnic and hypoxic patients with intrinsic lung disease cannot reverse hypoxia by assisted ventilation or noninvasive elimination of airway secretions. The typical patient in this category has chronic obstructive pulmonary disease (COPD) and a normal pH; hypoxia can be alleviated only by supplemental oxygen administration.

The term *respiratory failure* is reserved for acute decompensation in pulmonary function due to intrinsic lung or airways disease with deterioration in arterial blood gases and a decrease in blood pH to less than 7.25. Like patients who suffer primarily from ventilatory impairment, patients with respiratory insufficiency often develop acute respiratory failure during pulmonary infections because respiratory muscles experience fatigue and mucus retention worsens. Pulmonary vascular resistance increases in the presence of generalized or local ventilation-perfusion mismatching or pulmonary tissue hypoxia—especially in the presence of the acidosis that results from local or generalized hypercapnia. The severe hypoxia, hypercapnia, and acidosis that occur during acute respiratory failure can lead to pulmonary artery hypertension and right ventricular failure. Although such patients require ventilator use, hypoxia cannot be resolved simply by ventilator use or assisted coughing. This chapter considers the pathophysiology of such clinical entities.

For patients who suffer primarily from ventilatory impairment, respiratory morbidity and mortality are a direct result of inspiratory and expiratory muscle dysfunction and can be avoided by assisting respiratory muscles. For patients who suffer primarily from oxygenation impairment, the respiratory muscles, although not primarily involved, can be placed at a mechanical disadvantage by the development of lung and chest wall deformities, weakened by malnutrition and overuse, and strained to their limits by the need to ventilate stiff, noncompliant, diseased lungs or obstructed airways. Overwork, relative or absolute, can eventually lead to secondary respiratory muscle dysfunction and overt respiratory failure. Patients who suffer primarily from ventilatory impairment and also have bulbar muscle dysfunction so severe that maximal assisted peak cough flows (PCF) are less than 160 L/min have essentially irreversible upper airway obstruction. They develop hypoxia without hypercapnia and are managed like patients who suffer primarily from oxygenation impairment.

RESPIRATORY MUSCLES

The rib cage and abdomen are separated by the diaphragm. The diaphragm and abdominal muscles contract against essentially noncompressible abdominal contents. As the diaphragm contracts, the abdominal wall is displaced forward. Because its downward movement is resisted by the abdominal contents, diaphragm contraction also results in upward movement of the ribs. Because of their attachments to the thoracic vertebrae and sternum, upward movement of the ribs to a more horizontal position results in anterior and lateral expansion of the chest wall and negative intrapleural pressure and inspiration. Downward rib motion results in contraction of the chest wall and expiration. The muscles that raise the ribs are, therefore, primarily inspiratory, whereas the muscles that lower the ribs are primarily expiratory. The diaphragm is innervated by the phrenic nerve, which receives input from the cervical C3–C5 nerve roots.

The parasternal intercostal muscles, which elevate the ribs, extend from the sternum and proximal costal ridges to the costal cartilages. These muscles are always active when the diaphragm contracts. Their activity is essential during normal inspiration to prevent paradoxical inward movement of the chest and to increase thoracic volumes. The scalenes originate from the C2–C7 cervical vertebrae and insert into the first and second ribs. These muscles also lift and expand the rib cage and are active during normal inspiration.[1]

The internal and external intercostal muscles run at right angles to each other. Although it is commonly accepted that the external intercostals have an inspiratory function and the internal intercostals have an expiratory function, their mechanisms of action and respiratory significance remain uncertain.[2] The intercostal muscles are innervated by peripheral nerves from the thoracic nerve roots.

The accessory muscles of inspiration are quiet during normal tidal breathing but can increase tidal volumes in times of need. The pectoralis major, pectoralis minor, trapezii, serrati, parasternal, and sternocleidomastoid muscles are among the many muscles that extend from the shoulder girdle to the spine or rib cage and that can elevate the ribs. The sternocleidomastoids are the most important of these muscles. They extend from the manubrium and medial one-third of the clavicle to the lateral surface of the mastoid process and lateral one-half of the occipital bone. Sternocleidomastoid contraction can displace the sternum cranially and expand the upper rib cage.

The accessory muscles of inspiration also can assist expiration. The latissimus dorsi, serratus anterior, and trapezius can help to decrease chest diameter and assist coughing, especially in the sitting position. In this position the trapezius can raise the shoulders. The dropping back of the shoulders into place provides an expiratory pulse or cough assist. This action is particularly useful for tetraplegic patients with little expiratory reserve volume. The accessory muscles are innervated by peripheral nerves from cervical nerve roots.

The muscles of the pharynx and larynx are innervated by the lower cranial nerves. The pharyngeal dilator muscles, including the genioglossus, contract to decrease upper airway resistance and prevent pharyngeal collapse. Their contraction is synchronized with contraction of the diaphragm and intercostal muscles. Supralaryngeal resistance is increased during sleep, whereas laryngeal and pulmonary resistances remain unchanged.[3] The pharyngeal and laryngeal muscles also can be considered accessory muscles of inspiration when they are used for GPB. In the absence of other inspiratory or expiratory muscle function, GPB can be used to provide normal tidal volumes and normal minute ventilation or deep inspiratory volumes, often to 3 liters or more.[4] Weakness or dysfunction of bulbar musculature and decreased pulmonary compliance decrease the ability to breathe with the glossopharyngeal muscles (see Chapter 7).

The abdominal muscles include the rectus abdominis, internal and external obliques, and transversus abdominis. Abdominal muscle contraction increases intraabdominal pressure and retracts the abdominal wall. This action displaces the relaxed diaphragm into the thoracic cavity for expiration and coughing. The abdominal muscles also pull the lower ribs downward and inward.

Some patients ventilate the lungs by using abdominal muscles to elevate the diaphragm passively. Examples include patients with diaphragm and chest wall paralysis, such as poliomyelitis survivors. After the diaphragm is elevated by contractions of the abdominal muscles, air enters the lungs as gravity causes the abdominal contents and diaphragm to redescend.

LUNG PHYSIOLOGY AND PATHOPHYSIOLOGY

Gas Exchange

The respiratory exchange membrane is the gas exchange surface of the lungs. It is the membrane between alveolar air and capillary blood.[5] Gas exchange depends on alveolar ventilation, capillary blood perfusion, and diffusion of gases across the respiratory exchange membrane. The quantity of oxygen and carbon dioxide that diffuses across the membrane is a function of the oxygen and carbon dioxide partial pressure differentials across the membrane and its total surface area; it is an inverse function of membrane thickness. Exchange normally takes place in one-third of the pulmonary capillary blood transit time. It is effective in maintaining arterial blood gases within normal limits over a 20-fold range of metabolic demand. The gas exchange membrane is reduced in patients with intrinsic lung disease of any etiology. Alveolar ventilation, capillary blood perfusion, and diffusion of gases across the respiratory exchange membrane are also commonly affected in intrinsic lung diseases.

Gas exchange in the lung depends on the matching of lung ventilation with capillary blood perfusion and the gas diffusion capabilities of the gas exchange membrane. Even in normal lungs, the distribution of ventilation is not uniform. During inspiration this variance is caused by (1) the shape of the thoracic cage and the movement of the ribs, which increase lung volume proportionately more at the bases than at the apices; (2) the descent of the hemidiaphragms, which expand the lower lobes of the lungs more than the upper lobes; (3) the expansion of the peripheral lung more than the deeper tissues (in the upright position); and (4) less inflation of the lower lung regions because the degree of stretch of the lungs at any level is related to transpulmonary pressure.

Lung pathology exaggerates physiologic causes of nonuniform ventilation. For example, regional elasticity changes due to pulmonary fibrosis decrease local compliance and, thus, local lung inflation. Regional airway obstruction can also decrease local ventilation.

Intrathoracic fluid accumulation can limit regional expansion and decrease lung compliance. Variations in breathing rate, excision of lung tissue, and body positioning in patients with asymmetric lung disease also can affect local ventilation.

Despite nonuniformity of distribution and mismatching of ventilation and perfusion, the efficiency of gas exchange is normally 97–98% of the theoretic maximal value for both oxygen and carbon dioxide.[6] In people with ventilatory or respiratory impairment, mild normocapnic hypoxemia is common, however.[7] It is often due to decreased total oxygen diffusion across a respiratory exchange membrane that is diminished or blocked by microatelectasis, bronchial mucus accumulation, or scarring due to recurrent pneumonic infiltrations. In the absence of intrinsic lung disease or severe sudden bronchial mucus plugging, PaO_2 to levels less than 55 mmHg are uncommon without concomitant hypercapnia.

SpO_2 depends on lung ventilation-perfusion relationships. Increases in temperature, pCO_2, hydrogen ion concentration, and 2,3-diphosphoglycerate levels decrease hemoglobin affinity for oxygen and, therefore, SpO_2. A decrease in these levels and carbon monoxide poisoning increase hemoglobin affinity for oxygen.[8] Thus, provided that supplemental oxygen administration is avoided, decreases in SpO_2 result from hypoventilation or fever, ventilation-perfusion mismatching caused by bronchial mucus plugging or intrinsic lung disease, or perfusion impairment caused by vascular disease.

Lung Growth and Mechanics

The trachea divides into left and right mainstem bronchi, which normally divide 26 more times by age 8 years. The alveoli multiply, ultimately reaching 300,000,000 in number and 4 liters in volume. The respiratory exchange membrane grows, atttaining an area of 85 m^2 (the equivalent surface area of a tennis court) by late adolescence.[5] Lung growth peaks with the plateauing of vital capacity at 19 years of age. After the plateau, vital capacity then decreases by 1–1.2% (about 30 ml) per year throughout life.[9]

Sixty to 70% of vital capacity and tidal volumes is provided by the diaphragm. The percentage of the tidal volumes provided by the diaphragm increases greatly in patients with neuromuscular disease (NMD). With severe or advanced NMD, upper thoracic volumes can decrease during inspiration.[10] For infants with spinal muscular atrophy, the result may be underdevelopment of the lungs and chest wall and the skeletal deformity known as pectus excavatum.

Although expiration is passive at rest in normal people, in patients with bronchospasm and during exercise the abdominal muscles contract to generate high thoracoabdominal pressures to elevate the diaphragm and become the principal muscles of expiration. In the presence of emphysema, the diaphragm is so depressed that the costal margin or base of the thorax cannot be expanded. The patient tends to lean forward, tipping the diaphragm anteriorly to favor increased excursion. To increase tidal volumes, the accessory muscles expand the upper chest, particularly during exercise or in situations in which the work of breathing is increased.

Oxygen Cost of Breathing and Hypoventilation

The oxygen cost of breathing is normally about 2.5 ml/min or 1–2% of total body oxygen consumption. This amount increases to 30 ml/min or more (over 15% of total oxygen consumption)[11] at the high levels of ventilation that accompany pneumonia, pulmonary fibrosis, emphysema, and disorders of the chest wall, such as obesity and kyphoscoliosis. In inactive patients with NMD and generalized muscle weakness, overall oxygen consumption is decreased, and energy expenditure for breathing can exceed 15% of overall consumption.

Fatigue has been described as "failure to maintain the required or expected force."[12] Increasing the work of breathing, in absolute terms or relative to respiratory muscle strength and mechanical factors, can result in respiratory muscle decompensation. Because decompensation can lead to an acute decrease in blood pH and possibly death, respiratory muscle fatigue must be avoided. To accomplish this goal, the set point in the brain for control of ventilation changes to permit shallow breathing. This mechanism eases the load on the respiratory muscles at the expense of hypercapnia and diffuse lung hypoventilation[13]; it also explains the hypercapnia seen in patients with neuromuscular muscle weakness, severe vertebral or chest wall deformities, or advanced respiratory impairment. Hypercapnia is insidiously progressive with disease progression or (in patients with "static" NMDs) age.[14] Thus, hypercapnia results directly from the resort to shallow breathing to avoid overloading respiratory muscles.[15] Although hypercapnia is not considered a sign of respiratory muscle fatigue but rather a sign of minimal functional reserve, resting inspiratory muscles by use of ventilatory assistance on a daily and, most often, nightly basis can greatly improve diurnal blood gases without necessarily improving pulmonary function or muscle strength.

Pulmonary Defense Mechanisms and Peak Cough Flows

Pulmonary defense mechanisms include alveolar phagocytosis and lymphatic clearance, the mucociliary elevator, proteolytic enzymes and immunoglobins, and cough. Phagocytosis and ciliary action keep the normal lower respiratory tract almost sterile. Mucociliary clearance is decreased by hyperoxia, hypoxia, drying, smoke and other pollutants,[16] bacterial colonization, and airway trauma associated with the presence of an indwelling tracheostomy tube. It is at times increased by adrenergic bronchodilatation and can be increased by the generation of high cough flows (see Chapter 13).

A normal cough requires that the arytenoid cartilages and vocal folds enlarge the airway diameter to permit a precough inspiration to about 85-90% of total lung capacity.[17] Then a rapid and firm closure of the glottis is reinforced by the closure of the ventricular folds and epiglottis for about 0.2 seconds. Both glottic opening and closure require gross muscular movements, including active intentional movements of the intrinsic laryngeal muscles. Contraction of abdominal and intercostal muscles results in intrapleural pressures as high as 140 mmHg. On glottic opening, this pressure causes an explosive decompression that generates transient PCF of 6–20 L/sec. One of the most important variables in the clearing of mucus and foreign bodies from the airways is the velocity of the gas stream.[18] The expiratory flow is facilitated by active gradual abduction of the vocal cords.[19] The rapid air flows cause vibration of the soft structures of the larynx. The transient high and more prolonged lower flow rates traverse the partially collapsed trachea and other airways, reach the mucus layer adhering to the airway walls, and transfer a portion of its energy as momentum. This shearing force causes acceleration of the fluid layer, leading to transport of accumulated secretions.[20] Total expiratory volume during normal coughing is 2.3 ± 0.5 L.[17] It has been demonstrated that, regardless of expiratory muscle function, PCF is decreased in patients whose inspiratory muscles cannot generate tidal volumes over 1500 ml.[21] Thus, to optimize PCF for patients with low vital capacity, particularly for those with vital capacity below 1000 ml, coughing must be preceded by the delivery of maximal insufflations or maximal air stacking (see Chapter 7). The delivered air should be to the maximal insufflation capacity (MIC), which, even when no greater than 1500 ml, can greatly increase the pressure of the lung's recoil once the glottis is opened during the cough. This process can dramatically increase PCF even without application of an abdominal thrust to augment the flows manually (Fig. 1).[21]

Maximal inspiratory and expiratory pressures are direct measures of inspiratory and expiratory muscle strength. In patients who suffer primarily from ventilatory impairment, expiratory muscles are usually weaker than inspiratory muscles.[14,22,23] Expiratory muscle weakness not only decreases peak expiratory flows but also decreases PCF. Routine pulmonary function testing includes the measurement of maximal expiratory pressures and peak expiratory flow rates but not PCF. This omission is quite ironic because the importance of PCF has been recognized for some time.[17] Although expiratory flow rates are important for patients

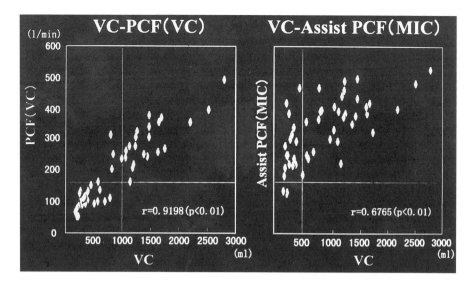

FIGURE 1. A comparison of peak cough flows (PCF) generated by patients taking a deep breath, essentially from vital capacitiy (VC), vs. PCF generated by the same patients from lung volumes increased by maximal air stacking, essentially to maximal insufflation capacity (MIC).

with bronchospasm, expiratory pressures and flow rates can be useless if they do not translate into effective cough flows to clear the airways. Normal peak expiratory flows range from 6 to 14 L/sec for adults and from 2.5 to 14 L/sec for children and adolescents, depending on gender, age, and height.[24,25] PCF may be 40–50% greater than peak expiratory flows in normal people as well as in patients with DMD.[26] In patients with severe bulbar ALS, however, PCF may not be measurable because of inability to close the glottis. PCF greater than 160 L/min (2.7 L/sec) is sufficient to eliminate secretions and debris from the airways.[27] Despite its importance, PCF has not been standardized.

In addition to inspiratory and expiratory muscle weakness, PCF also is decreased by bulbar muscle dysfunction that impairs glottic retention of an optimal breath; that impairs glottic patency, vocal cord movement, and pharyngeal dilator function; and that leads to aspiration of food or saliva. PCF is the best indication of the functional integrity of bulbar musculature. It is also decreased by upper or lower airway obstruction, anatomic or functional.

Excessive functional collapse of the upper airway during coughing and exsufflation can also render cough flows ineffective. After the glottis opens during the cough cycle, intrathoracic pressure remains momentarily higher than intraluminal pressure, causing the normal decrease in the caliber of the airways. Mild narrowing serves to increase cough flows, thereby making them more effective. A decrease greater than 50% in the cross-sectional lumen of the upper airways during coughing is considered abnormal and results in ineffective coughing.[28] Airways can collapse in the mediastinum (e.g., trachea and right and part of the left mainstem bronchus) and in proximal and distal areas (e.g., subpleural and intrapulmonary bronchi). The degree of bronchial collapse varies with the extent of pulmonary disease; in severe disease, all locations collapse. Tracheal collapse is usually caused by invagination of the posterior membrane. When tracheal collapse is complete, airways below this level do not collapse because of the increase in luminal pressure. When patients with chronic pulmonary diseases have greater than 50% luminal closing, PCF can be increased by huffing (see Chapter 13).

Airway obstruction can be considered reversible or irreversible, depending on whether it can be alleviated by the use of respiratory muscle aids or bronchodilators.

Essentially irreversible upper airway obstruction is most often due to tracheal stenosis, pharyngeal and laryngeal muscle dysfunction, or postintubation vocal cord adhesions or paralysis. Tracheomalacia, a frequent complication of tracheostomy (especially with an inflated cuff), occasionally causes excessive airway collapse and stridorous inspiration. Essentially irreversible lower airway obstruction is most often caused by COPD. Reversible airway obstruction results from acute bronchospasm, airway mucus accumulation, or the presence of a foreign body or granulation tissue in the airways of any patient without irreversible airway obstruction. Airway obstruction can vary from inspiration to expiration.

Ventilator weaning parameters include resting minute ventilation, maximal voluntary ventilation, tidal volume, vital capacity, maximal inspiratory force, arterial-alveolar oxygen gradient on 100% oxygen, ratio of dead space to tidal volume, and functional residual capacity. The parameters are so numerous because none of them is very useful. Most are related to inspiratory rather than expiratory muscle function. We demonstrated that PCF exceeding 160 L/min is the most important parameter for predicting successful extubation.[27] Patients whose spontaneous or assisted PCF cannot exceed 270–300 L/min when they are well[29] are at high risk of flows below 160 L/min during chest colds or after general anesthesia because of fatigue, temporary weakening of both inspiratory and expiratory muscles,[30] and bronchial mucus accumulation. For patients with NMD, vital capacity and maximal inspiratory and expiratory pressures decrease by 10–25% and $PaCO_2$ increases by 10% during the first day after onset of cold symptoms.[31] Concomitant weakness of oropharyngeal muscles exacerbates the problem. The attainment of adequate PCF is critical for preventing pneumonia and respiratory failure in such patients.[27,29,32] For patients whose assisted PCF is less than 160 L/min, even when they are well, airway collapse can prevent manually and mechanically assisted coughing from reversing mucus-associated oxygen desaturation in arterial blood and preventing pneumonia and acute respiratory failure. Such patients often require translaryngeal intubation during chest infections.[33]

Long-term aspiration of upper airway secretions and failure to eliminate airway mucus can lead to chronic ventilation perfusion imbalance, atelectasis, and lobar or segmental collapse. Bronchial mucus also can cause obstructive emphysema and a hyperinflated lung with the obstructive emphysema seen with foreign-body aspiration.[34] Patients also may experience lung collapse, loss of lung compliance with pulmonary infiltrates and subsequent scarring, cor pulmonale, and eventually cardiopulmonary arrest. Mucus plugging can simulate pulmonary emboli. Sudden, severe hypoxia, dyspnea, and chest pain can occur in the presence of normal chest radiographs and perfusion scintiscans that show diminished or absent perfusion of the involved portions of the lungs.[35] Flow-volume curves have been used to detect airway secretions in ventilator users.[36] Airway mucus accumulation is particularly dangerous when it causes SpO_2 to decrease suddenly below 95%. In patients with airway obstruction due to chronic plugging or aspiration of upper airway secretions, tracheostomy is needed when the SpO_2 baseline remains below 95% in the absence of hypercapnia and despite aggressive use of expiratory muscle aids. Tracheotomy should not be considered unless assisted PCF cannot exceed 160 L/min over the long term.[27,29,37]

Because the cough reflex is suppressed during sleep, mucus accumulation is more likely to cause sudden hypoxia and acute respiratory failure overnight— especially if the patient receives supplemental oxygen or sedatives. Many patients with myopathic disease have varying degrees of cardiomyopathy that render them particularly susceptible to arrhythmias and cardiac decompensation triggered by mucus-associated hypoxia.

REGULATION OF PULMONARY VENTILATION AND SLEEP

Hypoxia, hypercapnia, and changes in blood pH affect lung ventilation. Peripheral chemoreceptors in the aortic and carotid bodies sense pCO_2 and pH but are primarily sensitive to pO_2 levels. Chemodenervation of the peripheral chemoreceptors can result in a

12-20% reduction in ventilation with an increase in $PaCO_2$ of 5–10 mmHg.[38] Gamma afferents from the intercostal muscles, diaphragm, and pulmonary stretch receptors are also involved in regulating the timing and depth of breathing. Central receptors located on the surface of the medulla respond to the pCO_2 and hydrogen levels of the central spinal fluid and play an important role in regulating overall lung ventilation.[6] The controller in the brainstem generates respiratory rhythm and integrates input from the peripheral receptors and other parts of the CNS; its output is to the respiratory muscles. Emotional states also can alter ventilation. With the change in the set point of the control of ventilation to avoid fatigue for patients with respiratory muscle dysfunction, chronic hypercapnia results in the development of a compensatory metabolic alkalosis with retention of bicarbonate ions in both peripheral blood and cerebrospinal fluid. High cerebrospinal fluid bicarbonate levels decrease the ventilatory response to hypercapnia. Other factors that decrease the ventilatory response to hypercapnia are sedative and narcotic medications, heavy mechanical loads, oxygen administration, and sleep.

Ventilatory drive is assessed by instantaneously occluding the mouth during the onset of inspiration. Except for patients with very weak inspiratory muscles, the decrease in pressure during the 100 milliseconds of occlusion at the outset of inspiration is thought to reflect the level of neural drive that was present at the outset of the previous unoccluded breath.[39] Ventilatory drive appears to be intact for hypercapnic patients with NMD. A second measure of ventilator drive derives from expressing minute ventilation as the product of the mean inspiratory flow rate (tidal volume/inspiratory time) and the fractional duration of inspiration (inspiratory time/inspiratory plus expiratory time). The first term reflects neural drive to the inspiratory muscles, whereas the second term reflects timing. Minute ventilation can be altered by changes in either variable alone or, as is usually the case, simultaneous changes in both drive and timing.

The anatomic proximity of respiratory centers to the pontobulbar control system provides a foundation for central anatomic and functional connections between respiratory centers and sleep-related neuronal systems. Reticular activating system stimulation that results in or heightens alertness also stimulates phrenic nerve activity,[40] and neuronal discharge rates of the rostral pontine pneumotaxic center and the respiratory neurons of the ventral part of the medulla are diminished during non–rapid-eye-movement (non-REM) sleep and even more so during REM sleep.[41,42] Decreased rate of discharge of these respiratory centers may largely explain the ventilatory changes that occur during non-REM sleep.

The maintenance of normal arterial blood gas levels depends on automatic and behavioral systems. The automatic system depends on communication between dorsal and ventral groups of respiratory neurons in the brainstem. Input to these neurons comes from medullary and peripheral chemoreceptors as well as from stretch, irritant, and juxtacapillary receptors in the lungs via the vagus nerve and from chest wall receptors via the spinal nerves. Such input modulates breathing during non-REM sleep. The behavioral system modulates breathing through inputs to the brainstem from cortical or subcortical neurons.

During sleep the ventilatory response to blood gas alterations, the cough reflex, and accessory inspiratory muscle recruitment are decreased. Minute ventilation, functional residual capacity, and PaO_2 decrease, whereas upper airway resistance and $PaCO_2$ increase.[43] The set point for $PaCO_2$ at which ventilation begins to increase is higher than during wakefulness, and there is a decrease in sensitivity to hypercapnia. In addition, the ventilatory response to carbon dioxide during tonic REM sleep is equal to that during non-REM sleep, but during phasic REM sleep the ventilatory response to hypercapnia is virtually abolished. Thus, neural rather than metabolic factors maintain ventilation. During non-REM sleep the ventilatory response to hypoxia depends primarily on peripheral chemoreceptors, whereas during REM sleep the response is significantly decreased. Hypercapnia of 55–60 mmHg arouses normal subjects from non-REM sleep, whereas hypercapnia of 65 or 66 mmHg arouses them from REM sleep. Oxyhemoglobin desaturations also result in brief arousals.

For patients with NMD, hypercapnia begins during REM sleep and extends throughout sleep and then ultimately into daytime hours. During REM sleep tonic automatic activity of intercostal muscles and diaphragm is abolished, and phasic activity of the intercostals is diminished. Phasic diaphragm activity is preserved, and the diaphragm normally increases its contribution to tidal volume to compensate for decrease or loss of accessory and intercostal muscle activity. When the diaphragm is distorted or involved in the primary NMD process, it may be unable to increase its contribution. This inability can result in underventilation. The decrease in rib cage and accessory muscle tone during REM sleep may further reduce the FRC. The combination of reduced FRC and airway secretion retention can increase ventilation-perfusion mismatching. Indeed, nocturnal hypoventilation and hypoxia may be due to any combination of cardiopulmonary disease with diminished diffusion, shunting, and ventilation- perfusion inhomogeneities, respiratory muscle dysfunction, decreased lung compliance, central and obstructive apneas,[44] and bronchial mucus accumulation as well as to normal changes with sleep.

Arnulf et al. reported that, as diaphragm weakness progresses, REM sleep diminishes even though apnea and hypopnea are rare in patients with ALS.[45] Until recently, however, it was thought that only the primary inspiratory muscles functioned during REM sleep. Remarkably, phasic inspiratory sternocleidomastoid activation has been reported during REM and appears to permit REM sleep for some patients with ALS.[45] Another study recently suggested that 70% of patients with NMD have accessory muscle activity during REM and slow wave sleep.[46]

Hypoxic patients with intact respiratory musculature hyperventilate in an effort to normalize blood oxygen levels. Oxygen administration can decrease ventilation; relieve respiratory muscle strain; ease tachypnea, shortness of breath, and other symptoms of hypoxia and respiratory distress; and decrease pulmonary hypertension and the tendency to cor pulmonale. For hypercapnic patients, however, oxygen administration exacerbates hypoventilation and its symptoms. It also further impairs respiratory muscle function[47] and leads to carbon dioxide narcosis and ventilatory arrest. For patients with nocturnal SpO_2 between 70 and 80% and transcutaneous carbon dioxide of 72 mmHg, supplemental oxygen that increases SpO_2 to 90% has been reported to increase $PaCO_2$ levels to over 95 mmHg.[48] Thus, oxygen must be given with great care to hypercapnic patients who suffer primarily from oxygenation impairment. It must not be administered to patients who suffer primarily from ventilatory impairment except when ventilation is controlled by intubation to treat a complicating pneumonia.

The first blood gas abnormalities in people who suffer primarily from ventilatory impairment occur during REM sleep as short periods of hypoxemia.[49] Hypercapnia and hypoxemia generally extend throughout most of the sleep cycle before ventilatory insufficiency occurs with the patient awake.[50,51] Awake hypercapnia tends to occur when the vital capacity decreases below 40%[14] of predicted normal. In 91% of cases, sleep hypoventilation causes SpO_2 to be below 90% for more than 2% of sleeping time.[52] Daytime $PaCO_2$ greater than 45 mmHg[53] and base excess greater than 4 mmol/L also signal nocturnal hypoventilation 91% and 55% of the time, respectively.[52] Decreases in FRC and total lung volume also correlate with nocturnal desaturations. For the same decrement in PaO_2, patients who already have reduced daytime PaO_2 experience more profound desaturation because they are operating on the steeper portion of the oxyhemoglobin dissociation curve. Once daytime hypercapnia is present, a further reduction in ventilation during sleep greatly exacerbates desaturation. Because of the inverse hyperbolic relationship between alveolar ventilation and $PaCO_2$, a small decrease in ventilation in an already hypercapnic individual can result in a greater change in carbon dioxide tension than does a comparable decrease in ventilation in eucapnic subjects. For patients who have a $PaCO_2$ greater than 50 mmHg when awake, nocturnal periods of SpO_2 below 85% are common.[54] The rapid, shallow, irregular breathing of normal REM sleep also exacerbates dead-space ventilation and further reduces effective alveolar ventilation. Because the ventilatory responses to hypoxia and hypercapnia are diminished with hypercapnia[55] and the threshold for arousal is lower to hypoxia and higher to hypercapnia, more severe and prolonged blood gas alterations occur without arousing the patient. Increasing $PaCO_2$ and decreasing PaO_2 levels cross at about 60 mmHg, a point at which it is tempting (but erroneous) to provide supplemental oxygen.

Medications such as calcium channel blockers, aminoglycosides, steroids, and benzodiazepines can reduce the ventilatory response to hypercapnia and hypoxia and exacerbate hypoventilation, especially during sleep. Beta blockers can increase airway resistance. Malnutrition, acidosis, electrolyte disturbances, cachexia, infection, fatigue, and muscle disuse or overuse also can exacerbate ventilatory insufficiency. Hypokalemia, a common problem in patients with small muscle potassium reserves, especially during upper respiratory tract infections, can cause weakness, constipation, and abdominal distention and thereby exacerbate inspiratory muscle dysfunction.[56] The hypophosphatemia that commonly occurs during episodes of acute respiratory failure also decreases diaphragm contractility.[57] The risk of long-term pulmonary complications also is increased by oxygen administration[58] used to give the patient with ventilatory insufficiency "a comfortable night's rest."[51] Oxygen therapy also has been shown to prolong hypopneas and apneas by 33% during REM sleep and at other times by 19% in patients with DMD who still have good ventilatory function (average vital capacity: 1.4 L).[59] It also appears to suppress the CNS-mediated reflex muscular activity needed to support ventilation overnight by noninvasive IPPV methods.[13,60]

The muscle weakness that often results in chronic hypercapnia for most patients with NMD cannot explain the chronic hypercapnia seen in many patients with myotonic dystrophy, myasthenia gravis, and other conditions when respiratory muscle weakness is not severe. These cases are explained by the presence of primary central hypoventilation, disordered afferents from diseased muscle, upper airway muscle involvement, abnormal muscle tone, upper motor neuron dysfunction, concurrent sleep disordered breathing, and increased work of breathing caused by decreased pulmonary compliance.

Sleep-disordered Breathing

Sleep-disordered breathing is a common entity in the general population that can develop into or exacerbate ventilatory insufficiency and that often complicates COPD and NMD as well. It refers to the occurrence of central, obstructive, or mixed apneas, hypopneas, or both during sleep. Sleep apneas, hypopneas, and hypoventilation are pathophysiologically distinct. Apneas and hypopneas are associated with disturbed sleep architecture and recurrent arousals. The obstructive apneas are most commonly due to hypopharyngeal collapse from a transluminal pressure gradient across the airway during inspiration and failure of airway dilator muscles that are normally reflexively activated at the onset of inspiration. Obstructive apneas are often accompanied by central apneas. There may be an etiologic association between them. It is conceivable that for some patients with severe obstructive sleep apnea syndrome (OSAS), central apneas result at least in part from CNS desensitivity to hypoxia. This desensitivity also occurs in the presence of chronic respiratory muscle weakness. Patients with generalized or, especially, bulbar neuromuscular weakness are particularly susceptible to the development of obstructive and central sleep apneas or sleep-disordered breathing.[61,62] Many investigators now also believe not only that obstructive apneas associated with snoring and increased upper airway resistance can cause arousals, but also that obstructive apneas can be triggered by arousals and result from disturbed sleep architecture.[44]

Carskadon and Dement found that 37.5% of people older than 62 years had apneas or hypopneas.[63] Apneas were defined as cessation of airflow for 10 seconds or more and hypopneas as reductions in normal tidal volumes by more than 30%. Many apneas and hypopneas are associated with oxygen desaturation in arterial blood of 4% or greater.[64] At least 3% of the general population is symptomatic for this condition and has an average of five or more episodes of apnea and hypopnea per hour (apnea/hypopnea index [AHI]).[64] OSAS is diagnosed when such people become symptomatic and have an AHI of 10 or more.[64,65] Symptoms, which include hypersomnolence, morning headaches, fatigue, frequent nocturnal arousals with gasping or tachycardia, and nightmares, are similar to those of simple ventilatory insufficiency.[66] Sleep-disordered breathing alone can result in chronic ventilatory insufficiency, hypoxia, right ventricular strain, systemic hypertension, and, when severe, neuropsychiatric disturbances, cardiac arrhythmias, and acute cardiopulmonary failure.[67–69] Hypoventilation is a teleologic unloading of chronically overloaded respiratory muscles.

The risk of symptomatic sleep-disordered breathing is higher in men and increases with age, androgen therapy, obesity, brainstem or spinal cord lesions, hypothyroidism, generalized NMDs, and any condition that obstructs the airway.[70,71] The decrease in pharyngeal cross-sectional area associated with age, particularly in men, increases susceptibility to OSAS.[72] Sleep-disordered breathing also occurs in most patients who use negative-pressure body ventilators[67,73] or electrophrenic nerve pacing.[74] Patients with NMD may have a higher incidence of sleep-disordered breathing because of a higher incidence of bulbar muscle weakness and obesity.[75,76] Kimura et al. suggested that the incidence of sleep-disordered breathing increases with bulbar and diaphragm weakness for patients with ALS.[77] Bulbar dysfunction can increase susceptibility to hypopharyngeal collapse and, therefore, obstructive apneas during sleep.[61,76] Many patients with NMDs also have central hypoventilation. It has been suggested that patients with spinal cord injury also have a high incidence of sleep-disordered breathing.[78–80]

The cause of congenital central alveolar hypoventilation is unknown; apparently it is not genetically determined.[81] Typical patients maintain adequate ventilation when awake but hypoventilate severely during sleep and have absent or depressed ventilatory responses to hypercapnia and hypoxia when awake or asleep.[82] A similar ventilatory drive insensitivity to hypoxia and hypercapnia is seen in patients with familial dysautonomia, Down syndrome, or certain previously described NMDs as well as in some patients with diabetic microangiopathy.[83] The extent of central alveolar hypoventilation and sleep-disordered breathing and their effects on patients with respiratory muscle compromise has not been adequately studied.

Airway Resistance Syndrome

Airway resistance syndrome is characterized by repeated increases in upper airway resistance to airflow that result in symptoms of sleep-disordered breathing and often in systemic hypertension. Patients have a narrow posterior airway space behind the base of the tongue.[84] It is diagnosed when nocturnal esophageal pressure monitoring indicates crescendo changes in intrathoracic pressures, followed by arousals.[85] Because of the invasive nature of this procedure, the diagnosis is often made indirectly by clinical symptoms and polysomnographic evidence of sleep disruption. The AHI may be slightly increased but is usually less than 5.[86]

Although CPAP continues to be the conventional treatment, sleep quality can be improved and snoring, hypersomnolence, and AHI can be reduced significantly by wearing an oral appliance that advances the position of the mandible and tongue, as for OSAS (Fig. 2). Some patients experience temporary masticatory muscle or temporomandibular joint discomfort.[86]

PULMONARY FUNCTION OF PATIENTS WITH VENTILATORY MUSCLE IMPAIRMENT

Patients with ventilatory impairment develop a restrictive pulmonary syndrome with a reduction in total lung volumes, vital capacity (Fig. 3), expiratory reserve volume, and,

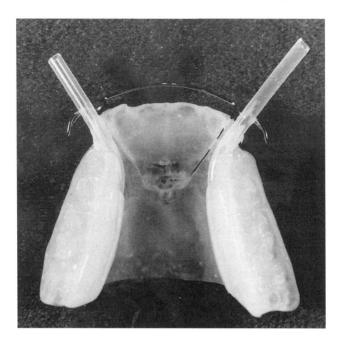

FIGURE 2.   An intra-oral appliance used to bring forward the jaw and open the airway in the treatment of obstructive sleep apneas (courtesy of Dr. John R. Haze, D.D.S., Montville, N.J.).

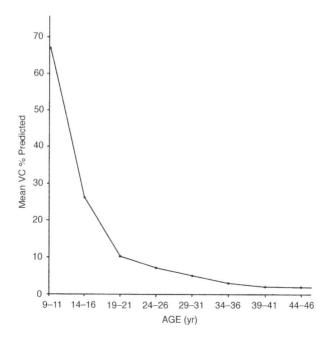

FIGURE 3.   Deterioration of vital capacity as a function of age for 29 patients with Duchenne muscular dystrophy who use ventilators. (From Bach J, Alba A, Pilkington LA, Lee M: Long-term rehabilitation in advanced stage of childhood onset, rapidly progressive muscular dystrophy. Arch Phys Med Rehabil 62:328–331, 1981, with permission.)

usually, FRC. Diaphragm weakness can result in paradoxical diaphragm movements in patients with NMDs. Supine posture then is associated with exacerbation of ventilatory impairment because of the effect of gravity on the contents of the abdomen. In the erect position, the abdominal contents exert hydrostatic pressure to displace the diaphragm caudally at end-expiration. This action opposes the tendency of the intercostal muscles to suck the diaphragm upward into the chest. In the supine position the opposite effect takes place. The hydrostatic forces displace the paralyzed diaphragm cranially, thereby working in conjunction with the action of the intercostal muscles and tending to decrease pulmonary volumes. In a study of 8 patients with severely paretic diaphragms, vital capacity was 30–65% of normal with patients in the sitting position and fell by half when they were supine.[87] The weaker the diaphragm in comparison with the chest and abdominal muscles, the higher the vital capacity will be when the patient first develops hypercapnia or breathing intolerance. The stronger the diaphragm in comparison with the chest and abdominal muscles, the lower the vital capacity will be when the patient first develops hypercapnia or breathing intolerance. In addition, decreases in vital capacity to 50% over a short time are likely to result in loss of breathing tolerance, whereas greater losses over longer periods are likely to result in good breathing tolerance in the face of increasing hypercapnia.[88]

In studying patients with ALS, we found that in 368 evaluations the mean vital capacity was 1749 ± 327 ml in the sitting position and 1475 ± 298 ml in the supine position. In some cases, the sitting values were as much as twice the supine values, and patients who had no difficulty with breathing in the erect or sitting position had no breathing tolerance in the supine position. In 647 measurements in patients with NMD who were old enough to cooperate with spirometry, the mean vital capacity was 1808.7 ml in the sitting position and 1582.8 ml in the supine position. In a small study of 24 patients with NMD (15 with muscular dystrophy, 8 with other myopathies, and 1 with polyradiculoneuritis), 11 of the 14 patients with clinically apparent paradoxical diaphragm movements had a greater than 25% drop-off in vital capacity when moving from the sitting to the supine position. The drop-off was less than 25% for 9 of the 10 patients without paradoxical diaphragm movement. The extent of the drop-off also was associated with a decrease in mouth pressure generated during a maximal static inspiratory effort (indicative of diaphragm weakness).[89]

Pulmonary compliance is a measure of the distensibility of the chest and lungs. Restriction and decreased compliance are due to any combination of respiratory muscle weakness, paralysis, and mechanical factors that stiffen the chest wall and lungs. Measurement of transpulmonary pressure—the difference between intrapleural and alveolar pressures—is needed to determine lung compliance. Dynamic compliance is reflected by the extent of lung volume change with changes in intrapleural pressure from the end of expiration to the end of inspiration. In a study of hypoventilated animals lying on their backs for as little as 2 hours, overperfusion of dependent portions of the lungs resulted in fluid accumulation and microatelectasis. When the animals were intermittently given insufflations to 40 cmH_2O, this overperfusion did not occur.[90] When human patients with diminished vital capacity do not receive maximal insufflations, they, too, develop a rapid, shallow breathing pattern and microatelectasis along with areas of compensatory emphysema. Such changes are often not seen on plain radiographs of the chest.[90] Microatelectasis can develop in 1 hour when tidal volumes cannot be increased.[91] Decreases in pulmonary compliance by 300% or more can occur in less than 3 months after loss of the ability to take deep breaths.[90] For children chronic underinflation results in underdevelopment of lung tissues as well as decreased chest wall elasticity[92,93] and static pulmonary compliance.[59,94,95] Diseases that destroy the lung's connective tissue (e.g., emphysema) increase compliance.

Mechanical problems associated with ventilatory impairment include obesity, improperly fitting thoracolumbar orthoses, sleep-associated hypopharyngeal collapse or other upper airway narrowing, and thoracic deformities.[13] Hypoxia and hypercapnia are exacerbated when intrinsic lung disease and concomitant mechanical conditions complicate inspiratory muscle weakness. Ultimately, right ventricular strain and serum acid-base imbalance develop but can be reversed by the effective use of inspiratory muscle aids.[96]

Kyphoscoliosis and Ventilatory Dysfunction

Idiopathic kyphoscoliosis reduces vital capacity and respiratory reserve independently of concomitant muscle weakness. Scoliosis can exacerbate the loss of pulmonary compliance, which, in turn, increases the work of breathing. This is not the case, however, for patients with scoliosis due to NMD; the decreases in vital capacity and respiratory reserve are due entirely to respiratory muscle weakness. Patients with kyphoscoliosis also develop ventilation-perfusion mismatching and have a higher incidence of obstructive sleep apneas when the skeletal deformities involve the upper cervical region and, therefore, the hypopharynx.

PULMONARY FUNCTION OF PATIENTS WITH RESPIRATORY IMPAIRMENT

COPD is characterized by low expiratory flow rates, normal or increased lung compliance, abnormal rib cage-abdominal motion from asynchronous breathing, rib cage-abdomen time lag, paradoxical breathing, and accessory muscle hypertrophy. Radiographic evidence indicates lung hyperlucency with flattening of the diaphragm and often lung bullae and blebs. Patients hyperventilate and have an increased oxygen cost of breathing. The maximal mid-expiratory flow rate is a most sensitive indicator of airway obstruction. Forced expiratory volume in one second (FEV_1) is decreased, and maximal mid-expiratory times are increased. Gas diffusion, although decreased in emphysema, is normal in pure bronchitis.

The chronic airflow obstruction of COPD results in an increase in FRC with air trapping as patients use active expiratory muscle contraction in an attempt to more completely exhale. Unfortunately, the greater thoracoabdominal pressures resulting from the expiratory muscle activity exacerbate airway collapse and air trapping. So much respiratory exchange membrane is blocked by airway collapse and obstruction that hypoxia results in a greater workload to increase lung ventilation in an attempt to normalize blood oxygen levels. With advanced disease, inadequate respiratory exchange membrane is ventilated to maintain normal carbon dioxide levels, and hypercapnia develops. The air trapping worsens whenever the patient must breathe more quickly, as when increasing skeletal muscle activity, or when bronchial mucus plugs block off airways. Ventilatory drive gradually resets to accommodate increasing hypercapnia and permit lower tidal volumes to avoid respiratory muscle fatigue, and a compensatory metabolic alkalosis develops.[14]

Hypercapnia is associated with increased morbidity and mortality in patients with COPD,[73] as in untreated patients with primarily ventilatory impairment.[7,97] There is a strong physiologic rationale to rest[22] the respiratory musculature of hypercapnic patients and normalize carbon dioxide levels.[98] The role of hypoxia in causing right ventricular decompensation is greatly diminished when acidosis is minimized by maintaining more normal $PaCO_2$ levels.[96] Although the use of noninvasive ventilation can relieve hypercapnia and rest inspiratory muscles in COPD, it also can increase air trapping. The use of ventilatory assistance by patients with normocapnic respiratory insufficiency may also be beneficial by reducing the oxygen consumption related to the increased work of breathing (see Chapters 4 and 11).

RESPIRATORY INSUFFICIENCY IN PATIENTS WITH BULBAR MUSCLE DYSFUNCTION

Patients with severe bulbar muscle dysfunction who have a long-term decrease in baseline SpO_2 below 95% because of chronic aspiration of upper airway secretions have respiratory rather than ventilatory insufficiency. Even when no pathology is visible on chest radiographs, such patients have microscopic atelectasis as well as assisted PCF less than 160 L/min. Thus, as in any other adult patients with assisted PCF below 160 L/min for whom respiratory muscle aids cannot effectively eliminate secretions and normalize baseline SpO_2,[27] pneumonia and respiratory failure are inevitable without tracheotomy. Because such patients are invariably averbal at this point, they can benefit from laryngeal diversion. This situation is rarely seen in patients other than those with severe bulbar-type ALS.

CONCLUSION

Two clinical syndromes have been defined. All patients with pulmonary disability present with either primarily ventilatory or primarily oxygenation impairment. The former develop hypoxia secondary to hypercapnia or reversible airway secretion encumbrance and can develop ventilatory impairment that necessitates ventilator use. The latter develop severe hypoxia without hypercapnia until the terminal stages of their disorder. Such patients are susceptible to respiratory insufficiency and failure.

Bronchial mucus accumulation during chest infections eventually results in pneumonia and respiratory failure for conventionally managed patients with ventilatory impairment— as it can for patients with primarily oxygenation impairment. Despite the eventual requirement of 24-hour noninvasive ventilatory support, patients with primarily ventilatory impairment who use respiratory muscle aids can avoid hospitalizations for ventilatory or respiratory failure.[99] Although patients with primarily oxygenation impairment at times can benefit from the use of respiratory muscle aids in both acute and long-term settings, episodes of respiratory failure and resort to intubation and tracheostomy cannot always be prevented by noninvasive approaches alone. Despite their widespread use, the conventional management approaches for patients with respiratory impairment are not indicated and often are harmful for patients with ventilatory impairment.

…no ande buscando tres pies al gato!

Miguel de Cervantes, *Don Quijote de La Mancha*

REFERENCES

1. De Troyer A, Estenne M: Coordination between rib cage muscles and diaphragm during quiet breathing in humans. J Appl Physiol 57:899–904, 1982.
2. De Troyer A, Estenne M: Functional anatomy of the respiratory muscles. Clin Chest Med 9:175–193, 1988.
3. Hudgel DW, Martin RJ, Johnson B, Hill P: Mechanics of the respiratory system and breathing pattern during sleep in normal humans. J Appl Physiol 56:133–137, 1984.
4. Bach JR, Alba AS, Bodofsky E, et al: Glossopharyngeal breathing and non-invasive aids in the management of post-polio respiratory insufficiency. Birth Defects 23:99–113, 1987.
5. West JB: Respiratory Physiology: The Essentials, 6th ed. Philadelphia, Lippincott Williams & Wilkins, 2000, pp 1–4.
6. Slonim NB, Hamilton LH (eds): Respiratory Physiology, 5th ed. St. Louis, Mosby, 1987, pp 123–130,281.
7. Inkley SR, Oldenburg FC, Vignos PJ Jr: Pulmonary function in Duchenne muscular dystrophy related to stage of disease. Am J Med 56:297–306, 1974.
8. Slonim NB, Hamilton LH (eds): Respiratory Physiology, 5th ed. St. Louis, Mosby, 1987, pp 143–149.
9. Bach JR: Pulmonary assessment and management of the aging and older patient. In Felsenthal G, Garrison SJ, Steinberg FU (eds): Rehabilitation of the Aging and Elderly Patient. Baltimore, Williams & Wilkins, 1993, pp 263–273.
10. Lissoni A, Aliverti A, Molteni F, Bach JR: Spinal muscular atrophy: Kinematic breathing analysis. Am J Phys Med Rehabil 75:332–339, 1996.
11. Levison H, Cherniack RM: Ventilatory cost of exercise in chronic obstructive pulmonary disease. J Appl Physiol 25:21–27, 1968.

12. Edwards RHT: Human muscle function and fatigue. In Human Muscle Fatigue: Physiological Mechanisms. London, Pitman Medical, 1981, pp 1–18.
13. Bach JR, Alba AS: Management of chronic alveolar hypoventilation by nasal ventilation. Chest 97:52–57, 1990.
14. Braun NMT, Arora MS, Rochester DF: Respiratory muscle and pulmonary function in polymyositis and other proximal myopathies. Thorax 38:616–623, 1983.
15. Begin P, Grassino A: Inspiratory muscle dysfunction and chronic hypercapnia in chronic obstructive pulmonary disease. Am Rev Respir Dis 143:905–912, 1983.
16. Slonim NB, Hamilton LH (eds): Respiratory Physiology, 5th ed. SXt. Louis, Mosby, 1987, pp 42–47.
17. Leith DE: Lung biology in health and desease: Respiratory defense mechainisms. Part 2. In Brain JD, Proctor D, Reid L (eds): Cough. New York, Marcel Dekker, 1977, pp 545–592.
18. Evans JN, Jaeger MJ: Mechanical aspects of coughing. Pneumonologie 152:253–257, 1975.
19. von Leden H, Isshiki N: An analysis of cough at the level of the larynx. Arch Otol 81:616–625, 1965.
20. Macchione M, Guimaraes ET, Saldiva PHN, Lorenzi-Filho G: Braz J Med Biolog Res 28:1347–1355, 1995.
21. Bach JR: Mechanical insufflation-exsufflation: Comparison of peak expiratory flows with manually assisted and unassisted coughing techniques. Chest 104:1553–1562, 1993.
22. Griggs RG, Donohoe KM, Utell MJ, et al: Evaluation of pulmonary function in neuromuscular disease. Arch Neurol 38:9–12, 1981.
23. Johnson EW (ed): Profiles of neuromuscular diseases. Am J Phys Med Rehabil 74:1–165, 1995.
24. Leiner GC, Abramowitz S, Small MJ, et al: Expiratory peak flow rate. Standard values for normal subjects. Use as a clinical test of ventilatory function. Am Rev Respir Dis 88:644, 1963.
25. Polgar G, Promadhat V: Pulmonary Function Testing in Children: Techniques and Standards. Philadelphia, W.B. Saunders, 1971.
26. Suarez AA, Pessolano F, Monteiro SG, et al: Peak flow and peak cough flow in the evaluation of expiratory muscle weakness and bulbar impairment of neuromuscular patients. Am J Phys Med Rehabil [in press].
27. Bach JR, Saporito LR: Criteria for extubation and tracheostomy tube removal for patients with ventilatory failure: A different approach to weaning. Chest 110:1566–1571, 1996.
28. Rayl JE: Tracheobronchial collapse during cough. Radiology 85:87–92, 1965.
29. Bach JR, Ishikawa Y, Kim H: Prevention of pulmonary morbidity for patients with Duchenne muscular dystrophy. Chest 112:1024–1028, 1997.
30. Mier-Jedrzejowicz A, Brophy C, Green M: Respiratory muscle weakness during upper respiratory tract infections. Am Rev Respir Dis 138:5–7, 1988.
31. Poponick JM, Jacobs I, Supinski G, DiMarco AF: Effect of upper respiratory tract infection in patients with neuromuscular disease. Am J Respir Crit Care Med 156:659–664, 1997.
32. King M, Brock G, Lundell C: Clearance of mucus by simulated cough. J Appl Physiol 58:1776–1785, 1985.
33. Hanayama K, Ishikawa Y, Bach JR: Amyotrophic lateral sclerosis: Successful treatment of mucus plugging by mechanical insufflation-exsufflation. Am J Phys Med Rehabil 76:338–339, 1997.
34. Cohn JR, Steiner RM, Posuniak E, Northrup BE: Obstructive emphysema due to mucus plugging in quadriplegia. Arch Phys Med Rehabil 68:315–317, 1987.
35. Dee PM, Suratt PM, Bray ST, Rose CE: Mucous plugging simulating pulmonary embolism in patients with quadriplegia. Chest 85:363–366, 1984.
36. Jubran A, Tobin MJ: Use of flow-volume curves in detecting secretions in ventilator-dependent patients. Am J Respir Crit Care Med 150:766–769, 1994.
37. Bach JR: Amyotrophic lateral sclerosis: Predictors for prolongation of life by noninvasive respiratory aids. Arch Phys Med Rehabil 76:828–832, 1995.
38. Lambertsen CJ: Chemical control of respiration at rest. In Mountcastle VB (ed): Medical Physiology, 14th ed. St. Louuis, Mosby, 1980, pp 1771–1827.
39. Milic-Emili J, Grassino AE, Whitelaw WA: Measurement and testing of respiratory drive. In Hornbein TF (ed): Regulation of Breathing. Lung Biology in Health and Disease, vol 17. New York, Marcel Dekker, 1981, pp 675–743.
40. Hugelin A, Cohen MI: The reticular activating system and respiratory regulation in the cat. Ann N Y Acad Sci 109:586–603, 1963.
41. Lydic R, Orem J: Respiratory neurons of the pneumotaxic center during sleep and wakefulness. Neurosci Lett 15:187–192, 1979.
42. Orem J, Montplaiser J, Dement WC: Changes in the activity of respiratory neurons during sleep. Brain Res 82:309–315, 1974.
43. Becker HF: Pathophysiology and clinical aspects of global respiratory insufficiency. Med Klin 92(Suppl 1):10–13, 1997.
44. Kohler D, Schonhofer B: How important is the differentiation between apnea and hypopnea? Respiration 64(Suppl):15–21, 1997.
45. Arnulf I, Similowski T, Salachas F, et al: Sleep disorders and diaphragmatic function in patients with amyotrophic lateral sclerosis. Am J Respir Crit Care Med 161:849–856, 2000.

46. Weinberg J, Klefbeck B, Borg J, Svanborg E: Respiration and accessory muscle activity during sleep in neuromuscular disorders. Eighth Journées Internationales de Ventillation à Domicile, abstract 150, March 7, 2001, Hopital de la Croix-Rousse, Lyon, France.
47. Juan G, Calverley P, Talamo C: Effect of carbon dioxide on diaphragmatic function in human beings. N Engl J Med 310:874–879, 1984.
48. Goldstein RS. Hypoventilation: Neuromuscular and chest wall disorders. Clin Chest Med 13:507–521, 1992.
49. Redding GJ, Okamoto GA, Guthrie RD, et al: Sleep patterns in nonambulatory boys with Duchenne muscular dystrophy. Arch Phys Med Rehabil 66:818–821, 1985.
50. Smith PEM, Edwards RHT, Calverley PMA: Ventilation and breathing pattern during sleep in Duchenne muscular dystrophy. Chest 96:1346–1351, 1989.
51. Soudon P: Ventilation assistee au long cours dans les maladies neuro-musculaire: Expérience actuelle. Réadaptation Revalidatie 3:45–65, 1987.
52. Hukins CA, Hillman DR: Daytime predictors of sleep hypoventilation in Duchenne muscular dystrophy. Am J Respir Crit Care Med 161:166–170, 2000.
53. Bradley TD, Mateika J, Li D, et al: Daytime hypercapnia in the development of nocturnal hypoxemia in COPD. Chest 97:308–312, 1990.
54. Ohtake S: Nocturnal blood gas disturbances and treatment of patients with Duchenne muscular dystrophy. Kokyu To Junkan 38:463–469, 1990.
55. Shneerson J: Disorders of Ventilation. Boston, Blackwell Scientific, 1988, p 43.
56. McDonald B, Rosenthal SA: Hypokalemia complicating Duchenne muscular dystrophy. Yale J Biol Med 60:405–408, 1987.
57. Aubier M, Murciano D, Lecocguic Y, et al: Effect of hypophosphatemia on diaphragmatic contractility in patients with acute respiratory failure. N Engl J Med 313:420–424, 1985.
58. Bach JR, Rajaraman R, Ballanger F, et al: Neuromuscular ventilatory insufficiency: The effect of home mechanical ventilator use vs. oxygen therapy on pneumonia and hospitalization rates. Am J Phys Med Rehabil 77:8–19, 1998.
59. Smith PEM, Edwards RHT, Calverley PMA: Oxygen treatment of sleep hypoxaemia in Duchenne muscular dystrophy. Thorax 44:997–1001, 1989.
60. Bach JR, Robert D, Leger P, Langevin B: Sleep fragmentation in kyphoscoliotic individuals with alveolar hypoventilation treated by nasal IPPV. Chest 107:1552–1558, 1995.
61. Guilleminault C, Motta J: Sleep apnea syndrome as a long-term sequela of poliomyelitis. In Guilleminault C (ed): Sleep Apnea Syndromes. New York, KROC Foundation, 1978, pp 309–315.
62. Steljes DG, Kryger MH, Kirk BW, Millar TW: Sleep in postpolio syndrome. Chest 98:133–140, 1990.
63. Carskadon M, Dement W: Respiration during sleep in the aged human. J Gerontol 36:420–425, 1981.
64. George CF, Millar TW, Kryger MH: Identification and quantification of apneas by computer-based analysis of oxygen saturation. Am Rev Respir Dis 137:1238–1240, 1988.
65. He J, Kryger MH, Zorick FJ, et al: Mortality and apnea index in obstructive sleep apnea. Chest 94:9–14, 1988.
66. Bach JR: Inappropriate weaning and late onset ventilatory failure of individuals with traumatic quadriplegia. Paraplegia 31:430–438, 1993.
67. Levy RD, Bradley TD, Newman SL, et al: Negative pressure ventilation: Effects on ventilation during sleep in normal subjects. Chest 65:95–99, 1989.
68. Katsantonis GP, Walsh JK, Schweitzer PK, Friedman WH: Further evaluation of uvulopalatopharyngoplasty in the treatment of obstructive sleep apnea syndrome. Otolaryngol Head Neck Surg 93:244–250, 1985.
69. Bradley TD, Phillipson EA: Pathogenesis and pathophysiology of the obstructive sleep apnea syndrome. Med Clin North Am 69:1169–1185, 1985.
70. Bonekat HW, Andersen G, Squires J: Obstructive disorder breathing during sleep in patients with spinal cord injury. Paraplegia 28:392–398, 1990.
71. Lombard R Jr, Zwillich CW: Medical therapy of obstructive sleep apnea. Med Clin North Am 69:1317–1335, 1985.
72. Brown IG, Zamel N, Hoffstein V: Pharyngeal cross-sectional area in normal men and women. J Appl Physiol 61:890–895, 1986.
73. Bach JR, Penek J: Obstructive sleep apnea complicating negative pressure ventilatory support in patients with chronic paralytic/restrictive ventilatory dysfunction. Chest 99:1386–1393, 1991.
74. Bach JR, O'Connor K: Electrophrenic ventilation: A different perspective. J Am Paraplegia Soc 14:9–17, 1991.
75. Hodes HL: Treatment of respiratory difficulty in poliomyelitis. In Poliomyelitis: Papers and Discussions Presented at the Third International Poliomyelitis Conference. Philadelphia, J.B. Lippincott, 1955, pp 91–113.
76. Bach JR, Tippett, DC, McCrary MM: Bulbar dysfunction and associated cardiopulmonary considerations in polio and neuromuscular disease. J Neuro Rehab 6:121–128, 1992.
77. Kimura K, Tachibana N, Kimura J, Shibasaki L: Sleep-disordered breathing at an early stage of amyotrophic lateral sclerosis. J Neurol Sci 164:37–43, 1999.

78. Bonekat HW, Andersen G, Squires J: Obstructive disordered breathing during sleep in patients with spinal cord injury. Paraplegia 28:392–398, 1990.
79. Flavell H, Marshall R, Thornton AT, et al: Hypoxia episodes during sleep in high tetraplegia. Arch Phys Med Rehabil 73:623–627, 1992.
80. Keenan SP, Ryan CF, Fleetham JA: Sleep disordered breathing following acute spinal cord injury. Am Rev Respir Dis 147:A688, 1993.
81. Marcus CL, Livingston FR, Wood SE, Keens TG: Hypercapnic and hypoxic ventilatory responses in parents and siblings of children with congenital central hypoventilation syndrome. Am Rev Respir Dis 144:136–140, 1991.
82. Oren J, Kelly DH, Shannon DC: Long-term follow-up of children with congenital central hypoventilation syndrome. Pediatrics 80;375–380, 1987.
83. Silverstein D, Michlin B, Sobel HJ, Lavietes MH: Right ventricular failure in a patient with diabetic neuropathy (myopathy) and central alveolar hypoventilation. Respiration 44:460–465, 1983.
84. Guilleminault C, Stoohs R, Kim Y, Chervin R, et al: Upper airway sleep-disordered breathing in women. Ann Intern Med 122:493–501, 1995.
85. Guilleminault C, Stoohs, Clerk A, Cetel M, Maistros P: A cause of excessive daytime sleepiness: The upper airway resistance syndrome. Chest 104:781–787, 1993.
86. Yoshida K: Oral appliance therapy for upper airway resistance syndrome. Neurology [in press].
87. Newsom Davis J, Goldman M, Loh L, Casson M: Diaphragm function and alveolar hypoventilation. Q J Med 45:87–100, 1976.
88. Dail CW, Affeldt JE: Vital capacity as an index of respiratory muscle function. Arch Phys Med Rehabil 38:383–391, 1957.
89. Fromageot C, Lofaso F, Annane D, et al: Supine fall in lung volumes in the assessment of diaphragmatic weakness in neuromuscular disorders. Arch Phys Med Rehabil 82:123–128, 2001.
90. Conference on Respiratory Problems in Poliomyelitis, March 12–14, 1952, Ann Arbor, National Foundation for Infantile Paralysis–March of Dimes, White Plains, NY.
91. Miller WF: Rehabilitation of patients with chronic obstructive lung disease. Med Clin North Am 51:349–361, 1967.
92. De Troyer A, Deisser P: The effects of intermittent positive pressure breathing on patients with respiratory muscle weakness. Am Rev Respir Dis 124:132–137, 1981.
93. Estenne M, De Troyer A: The effects of tetraplegia on chest wall statics. Am Rev Respir Dis 134:121–124, 1986.
94. De Troyer A, Borenstein S, Cordier R: Analysis of lung volume restriction in patients with respiratory muscle weakness. Thorax 35:603–610, 1980.
95. Gibson GJ, Pride NB, Newsom-Davis J, Loh LC: Pulmonary mechanics in patients with respiratory muscle weakness. Am Rev Respir Dis 115:389–395, 1977.
96. Enson Y, Giuntini C, Lewis ML, et al: The influence of hydrogen ion concentration and hypoxia on the pulmonary circulation. J Clin Invest 43:1146–1162, 1964.
97. Boushy SF, Thompson HK Jr, North LB, et al: Prognosis in chronic obstructive pulmonary disease. Am Rev Respir Dis 108:1373–1383, 1973.
98. Stoller JK, Ferranti R, Feinstein AR: Further specification and evaluation of a new clinical index for dyspnea. Am Rev Respir Dis 134:1129–1134, 1986.
99. Bach JR, Ishikawa Y, Kim H: Prevention of pulmonary morbidity for patients with Duchenne muscular dystrophy. Chest 112:1024–1028, 1997.

3 —— The History of Mechanical Ventilation and Respiratory Muscle Aids

JOHN R. BACH, M.D.

All truth passes through three stages. First it is ridiculed.
Second, it is violently opposed. Third, it is accepted as
being self-evident.

Arthur Schopenhauer (1788–1860)

In 1852, the English physician Meryon described how a 16-year-old boy with what became known as Duchenne muscular dystrophy (DMD) died from acute respiratory failure during a febrile episode with "profuse secretion of mucus from the trachea and larynx."[1] One hundred fifty years later, most patients with progressive neuromuscular diseases (NMDs) still die prematurely or are unnecessarily hospitalized and undergo tracheotomy because of failure to aid the respiratory muscles. This chapter puts the development of invasive mechanical ventilation and noninvasive respiratory muscle aids into historical perspective.

EARLY IDEAS

Mechanical ventilatory assistance may have been first attempted by Theophrastus Paracelsus in 1530. Paracelsus used his chimney bellows to ventilate patients' lungs via the mouth. This technique of respiratory resuscitation continued to be used in Europe through the 1830s.[2]

The effect of electrical stimulation of the phrenic nerve on diaphragm motion was first reported by Caldani in 1786.[3] Numerous reports of resuscitation by restoration of respiration with electrical stimulation of the phrenic nerves followed.[4,5] Phrenic nerve stimulation was abandoned as a method of ventilatory assistance when negative pressure body ventilators (NPBVs) became available in the mid-19th century.[5] The technique was resuscitated in 1948 when Sarnoff and associates demonstrated that adequate ventilation could be obtained by unilateral stimulation of a phrenic nerve.[6] Emerson put phrenic pacemakers on the American market in 1956. Since 1972, over 1000 phrenic nerve pacemakers have been implanted with variable success (see Chapter 7).[5,7,8] In essence, Paracelsus and Caldani attempted to assist the inspiratory muscles by mechanical or electrical methods. Inspiratory and expiratory muscle aids involve the application of forces to the body or pressure changes to the airway to assist inspiratory or expiratory muscle function.

BODY VENTILATORS

The tank-style ventilator was the first device used for effective mechanical ventilatory support. Tank ventilators continue to be used for both acute and long-term ventilatory support. They consist of a chamber that contains the patient with only the head protruding. Negative pressure is generated in the chamber by a bellows, negative pressure pump, or ventilator. This device creates a negative intrapleural pressure that results in lung insufflation.

The first tank ventilator was described by the Scottish physician, John Dalziel, in 1838.[9] The negative pressure was created in the tank by a pair of bellows worked from outside the tank by manual operation of a piston rod. A one-way valve prevented positive pressure in the tank. This device was used on at least one drowned victim, as demonstrated by a letter to the editor of the *Edinburgh Medical and Surgical Journal* in 1840.[10] The writer noted:

> In consequence of the patient's body being enclosed in the interior of the apparatus (in the sitting position), the elevation and depression of the chest were not perceptible, but the effects of air entering into and returning from the lungs were very visible on the cheeks, and lips, and also the nose. A lighted candle was extinguished by being held under one nostril, and again lighted by being placed opposite the other. The dead body was made to breathe in such a manner as to lead the bystanders to suppose that the unfortunate individual was restored to life.

An almost identical device was constructed and patented (no. 44,198) by Alfred F. Jones of Kentucky in 1864 (Fig. 1). The U.S. patent indicated that it could be used to "cure paralysis, neuralgia, rheumatism, seminal weakness, asthma, bronchitis, and dyspepsia. Also deafness . . . ."

Other tank ventilators of note included Woillez's first workable iron lung, which he called a "spirophore" (Fig. 2). A colleague suggested placing spirophores all along the Seine for drowning rescues, but public financing was not available.[11] For "resuscitating asphyxiated children," Egon Braun of Vienna devised a small wooden box in which pressure and suction were created by the doctor's breathing and sucking forcefully through a tube. The infant was supported in a plaster mold with the nose and mouth pressed against an opening (Fig. 3). Braun reported 50 consecutive successful cases.[11]

A prototype respirator room was patented by Peter Lord of Worcester, Massachusetts in 1908 (Fig. 4). He pictured huge pistons to create the pressure changes and to supply fresh

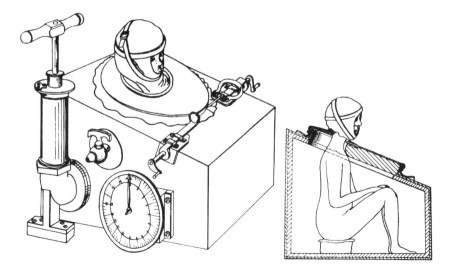

FIGURE 1. Body-enclosing iron lung described by Alfred F. Jones of Lexington, Kentucky, in 1864.

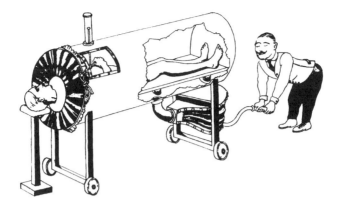

FIGURE 2.   The 1876 Woillez "spirophore" tank ventilator. (Courtesy of the J.H. Emerson Company.)

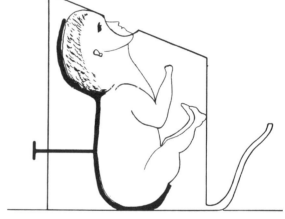

FIGURE 3.   A tank ventilator for "resuscitating asphyxiated children," made by Egon Braun of Vienna in 1889.

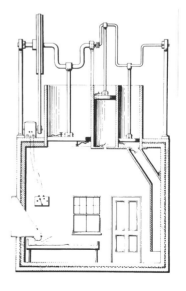

FIGURE 4.   The first design of an iron lung room by Peter Lord of Worcester, Massachusetts, in 1908.

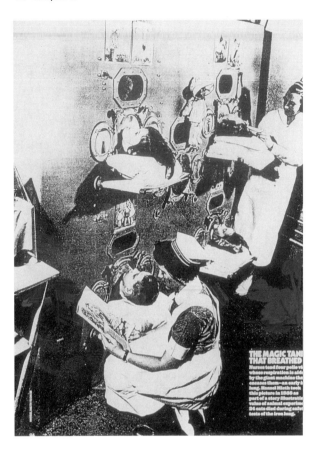

FIGURE 5. Thirty years after Lord's design of an iron lung room, the above chamber was created to provide simultaneous ventilatory support for patients and facilitate nursing care.

air. Since the use of a respirator room would facilitate nursing care, multiple patient respirator rooms were developed by James L. Wilson in the 1930s (Fig. 5).

H. H. Janeway, a chest surgeon, used a miniature iron lung that enclosed only the patient's head to maintain alveolar ventilation during surgery.[12] The Schwake "pneumatic chamber,"[11] developed in 1926, was concerned with portability and with matching the patient's breathing depth and rhythm. Schwake of Oranienburg-Eden, Germany, also believed that the "negative pressure upon the skin . . . draws out . . . the gaseous by-products." His device not only eliminated the need to have a care provider's manual assistance but also allowed the user to exercise his own limbs to ventilate his lungs (Fig. 6).

In 1927 Philip Drinker and Louis Agassiz Shaw at Harvard University paralyzed a cat, placed it in an airtight box, and alternated air pressure inside using a vacuum cleaner. In 1929 they developed an "iron lung" for humans (Fig. 7).[13] It had a sliding bed with headwall attached and a rubber collar. Pressure changes were created by an electrically powered rotary blower (the first electrically powered ventilator) and an alternating valve. This device was donated by Harvard University to Bellevue Hospital in New York City and was subsequently presented to the Beijing Medical College in China as a gift of the Rockefeller Foundation. Ultimately, it was used to sustain people who were recovering from opium overdoses in Beijing opium dens.

In 1931 John Emerson of Cambridge, Massachusetts, built a simplified, inexpensive, and more convenient iron lung that operated quietly, permitted speed changes, and could be operated by hand if electricity failed (Fig. 8). In 1936 Fred Snite, Jr., aged 25 years, son of Colonel Frederick Snite, a prominent Chicago financier, was stricken with poliomyelitis

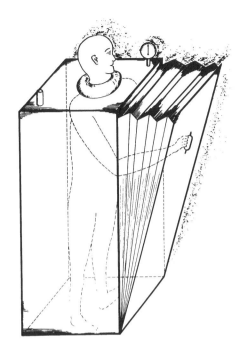

FIGURE 6. The "pneumatic chamber" made by Wilhelm Schwake of Germany was a tank ventilator designed to be operated by the patient.

while traveling with his family in Beijing. The Drinker iron lung, one of only 222 iron lungs in the world in 1936, was used by Mr. Snite for 1 year. He then returned to the United States via truck, ocean liner, and train along with a physician, seven Chinese nurses, a Chinese physiotherapist, two American nurses, and his family.[14,15] The fanfare, including the fact that he married and fathered three daughters, stimulated public awareness and resulted in mass production of Emerson iron lungs in time for the future poliomyelitis epidemics (Fig. 9). Mr. Snite lived using the iron lung continuously until 1954 when he died from cor pulmonale.

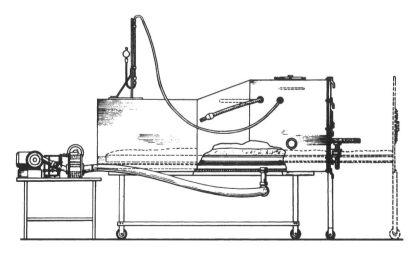

FIGURE 7. The Drinker and Shaw iron lung of 1928 was the first iron lung to receive widespread use.

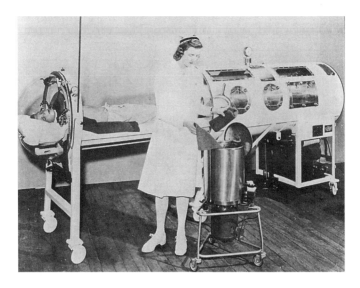

FIGURE 8. While nursing care was performed on their bodies, iron lung users received ventilatory support via a dome that covered their heads (J.H. Emerson Company's iron lung of 1932).

In 1947 Emerson placed transparent glass domes that enclosed the user's heads and were sealed at the neck collar of the iron lung. The iron lung bellows created both negative and positive pressure in the cylinder, and after 1947 the bellows could create positive pressure under the dome. Just as the negative tank pressure insufflated the lungs, the subsequent positive pressure forcibly exsufflated the patient, increasing tidal volumes. When iron lungs had to be opened to permit access to the body, patients with no breathing tolerance received intermittent positive-pressure ventilation (IPPV) via the dome (see Fig. 8).

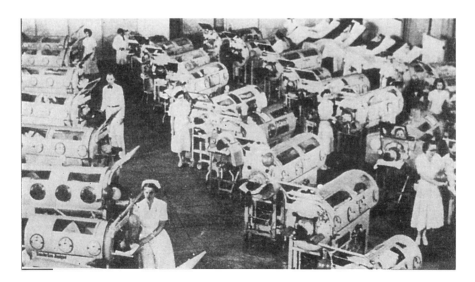

FIGURE 9. Iron lung wards that managed tens of patients during the mid-20th century poliomyelitis epidemics.

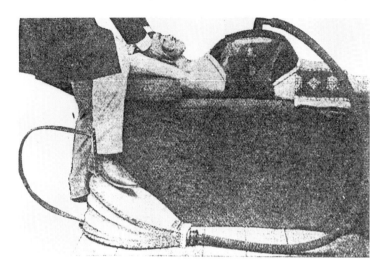

FIGURE 10.   The Eisenmenger chest shell ventilator of 1904.

The first chest-shell ventilator was developed by Ignez von Hauke of Austria in 1876.[16] He had used continuous positive airway pressure (CPAP) via an oral-nasal mask to treat atelectasis and was trying continuous negative airway pressure for the same reason when he realized that applying intermittent negative pressure to the chest and upper abdomen would assist lung ventilation.[17] The Eisenmenger chest shell of 1904 is essentially identical to the devices that later were mass-produced and used during the mid-century poliomyelitis epidemics[18] (Fig. 10). For the 1904 model, however, the cuirass was evacuated by a foot-powered bellows pump. Eisenmenger devised a motorized fan to evacuate the cuirass intermittently in 1927.

The Fairchild-Huxley chest respirator[19] and Monaghan Portable Respirator[20] were introduced in 1949 and became the first mass-produced chest shells. The Monaghan MRH ventilator had two outlets that could provide ventilation for two patients simultaneously. The machine was the size of a large desk on rollers. It could provide both negative and positive pressures to 30 mmHg. Adjustable pop-off valves set the delivered pressures. Like the iron lung bellows, the Monaghan device could provide both negative and positive pressures. Shortly afterward, Monaghan produced the ARG, a much smaller but still not very portable ventilator. It was about $30 \times 15 \times 15$ inches. It was sufficiently powerful to deliver positive and negative pressures to 40 mmHg in a tank half the size of an iron lung. It had a rate indicator and could be set from 10 to 50, and inspiratory/expiratory ratios were adjustable. Like the earlier Monaghan machine, it could be powered by a 24-volt battery and had a light that indicated when it was powered by battery as opposed to 110-volt alternating current. Emerson developed a negative-pressure cycling generator for chest shells in 1950. Thompson manufactured a chest-shell ventilator in 1956. Although the shells were portable, the negative pressure generators were not. These devices were built by hand and quite expensive. Because there were no filters, patients inhaled a great deal of dust and particles from the ventilator itself. The piston was too small for the ventilator to work with an intermittent abdominal pressure ventilator (IAPV). The pistons also shook during use and wore out quickly. They were covered by thin, fragile plastic cases. In 1960 Thompson created an IAPV attachment so that the ventilators could drive both chest shells and exsufflation belts.

Chest shells were used over the long term for daytime ventilatory support (with the user in the sitting position) as well as for nocturnal support (with the user in the supine position). Similar chest shells are manufactured today and are used predominantly for nocturnal ventilatory assistance (Respironics, Inc., Murrysville, PA; J. H. Emerson Company, Cambridge, MA). Custom-molded designs were made for patients with scoliosis.[21] The use of chest-shell ventilators for daytime aid was supplanted largely by more practical and effective methods, including mouthpiece IPPV, IAPV, and glossopharyngeal breathing (GPB).[22]

After successfully resuscitating drowned cats with a negative-pressure body jacket, Alexander Graham Bell developed a similar negative-pressure jacket to assist ventilation in premature infants in 1881. However, Bell's invention was not appreciated by the medical community until the British Tunnicliffe breathing jacket was described in 1955 and Jack Emerson put the Poncho "wrap" style ventilator on the market in 1957.[23] These ventilators—and the wrap ventilators that followed them—consist of a firm grid covering at least the thorax and upper abdomen. The grid and the body beneath it are covered by a windproof jacket that is sealed around the neck and extremities. As negative pressure is cycled under the wrap and grid, air enters the upper airway to ventilate the lungs. The only significant changes from the original designs in modern wrap ventilators are the plastics used to fabricate the jacket and grid and the length and form of the extremity sleeves (Fig. 11).

The Rocking Bed Ventilator (J. H. Emerson Company, Cambridge, MA) has been used for ventilatory assistance since 1932 (Fig. 12).[24] It rocks the patient 15–30°, thereby using gravity for cyclical displacement of abdominal contents and diaphragmatic excursion. It was used until the late 1950s, predominantly by patients with poliomyelitis and muscular dystrophy, and is still used occasionally today. This device is generally less effective than other body ventilators but can be adequate for some patients.[25]

The prototype IAPV was the Bragg-Paul Pulsator, described by C.J. McSweeney in 1938 (Fig. 13): "The apparatus . . . consists of a distensible rubber bag applied around the patient's chest in the form of a belt, this belt being rhythmically filled with, and emptied of, air."[26] The IAPV was developed by Alvin Barach in the United States in 1955 (Fig. 14). Barach, the author of the first comprehensive book on respiratory therapy,[27] used a pump made by the Gast Rotary Pump Company to pump air from an air reservoir into the sack inside the belt. This essentially modern IAPV[28] consisted of an elastic inflatable bladder incorporated within an abdominal corset worn beneath the patient's outer clothing. In the modern Exsufflation-belt (Respironics, Inc., Murrysville, PA), the action of the bladder

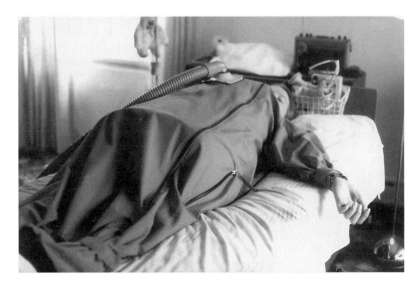

FIGURE 11. The pneumowrap ventilator (Respironics, Inc., Murrysville, PA) used by a patient with late-onset chronic ventilatory failure secondary to spinal cord injury.

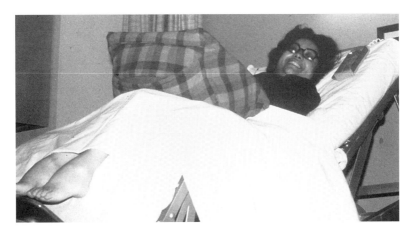

FIGURE 12. The rocking bed ventilator (J.H. Emerson Company, Cambridge, MA) used by a patient with poliomyelitis and no autonomous breathing tolerance since 1952.

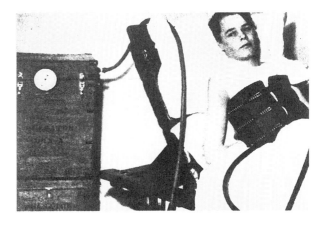

FIGURE 13. The prototype intermittent abdominal pressure ventilator was the Bragg-Paul Pulsator described by C.J. McSweeney in 1938.

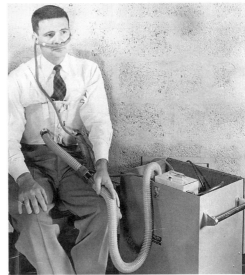

FIGURE 14. William H. Smith, Alvin Barach's engineer, modelling a prototype American intermittent abdominal pressure ventilator in 1952.

moves the abdominal contents and, therefore, the diaphragm. If the patient has any inspiratory capacity or is capable of effective GPB, he or she can add autonomous tidal volumes to the mechanically assisted inspirations. The Huxley Multilung, which became available in the late 1950s, was a powerful ventilator designed to inflate the air sac of the IAPV. It was essentially a double positive-pressure ventilator that could alternately operate an IAPV and cycle positive pressure separately for mouthpiece IPPV. It also had negative-pressure capabilities.

A device that is much like a combination of the IAPV and a chest shell consists of a wooden plate that covers the chest with an underlying bag, which is inflated by a motorized piston. This device was reportedly used successfully by a patient with DMD in 1995.[29]

POSITIVE-PRESSURE VENTILATORS FOR NONINVASIVE IPPV

In 1899 Bernard Dräger developed a miniature high-pressure gauge and manufactured the Dräger Oxygen Unit. By means of gas extraction, this unit could provide a constant working gas pressure in the cylinder, regardless of the pressure drop. Dräger produced a portable oxygen unit in 1902, and in 1909 he developed a clockwork-operated valve mechanism that controlled the flow of oxygen to the patient via an anesthesia mask attached to a cylinder called the Pulmotor. The Pulmotor, gas-operated and pressure-limited, was the first machine to use the pressure of gas for automatic operation. By 1913, 2000 Pulmotor units had been distributed. Railway rescue squads in special Pullman carriages were equipped with Pulmotor units. By 1914 more than 100 rescue stations in the United States were equipped with them, and by 1929 there were 6500 Pulmotors worldwide. On January 6, 1916 in New York City, 200 people who suffered from smoke inhalation were resuscitated using some of New York's 150 Pulmotor units.[30]

In 1915 J. H. Emerson developed and patented a similar device, called the Lungmotor (Fig. 15). It was much like a bicycle pump to which an oxygen tank could be attached. The pressure delivery settings could be adjusted so that, by manually activating the pump,

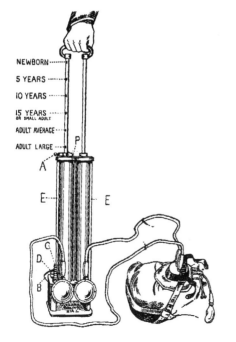

FIGURE 15. The Emerson Lungmotor of 1915.

appropriate tidal volumes could be provided for patients of any size. A smaller "Baby Lungmotor" was also available. Police and fire squads used these and similar devices powered by self-contained oxygen cylinders for resuscitation. The medical profession took no interest in such devices.

As aircraft began to reach higher altitudes, an oxygen supply became necessary. In 1914, Linnekogel achieved the world altitude record of 6300 meters using a Dräger high-altitude breathing apparatus with a rudimentary "demand regulator" that made it possible to supply exactly the amount of air required by the user.[30] In the United States, on the other hand, as late as World War II oxygen from a bag strapped to the head was delivered to pilots via Boothby-Lovelace-Bulbulian (BLB) masks or "horse masks" (so-called because the mask-bag assembly resembled a horse's feed bag). The BLB mask operated on a continuous-flow basis and was controlled by the A3A regulator. This regulator allowed air flow to increase automatically as the plane ascended.

Toward the end of World War II Forest Bird gained access to a German demand regulator and described it as the "first demand-flow device I had ever encountered. The only problem was you had to suck your guts out to turn the flow on."[30] He modified the regulator and added a diaphragm to create a demand valve that would trigger with a negative-pressure effort of 1–2 cmH$_2$O.[31] Barach insisted that CPAP would have important therapeutic applications; thus, Bird created a "pressure head" that maintained slight CPAP. By poking "the diaphragm forward with a pencil, providing pressure only during inspiration . . . [and] placing a doorknob on the handle of the demand regulator," he essentially created a hand-operated pressure-limited IPPB machine in 1949. In 1952, these prototypes developed into his Mark Series of IPPB machines, which permitted flow control.

Late in the 19th century, Friedrich Trendelenburg, a professor of surgery in Leipzig, realized that patients were dying from ventilatory failure when their chests were opened. His assistants designed a pump-type ventilator similar to the Engstrom device developed in the early 1950s.[12] The next pneumatically operated pressure-limited ventilator was the Spiropulsator, which was used during chest surgeries in Sweden in 1940. A similar unit was used by Mautz in Cleveland.[12] Blease, a British engineer, introduced a pressure-limited control mode ventilator called the Pulmoflator in 1944–1945. The first American-made ventilator available for controlled ventilation during anesthesia was the pressure limited Emerson Assistor, released in 1951. By 1952 Air Shields, Dräger, and Monaghan had IPPB machines on the market.[32]

Although a large number of iron lungs were available in the United States in the 1950s, there was a shortage of NPBVs and anesthesia ventilators when the polio epidemic broke out in Denmark in 1952. As a result, patients underwent tracheotomy and were ventilated around the clock by the manual squeezing of a rubber bag. Modern manual resuscitators became available in the following year, when the Ohio Chemical and Surgical Equipment Company of Madison, Wisconsin, released the Kreiselman Model 116, an accordion-style manual resuscitator. It came with a portable suction unit in a box (Fig. 16). Emerson put a hand-operated resuscitator "bag" on the market in 1954, and the Rubin resuscitator "bag" became available in 1955.[33]

As a result of the polio epidemic in Europe, rugged volume-limited and electrically powered mechanical pumps were developed. The Engstrom ventilator appeared in Sweden and the Morch piston ventilator in the U.S. in 1954. These devices had large electrical motors with variable speed drives to a large volume piston. The Morch ventilator delivered much larger air volumes than necessary for closed-system ventilation. They were needed to provide adequate alveolar ventilation despite the air leakage around cuffless silver tracheostomy tubes. The Engstrom unit was a more refined machine that provided more precise tidal volumes and used a large piston to compress a bag-in-bottle device. This machine provided a pressure plateau for more smooth delivery of air to the lungs.

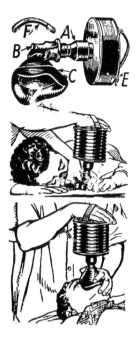

FIGURE 16. Kreiselman accordion-style manual resuscitator of 1953.

Until this time, however, most long-term ventilator users were still in iron lungs; the chest shell was often used for daytime support. Jack Emerson in 1955 and Ray Bennett in 1957 manufactured assist controllers (PR 1A) that, along with the Bird Mark VII, were used for surgical and postoperative assisted ventilation. These ventilators required constant supervision because they responded to decreases in compliance or increases in resistance by reducing delivered volumes. In 1957 the Bennett pressure- or volume-limited BA-2 anesthesia ventilator introduced a controller assistor combined with a "bag-in-bottle" device. If the inflation pressure was set high enough, the ventilator would deliver the chosen volume despite any decrease in compliance. For this reason, Bendixen used the BA-2 in the polio unit at Massachusetts General Hospital during the last of the respiratory polio epidemics in Boston in the 1950s.[12]

Meanwhile, ventilators were becoming more portable as patients wished to leave iron lungs and use IPPV. Harris Thompson left the J. J. Monaghan Company in 1955 to create the Thompson Engineering Company and, shortly thereafter, Thompson Respiratory Products. In 1957 Thompson released a small, 25-pound, pressure-limited control ventilator called the Bantam. It was not much larger than a bread box. It contained a simple 12-volt motor blower about 6 inches long and 5 inches in diameter that could be used with an air tube as long as necessary. The plastic tube ended in a flattened plastic mouthpiece that was held in the mouth and cycled by the patient's tongue, which blocked the tube in an alternating pattern. While the patient was sleeping, the blower and mouthpiece cycled the air on and off with the patient's tongue. When the tubing was constricted to decrease airflow to the patient's lungs, the patient would automatically increase the insufflation time to compensate for the decrease. The Bantam was used most often with a short, 5- to 6-foot tube to optimize portability. During swimming pool therapy, the patient could lengthen the inspiratory cycle by delaying blockage of the tube with the tongue and thereby deeply insufflate the lungs, which facilitated floating. The Bantam operated on both alternating current and 12-volt batteries and could be used with a car battery. It had a Samsonite case, and filters were changed every 3–6 months. The Bantam was ideal for mouthpiece IPPV and sufficiently powerful to operate IAPVs.

In 1964, Jack Emerson introduced the American equivalent of the Engstrom ventilator without the bag-in-bottle device. The air delivery was controlled by directly varying the piston's stroke, and, for the first time, electronic speed controls varied the inspiratory and expiratory phases. This device reliably delivered set volumes regardless of changes in lung compliance and airway resistance. In 1967 the Bennett MA-1 used a small compressor to provide air under high pressure. It had a potentiometer to control tidal volume, and safety alarms were introduced.[12] The MA-1 became the benchmark against which other intensive care unit (ICU) ventilators were measured and in a real sense was the first modern ICU ventilator.

The pressure-cycled Bantam and the later ST and GT model Bantams were the only truly portable ventilators until 1976, when Borg, an electrical engineer, released the first portable volume-cycled ventilator. The Thompson Mini-lung volume-cycled ventilator quickly followed in 1978. Because of their alarm systems, smooth and adjustable flow rates, "sigh" capabilities, internal batteries, and economic use of electricity, portable volume-cycled ventilators quickly captured the market. Portable pressure-cycled machines disappeared until the advent of bilevel positive airway pressure (BiPAP) machines in 1990. Many Bantam users, however, refused to switch to volume-cycled ventilators, and some continue to use Bantams today.

SWITCH TO TRACHEOSTOMY

In 1869 Trendelenburg first described the use of a tracheostomy tube with an inflated cuff for manual application of positive-pressure ventilatory assistance during anesthesia of a human.[34] The use of transoral intubation for ventilatory support during anesthesia was described soon afterward.[35] In 1893 a hand-powered bellows was devised for delivering IPPV. Rubber tubing connected it to the patient via either a tight-fitting oral-nasal interface or a tracheostomy tube.[36,37] Tracheostomy and the use of a mechanical bellows for ventilatory support became widely used for anesthesia during World War I.[38] The use of tracheostomy tubes specifically to facilitate the suctioning of airway secretions led to modification of iron lungs to accommodate patients with indwelling tracheostomy tubes after 1943. Tracheostomy tubes were not used for long-term ventilatory support, however, until the inadequate supply of NPBVs necessitated long-term use during the 1952 Danish polio epidemic.[39]

Although iron lungs provided adequate ventilatory support, their use was not without difficulty:

> In the beginning, doctors sometimes delayed too long before committing a patient to the iron lung but as the procedure became less threatening, ventilation was started earlier—a fact that allowed patients to adjust before the onset of total paralysis. Once patients had been placed in the lung, technical questions arose—how much positive or negative pressure, what rate to set, and the often emotional issue of how and when to begin the process of weaning the patient off mechanical support.[40]

Weaning was often considered the obligation of the patient. Patients were typically encouraged to breathe on their own: "One day a doctor and a nurse decided to give him a treat and take him for a car ride. He still remembers the sheer terror invoked by his very real air hunger and the reassurance of the doctor and the nurse not to worry—his lips weren't blue!"[40]

Likewise, patients had to remain immobile and recumbent when using iron lungs. Evacuation of airway secretions was quite difficult for supine patients without tracheal intubation and with limited access to the body for manually assisted coughing. Noninvasive IPPV had not yet been reported, and mechanical forced exsufflation devices to assist cough were not widely available until after 1953.[41–43] Furthermore, during the Danish epidemic the mortality rate was 94% for patients with respiratory paralysis and concomitant bulbar muscle involvement and 28% for patients without bulbar involvement.[39] Three hundred forty-five of 2300 patients (15%) had some combination of ventilatory failure and impaired swallowing. Lassen reported that mortality figures for ventilator-supported patients decreased from 80% to 41%, or to about 7% for the entire Danish acute paralytic poliomyelitis population. This decrease was in part due to more frequent use of tracheostomy, particularly for patients with severe bulbar involvement.

Tracheostomy, however, was not without its difficulties:

> There was preoccupation and uncertainty about the place of tracheostomy. This operation may have created more problems than it solved. Nurses and doctors alike were unfamiliar with tracheobronchial hygiene, nebulization was primitive and each "trach" brought in its wake a nightmare of "plugs"—hard excrescences of blood and mucus that formed and reformed in the trachea and mainstem bronchi. So universal was this complication that the regular staff became quite expert at emergency bronchoscopy and forceps removal of inspissated debris.[40]

In the meantime, specialized centers in the United States were reporting equally impressive decreases in mortality by "individualizing" patient care. From 1948 to 1952, 3500 patients were treated at Los Angeles General Hospital; 15–20% required ventilatory support. The mortality rate of acute poliomyelitis decreased from about 15% in 1948 to 2% in 1952 without the use of tracheostomy for ventilatory support.[44] Although many patients at Los Angeles General Hospital, particularly those with bulbar polio, underwent tracheotomy for management of secretions while they were ventilated by NPBVs, in other centers, where few tracheotomies were performed, the mortality rate also decreased to about 2%.[44] It was concluded that the previously high fatality rate was not because of inadequacy of NPBVs but because of bulbar insufficiency and aspiration of secretions.[44] Better nursing care and attention to managing airway secretions, including the use of devices to help eliminate them, were major factors in decreasing mortality rates.[45]

A long debate ensued about whether tracheostomy, IPPV, or body ventilators were preferable for ventilatory support. In 1955, an International Consensus Symposium defined the indications for tracheostomy as the combination of respiratory insufficiency with swallowing insufficiency and disturbance in consciousness or vascular disturbances:

> If a patient is going to be left a respirator cripple with a very low VC [vital capacity], a tracheotomy may be a great disadvantage. It is very difficult to get rid of a tracheotomy tube when the VC is only 500 or 600 cc and there is no power of coughing, whereas, as we all know, a patient who has been treated in a respirator [NPBV] from the first can survive and get out of all mechanical devices with a VC of that figure.[44]

In 1958 Forbes wrote:

> Tracheotomy, which is designed to provide a more efficient airway and access to the trachea in certain patients, does not materially assist in ridding the bronchi of secretions which must migrate to the upper bronchi and trachea before they become accessible to suction through the tracheotomy tube. The inaccessibility of these secretions in the lower bronchial tree even to bronchoscopy makes it necessary to provide indirect means for their mechanical expulsion.[46]

Forbes noted that the published mortality figures in six studies of acute patients were lower with tank respiration than with tracheostomy IPPV. He also noted that in patients with respiratory paralysis without pharyngeal paralysis, tracheostomy led to tracheal damage, loss of capability for GPB, and loss of "the routine application of chest compression" to help clear airway secretions. The result was a worse prognosis compared with patients managed by noninvasive methods.[46]

Nonetheless, tracheostomy IPPV became the standard for long-term ventilatory support in the 1960s for the following reasons: (1) NPBV use severely restricted patient mobility; (2) uncooperative patients and patients with severe bulbar muscle dysfunction could not effectively use noninvasive inspiratory muscle aids indefinitely; and (3) oximeters were not available to guide use of noninvasive respiratory aids.[47] Tracheostomy also provided a closed system of ventilatory support that was amenable to precise monitoring of ventilatory volumes and pressures and oxygen delivery and to the use of the high-technology respirators and alarm systems that were to come.

As the use of endotracheal methods became widespread, manually assisted coughing was no longer taught in medical, nursing, and respiratory therapy curricula and clinicians lost familiarity with body ventilators. Noninvasive IPPV methods[48] were not to be described until 1969[49] and 1973,[50] and their 24-hour use was not reported for a large population until 1993.[51] Furthermore, the only studies of the use of MI-E devices had been in patients with acute poliomyelitis and patients with severe intrinsic pulmonary disease.[45] The former were felt to be a transient population and the latter a population for which the use of noninvasive respiratory muscle aids was not ideal. Although MI-E devices disappeared from the market in the 1950s and early 1960s, they continued to be used by patients who had access to them.[47] Meanwhile, with widespread use of translaryngeal intubation and tracheostomy, numerous reports of complications appeared (see Chapter 6).

RETURN TO NONINVASIVE IPPV

In the 1870s Ignez von Hauke of Austria may have become the first person to deliver IPPV via a face mask.[52] By the 1930s, "the OEM face mask was in common usage all over the world" for delivering anesthesia and ventilatory assistance during surgery and for other acute care needs.[53] Although noninvasive IPPV is now delivered via oral,[54–56] nasal,[57–59] or oral-nasal interfaces for both acute and long-term ventilatory support,[60,61] long-term noninvasive IPPV was first delivered for these purposes via a simple mouthpiece.

Mouthpiece IPPV

Ironically, what may seem like the simplest solution to the problem of providing ventilatory support—delivery of positive-pressure ventilation via a simple mouthpiece—continues to be the last option to be considered. In 1947, when the tank was opened to provide nursing care, the iron lung bellows ventilated patients by delivering positive pressure intermittently under the domes that surrounded the patient's head. As noted, Emerson delivered bellows-generated positive pressure to patients via a face mask in 1947, and in 1951 the IPPB machine became available.[62] Meanwhile, Huxley and Monaghan negative-positive pressure pumps were already available to operate chest shells and could be used for mouthpiece IPPV as well.

In 1953, John E. Affeldt of Rancho Los Amigos Hospital in Los Angeles made the following report at a conference on postpoliomyelitis respiratory equipment:

> There is just one point I would like to mention, which has just come along, which, I think, makes it [noninvasive positive pressure ventilation] even more feasible. It is so simple that why it wasn't thought of long ago I don't know. Actually, some of our physical therapists, in struggling with the patients, noticed that they could simply take the positive pressure attachment, apply a small plastic mouthpiece... and allow that to hang in the patient's mouth. You can take him to the Hubbard tank by such means and you can do any nursing procedure, if the patient is on the rocking bed and has a zero vital capacity, if you want to stop the bed for any reason, or if you want to change him from the tank respirator to the bed, or put the cuirass respirator on, or anything to stop the equipment, you can simply attach this, hang it by the patient, he grips it by his lips, and thus it allows for the excess to blow off which he doesn't want.
>
> It works very well. We even had one patient who has no breathing ability who has fallen asleep and been adequately ventilated by this procedure, so that it appears to work very well, and I think does away with a lot of complications of difficulty of using positive pressure. You just hang it by the patients and they grip it with their lips, when they want it, and when they don't want it, they let go of it. It is just too simple.[62]

Most often the positive-pressure attachment used to deliver IPPV was the simple mouthpiece used for pulmonary function testing. Patients intermittently blocked the mouthpiece to cycle adequate tidal volumes into their lungs. Although in 1950 patients had received noninvasive IPPV via a face mask circuit attachment to the iron lung bellows, Affeldt noted that "you don't have to have an attachment made for the tank respirator. We took the cuirass respirator pump and by just putting a filter in the line attaching this at the other end, you have got a pump right there . . . simply set up a gauge, a filter, and you have got that to use any place you want with the patient, and you have got positive pressure." David D. Dickinson, Medical Director of the Poliomyelitis Respirator Center of Ann Arbor, Michigan, added that he used "a vacuum cleaner and a glass jugful of water with a glass tube that can be raised or lowered so that you have an automatic stop for pressure in the mask. It can roll around and you can breathe the patient. It costs about four dollars for the whole outfit exclusive of the vacuum cleaner, which you can swipe from the house-keepers around the hospital." Likewise, Benjamin Ferris of the Harvard School of Public Health reported that a "vacuum cleaner and positive pressure is applied by a face mask and a thumb leak which controls your pressure. By merely sliding the thumb over the aperture the pressure is allowed to build up in the patient and then released by just drawing the thumb back across the thumb hole." David Dickinson of the Polio Respiratory Center of Ann Arbor added, "We have used vacuum cleaner and a mask over the face for all patients only because we felt it was simpler...for giving each person a deep breath."[62] Not only were positive-pressure pumps available for noninvasive IPPV, but also the exhaust from negative-pressure pumps could be used for the same purpose.

The ventilator unit of Goldwater Memorial Hospital in New York City was opened in 1955. In a short time the 80-bed unit was filled mostly with post-poliomyelitis patients who used NPBV. Most patients had been recumbent in iron lungs in local hospitals since contracting poliomyelitis. Patients at Goldwater Hospital, who often had no breathing tolerance, were encouraged to leave their iron lungs during daytime hours and to use the chest-shell ventilator or IAPV when sitting. Although these body ventilators were not optimal for every patient, most patients learned that they could receive optimal tidal volumes via a mouthpiece from the positive cycling of the ventilators. Patients could be placed in wheelchairs using chest shells, IAPVs, or IPPV via mouthpieces, and the "portable" negative-positive pressure ventilators were rolled behind them until smaller machines, such as the Bantam, became available in 1957.

Because mouthpiece IPPV can provide much greater air volumes directly to the lungs than IAPV or chest shells, it became the mode of ventilatory support during chest infections and other times of stress. The mouthpieces were held in the mouth or fixed onto motorized wheelchair controls (sip and puff, chin, or tongue control) adjacent to the mouth for easy access by the patient (Fig. 17). The Thompson Bantam was mounted directly onto the wheelchair, allowing patients to be much more mobile than when they used the heavier negative-positive pressure ventilators to operate chest shells. Although still using body ventilators overnight, the great majority of Goldwater patients switched to Bantams for IAPVs as well as mouthpiece IPPV during daytime hours. Despite the fact that mouthpiece IPPV was used routinely for daytime ventilatory support at both Goldwater Memorial Hospital and Ranchos Los Amigos Hospital in California by 1957,[51] its use was first reported in the medical literature in 1969.[50]

Along with the Bantam, Thompson produced a mouthpiece that was flattened on the open end. Its lower edge folded down so that it could hook over the lower lip or teeth to minimize the effort needed to grip it (see Fig. 17). Some mouthpieces had flanges between the lips and teeth and were precursors to the Bennett lipseal. Thompson found that the butyrates in vacuum cleaner tubing were the ideal material for mouthpieces—much better than hard, slippery, transparent acrylic. They were gray, softer to the tongue, more comfortable to the teeth, and not slippery; they also lasted much longer.

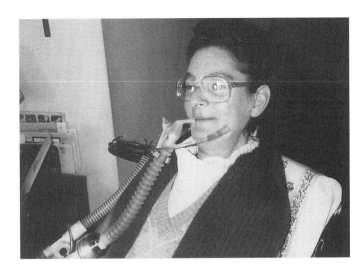

FIGURE 17. IPPV delivered via a mouthpiece fixed adjacent to sip-and-puff controls of a motorized wheelchair for a patient with no autonomous breathing tolerance since 1954.

At the same time, across the United States body ventilator users were told to undergo tracheotomy so that they could benefit from the enhanced mobility permitted by mounting the Bantam onto the wheelchair and because it was thought that a tracheostomy was needed for airway secretion management. Although in centers other than Goldwater Hospital the great majority of ventilator users were switched to tracheostomy IPPV, isolated patients around the country refused tracheotomy, and some reported that they had the idea to ventilate their lungs via mouthpieces.

When Augusta Alba took charge of the Goldwater Memorial Hospital ventilator unit in 1956, she encouraged patients to use mouthpiece IPPV for daytime ventilatory support. Like Dr. Affeldt before her, she soon discovered that mouthpiece IPPV users could nap during the daytime without displacement of the mouthpiece. This observation was remarkable for several reasons: (1) many patients had little or no autonomous breathing ability; (2) the ventilators did not have alarms; (2) there was nothing to hold the mouthpiece in place other than the patient's own oropharyngeal muscles, which are not thought to function during REM sleep; and (3) because patients had little or no extremity function, they could not have replaced the mouthpiece if it fell out of their mouth. In 1964 she permitted a number of patients to use mouthpiece IPPV overnight rather than return to body ventilators.[54,55] Few, if any, patients died from losing the mouthpiece during sleep. No patients were admitted to or managed with tracheostomy tubes on the Goldwater Memorial Hospital ventilator unit until 1968. From the mid-1960s until nocturnal nasal IPPV was described in 1987, simple mouthpiece IPPV was the only method of daytime or nocturnal noninvasive IPPV. Only when oximeters became widely available in the early 1980s was it discovered that patients experienced frequent, and at times, severe desaturation in arterial oxygen, which was associated with periods of leakage of ventilator-delivered air (insufflation leakage) during sleep.

The Bennett mouthpiece with lipseal retention (Mallincrodt, Pleasanton, CA) entered the market in 1968 (Fig. 18). It was designed to be used for pulmonary function testing. To prevent the mouthpiece from falling out of the mouth during sleep, Alba convinced many of her patients to use mouthpiece IPPV with lipseal retention. By sealing the lips, this device not only ensured mouthpiece retention but also greatly reduced insufflation leakage out of the mouth.

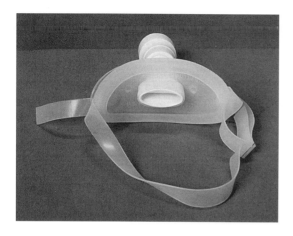

FIGURE 18. Mallincrodt Puritan-Bennett Lipseal.

By 1980, mouthpiece IPPV was used as ventilatory support for up to 24 hours by 270 patients at the Goldwater Memorial Hospital Ventilator Unit alone. Other patients using mouthpiece IPPV around the country shared their knowledge and experiences in patient support organizations such as the Gazette International Network and the International Ventilator Users' Network (St. Louis, MO). In addition to mouthpieces designed for pulmonary function testing, patients used oral interfaces that they devised from scuba diving equipment and tygon tubing and made custom-molded acrylic mouthpieces (Fig. 19) with bite-plate retention (Fig. 20). In 1981, Bach and Alba published the first study in which ventilator users with DMD ventilated their lungs around the clock by using only mouthpiece/lipseal IPPV.[63]

The creation of the medical specialty of respiratory therapy in 1961 and the training of respiratory therapists have been of paramount importance in the noninvasive management of patients with ventilatory impairment.[61] Respiratory therapists continue to be essential for evaluating and training patients in the use of noninvasive ventilation and expiratory muscle aids.

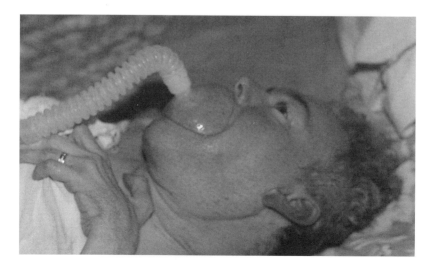

FIGURE 19. Custom acrylic mouthpiece with orthodontic bite plate and lipseal used by a patient with no breathing tolerance since 1955. (Photograph courtesy of G. McPherson.)

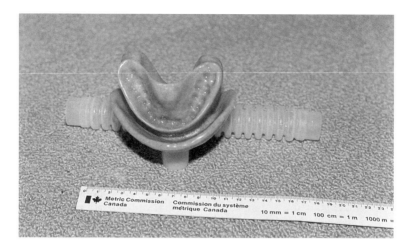

FIGURE 20.   Bite plate for acrylic lipseal.

Nasal Intermittent Positive-pressure Ventilation

And the Lord God formed man of the dust of the ground, and gave him intermittent positive-pressure ventilation via nasal access, the breath of life.

In 1981, as a technical advisor to Yves Rideau of the University of Poitiers, Bach introduced mouthpiece and lipseal IPPV into France. In the winter of 1981–1982, Rideau suggested to Bach and Delaubier that ventilation should be attempted via nasal access. He believed that humidification would be facilitated and that the nasal route would prove a more physiologic alternative for IPPV. Bach and Delaubier first used urinary drainage catheters with the cuffs inflated in each nostril to deliver nasal IPPV to themselves and then to French patients with muscular dystrophy for daytime and nocturnal ventilatory assistance.[64,65] Nasal IPPV was first used as an alternative to airway intubation for 24-hour ventilatory support in 1984, and its use was first reported in 1987.[66] In 1984, nasal CPAP masks became commercially available and could be used as IPPV interfaces.[67] This technique permitted rapidly expanding application of nasal ventilation.

Excessive nasal bridge pressure and insufflation leakage into the eyes were common complaints when nasal IPPV was used with the first commercial CPAP "masks." Attempts at customizing nasal interfaces for IPPV were first described in 1987.[66] Custom-molded nasal interfaces eventually became available both commercially and individually.[61]

Sleep-disordered Breathing and Bilevel Positive Airway Pressure

Sleep-disordered breathing was essentially "discovered" in the late 1970s (see Chapter 2). The conventional treatment quickly became the delivery of CPAP. CPAP, however, is of little use for patients who suffer primarily from ventilatory impairment, such as those with obesity-hypoventilation syndrome or NMD. Since 1990, by permitting the independent adjustment of inspiratory (IPAP) and expiratory positive airway pressures (EPAP), bilevel positive airway pressure (BiPAP) machines have provided pressure spans (IPAP minus

EPAP) that assist inspiratory muscle function. Thus, pressure-cycled ventilators, albeit not powerful ones, were again on the market.

Oral-Nasal Interfaces

During the 1952 polio epidemics, the most popular and practical way for delivering IPPV via anesthesia masks was with the exhaust from vacuum cleaners adapted with safety relief valves.[68] Intensive care developed out of the use of ventilatory support during the epidemics. In 1965, four publications reported an 85% success rate in avoiding intubation for 257 patients with COPD in respiratory failure ($PaCO_2 > 70$ mmHg; mean reported pH 7.27–7.36) with the use of oral-nasal IPPV. However, the medical personnel required special training, the patients were not always cooperative, and they required much attention. Thus, ultimately, the technique was forgotten.[68a]

In the late 1980s Adolphe Ratza, a Swedish survivor of poliomyelitis, experimented with the construction of strap-retained custom nasal and oral-nasal interfaces (Fig. 21). His oral-nasal interfaces, with strap retention systems much like those used for lipseal and nasal IPPV, were described for long-term supported ventilation in 1989.[69] Over the past 6 years, strap-retained oral-nasal interfaces have been marketed by Respironics, Inc., and Mallincrodt, Inc.

In 1985, Bruni Bung, a German survivor of poliomyelitis who had been symptomatic for chronic alveolar hypoventilation, hired her dentist to custom-mold an acrylic oral-nasal shell that was retained by an acrylic bite-plate (Fig. 22).[69] The bite-plate retention was important for Bung because she lived alone and could not don a strap-retention system because of limited upper limb strength and range of motion (Fig. 23).[61] This style of strapless custom-molded acrylic low-profile oral-nasal interface with bite-plate retention became the main interface constructed and used at Dallas Rehabilitation Institute for the nocturnal ventilatory support of decannulated patients with high-level traumatic spinal cord injury.[61]

HOME MECHANICAL VENTILATION

By 1949, over 400 survivors of respiratory polio were using ventilators in the United States in custodial care at over 100 hospitals scattered around the country. They were funded by the National Foundation for Infantile Paralysis (March of Dimes), which President Franklin Roosevelt had founded. The hospital charges were so high that the March of Dimes funded a study to find ways to reduce the cost. The study showed that it

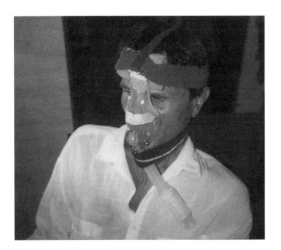

FIGURE 21. Early custom-made strap-retained oral-nasal interface.

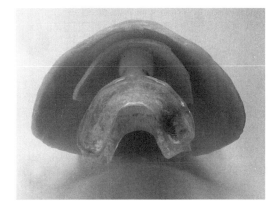

FIGURE 22. Bite-plate retention for a strapless oral-nasal interface (SONI).

would be far more economic to move patients to regional centers with multidisciplinary professional teams. Thus, 16 polio respiratory and rehabilitation centers with 15–160 patients were created at the teaching hospitals of 16 medical schools. The first two centers were established at Boston and Houston in 1950. Most of the centers lasted less than 10 years, but their impact on physical medicine, independent living, and vocational rehabilitation of ventilators users and others with disability was tremendous. As money poured in, the March of Dimes paid for the centers' professional staff, patient care, equipment, research, and, ultimately, for home care, home modifications, and personal care attendants.[15] Of interest, no pulmonologists or respiratory therapists existed at that time. The patients and their families were taught how to ventilate lungs and how to facilitate airway secretion elimination and became key participants in the rehabilitation team.

In 1953 a home-care plan was developed at Rancho Los Amigos Hospital in California when it was shown that deinstitutionalization with home care by attendants could result in 75% cost savings.[15] The first attendants were trained by the centers, but ultimately attendants were hired and trained by the patients and families themselves. In 1953 it was estimated that 1800 patients with poliomyelitis had been respirator (iron lung)-supported for 1 month or more and that 20% of these patients had already been discharged home. Forty-four percent of the users of home mechanical ventilation were cared for solely by their families, and 15% were under 9 years of age.[70] Over 50% of patients required ventilatory support over 16 hours per day. At that time, "[t]he average cost of hospital per diem was $20/day. At home we estimated $5/day."[70] By 1956, 92% of permanently ventilator-dependent patients had been discharged to their homes.[15] In the late 1950s, however, with the

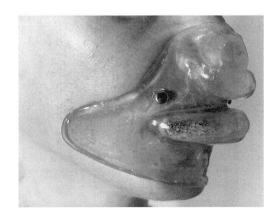

FIGURE 23. The first strapless oral-nasal interface (SONI) made of acrylic from a plaster moulage with bite-plate retention used by a patient who cannot independently don a strap-retained interface.

success of the polio vaccines and the drying up of public support, funding for attendant care was no longer available. The cessation of attendant care in 1959 stimulated the disability movement and the beginning of some federal funding of attendant care in 1960.

MANAGEMENT OF AIRWAY SECRETIONS

Patients with weak inspiratory muscles usually have weak expiratory muscles and difficulty in coughing and clearing airway secretions. When only body ventilators were available for noninvasive ventilatory support, the importance of manually assisted coughing (see Chapter 7) was greatly appreciated. Quantification of manually assisted PCF and the importance of generating maximal cough flows were reported in 1966.[71]

The importance of deep GPB-assisted breaths on cough effectiveness was also described in 1956.[72] In addition to being useful for providing a deep breath before spontaneous or manually assisted coughing, GPB was recognized as an alternative method of ventilating the lungs in the event of ventilator failure. It was first described for 15 patients with polio in 1951,[73] and an excellent educational video was made in 1954.[74]

Many patients used manual resuscitators or volume-cycled ventilators to fill their lungs with air. They then turned to vacuum cleaners to exsufflate their lungs! Another technique was nicely described by Harris Thompson:

> Probably the most effective method for coughing a post-polio that I saw was to turn the pressure up on a Bantam (or other small blower) to give a comfortable deep breath. Slow the rate as low as possible on the Bantam. Tie a towel around the abdomen to restrict diaphragm movement. The patient was usually lying on his chest with his head hanging over the edge of a table or bed. The chest was decompressed when simultaneously a person pressed firmly down on the back of the chest with the patient trying to cough.

Mechanically Assisted Coughing

In the late 1940s, Henry Seeler, working for the U.S. Air Force, developed a mechanical insufflator-exsufflator designed to deliver alternating positive and negative pressures to ventilate and exsufflate people suffering from exposure to "chemical weapons" and "nerve gas."[75] In 1951, Barach et al. described an exsufflator attachment for iron lungs. The device used a vacuum cleaner motor with a 5-inch solenoid valve attached to an iron lung portal. With the valve closed, the motor developed a negative intratank pressure to – 40 mmHg. At peak negative pressure the valve opened, triggering a return to atmospheric pressure in 0.06 sec and causing passive exsufflation.[76] This technique increased PCF by 45% for six ventilator-supported patients with poliomyelitis. An additional increase was obtained by timing an abdominal compression with valve opening.[77] These techniques were sufficiently effective for the investigators to report that the exsufflation produced by the device "completely replaced bronchoscopy as a means of keeping the airway clear of thick tenacious secretions." Another patient "would have required bronchoscopy or re-opening of the tracheotomy if the exsufflator had not been successful in clearing the airway."[76]

In the late 1940s, Barach, Beck, and their engineer Gutterman developed a "mechanical cough chamber." A pressure change of 110 mmHg was induced 25 times per minute. A close-fitted baffle around the neck split the chamber into two parts. A blower applied positive pressure to the head chamber, which resulted in a higher pressure in the head chamber than in the body end of the chamber. When the pressure rose 110 mmHg above the atmosphere in the head chamber, a differential head-body pressure gradient up to 40 mmHg caused air to enter the lungs. The sudden opening of the 5-inch valve in the head compartment resulted in a 100-mmHg explosive decompression and a head-body pressure differential shift of + 40 mmHg to a level of about – 40 mmHg, which created forced exsufflation. The expiratory flows were enhanced by the perceptible forward shift of the

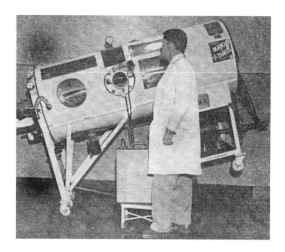

FIGURE 24. The Exsufflator, seen on the stool on the floor, applies exhaust to the iron lung portal for forced exsufflation.

body as the positive differential pressure in the body compartment dropped to 0 mmHg with the return of atmospheric pressure on both sides of the baffle.[78,79]

In 1951 the same group began to apply vacuum cleaner suction to an iron lung portal to increase negative-pressure lung insufflation. William Smith replaced Gutterman as the engineer and, at the urging of Gustav Beck, also applied a positive-pressure exhaust to the portal to augment the forced exsufflation (Fig. 24). This addition, combined with the patient's cough efforts, increased cough flows. Smith then developed a much more compact exsufflator that could be carried by hand. Also in 1951, he built an additional valve into the auxiliary dome of the iron lung and applied – 20 mmHg to the dome during the expiratory cycle, using the same exsufflation source and a T connector. Emerson supplied the iron lungs for these endeavors and began to apply vacuum cleaner suction to the portals.

In 1952, Barch, Beck, and Smith began to apply negative pressure to patient airways via a face mask. Smith developed the first "exsufflation with negative pressure" device in a steel box; the pressures were adjusted by controlling pump speeds. At Beck's urging, positive pressure was applied to the airway before the forced exsufflation. Using his aunt's Eureka Hand Vacuum, a small air pump that worked perfectly, Smith completed the first exsufflation with negative pressure device designed for use via a face mask in June 1952. Later in 1952, Smith helped Rudy Frohner of O.E.M. build the first preproduction prototype for the American market.

In May of 1953, John Affeldt of Rancho Los Amigos noted that his patients had tried many methods to maximize cough flow, including Barach's mechanical cough chamber, vacuum cleaner suction, manual chest and abdominal compression, and maximal insufflation in an iron lung, followed by closing of the glottis until positive pressure peaks were created in the tank. He reported being disappointed that he was unable to clear atelectasis in a number of patients with these methods. Emerson, however, noted that it made much more sense to apply positive and then negative pressure to a face mask to increase cough flows than it did to place patients in the mechanical cough chamber.[62] Five months later, OEM, the company of Fagin and Barach's brother Edward, marketed the exsufflation with negative pressure device called a "Cof-flator."

The Cof-flator delivered MI-E directly to the airway via a mouthpiece, mask, or endotracheal tube[43,80] (Fig. 25). The Cof-flator consisted of a two-stage axial compressor that gradually inflated the lungs at positive pressures up to 40 mmHg over 2 seconds. The pressure in the upper respiratory passageway was then dropped to 30–40 mmHg below atmosphere in 0.02 seconds by the swift opening of a solenoid valve connected to a negative

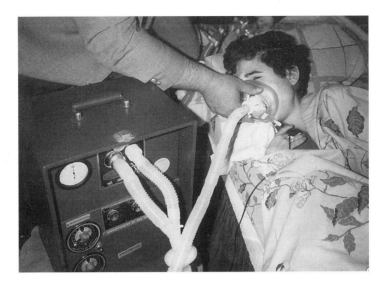

FIGURE 25. Cof-flator, OEM Company, New Haven, CT (circa 1952), used by a patient with Duchenne muscular dystrophy in 1992.

pressure blower. Insufflation and exsufflation pressures were independently adjusted for comfort and efficacy. The negative pressure was maintained for 1-3 seconds.[81,82]

In 1954 Beck and Barach wrote of the Cof-flator: "The life-saving value of exsufflation with negative pressure was made clear through the relief of obstructive dyspnea as a result of immediate elimination of large amounts of purulent sputum, and, in a second episode, by the substantial clearing of pulmonary atelectasis after 12 hours' treatment."[83] Although many studies demonstrated its efficacy and no major untoward effects were described with its use, the Cof-flator was abandoned because of the increasing use of tracheostomy. However, patients who had access to the original Cof-flators kept and used them effectively as needed. Occasional medical publications continued to refer to its effective use, even though it was no longer on the market.[55,57,79,84–87] Patients without access to the Cof-flator not uncommonly air-stacked to maximal insufflations, using ventilators or GPB, then exsufflated the airways, using vacuum cleaners.

In February of 1993, a new mechanical insufflator-exsufflator (In-Exsufflator, J. H. Emerson Co., Cambridge, MA) was marketed. The In-Exsufflator operated like the Cof-flator except that cycling between positive and negative pressure had to be done manually. The manual cycling feature facilitated care giver-patient coordination of inspiration and expiration with insufflation and exsufflation, but it also required an additional hand to deliver an abdominal thrust. Then, in 1995, an automatically cycling device became available. In 2001 it was renamed the Cough-Assist™.

Mechanical Oscillation Techniques

In 1939 it was recognized that alveolar ventilation and blood circulation could be assisted by rapidly alternating negative and positive pressure under a chest shell.[88] In the early 1950s, J.H. Emerson developed the first high-frequency chest wall oscillation jacket, the Ucyclist-B Vest, to facilitate bronchial secretion clearance, but he provided oscillation only during part of the breathing cycle.[32] Barach described use of a similar unit by patients with chronic bronchial asthma and emphysema in 1966.[89] Oscillation can be applied externally to the chest wall or abdomen or directly to the airway as high-frequency positive-pressure ventilation, jet ventilation, or oscillation with rapid, small-amplitude pressure swings above and below atmospheric pressure.[90] In the 1960s Bird operated the Mark II at cycling frequencies near 20 Hertz during anesthesia in conjunction with the pneumobag. The pneumobag was a bag within a bag. The inside bag contained the anesthetic agents, and lung volume and oxygenation were maintained by rapid cycling of the Mark II. This technique was called "diffusive respiration," a harbinger of jet ventilation. To eliminate carbon dioxide, the outer bag was squeezed to provide "convective ventilation."[31] In addition to assisting gas exchange, all of these techniques have some effect on mucociliary transport (see Chapter 13).

ACKNOWLEDGMENTS

The author thanks John Weissleder, R.T., Mr. Harris Thompson, and Mr. William Smith for their valuable input.

~~~~

Vivo de la mia morte e, se ben guardo,
Felice vivo d'infelice sorte;
E chi viver non sa d'angoscia e morte,
Nel foco venga, ov'io mi struggo e ardo.

Michelangelo Buonarrotte, 1532

~~~~

REFERENCES

1. Meryon E: On granular or fatty degeneration of the voluntary muscles. Medico-Chirurg Trans 35:73–85, 1852.
2. Gordon AS: History and evolution of modern resuscitation techniques. In Gordon AS (ed): Cardio-pulmonary Resuscitation Conference Proceedings. Washington, DC, National Academy of Sciences, 1966, pp 7–32.
3. Caldani LMA: Institutiones Physiologicae. Venezia, Pezzana, 1786. [Cited by Schecter DC: Application of electrotherapy to non-cardiac disorders. Bull N Y Acad Med 46:932–951, 1970.]
4. Duchenne G: De l'electrisation localise et de son application la pathologie et la thérapeutique. Paris, Bailliere, 1872, p 914. [Cited in Vanderlinden RG, Epstein SW, Hyland RH, et al: Management of chronic ventilatory insufficiency with electrical diaphragm pacing. Can J Neurol Sci 15:63–67, 1988.]
5. Glenn WWL, Phelps ML: Diaphragmatic pacing by electrical stimulation of the phrenic nerve. Neurosurgery 17:974–984, 1985.
6. Sarnoff SJ, Hardenbergh E, Whittenberger JL: Electrophrenic respiration. Am J Physiol 155:1–9, 1948.
7. Glenn WWL, Hogan JF, Loke JSO, et al: Ventilatory support by pacing of conditioned diaphragm in quadriplegia. N Engl J Med 310:1150–1155, 1984.
8. Stauffer ES, Bell GD: Traumatic respiratory quadriplegia and pentaplegia. Orthop Clin North Am 9:1081–1089, 1978.
9. Dalziel J: On sleep and an apparatus for promoting artificial respiration. Br Assoc Adv Sci 2:127, 1838.
10. Lewins R: Apparatus for promoting respiration in cases of suspended animation. Edinburgh Med Surg J 53:255, 1840.
11. Emerson JH, Loynes JA: The Evolution of Iron Lungs: Respirators of the Body-Encasing Type. Cambridge, MA, J.H. Emerson Company, 1978.
12. Rendell-Baker L: Principles in design and function of mechanical ventilators. Respir Ther 9:63–69, 1979.
13. Drinker PA, McKhann CF: The iron lung: First practical means of respiratory support. JAMA 255:1476, 1986.
14. Gorham J: A medical triumph: The iron lung. Respir Care 9:71, 1979.
15. Laurie G: Ventilator users, home care, and independent living: An historical perspective. In Kutscher AH, Gilgoff I (eds): The Ventilator: Psychsocial and Medical Aspects. New York, Foundation of Thanatology, 2001, pp 147–151.
16. Von Hauke I: Der Pneumatische Panzer. Beitrag zur mechanischen Behandlung der Brustkrankheiten. Wiener Medizinische Presse 15:785, 836 ,1874.

17. Waldenburg L: Die pneumatische Behandlung der Respirations und Circulationskrankheiten im Anschluss an die Pneumatometrie und Spirometrie. Hirschwald, Berlin, 1880, p 420. [Cited in Woollam CHM: The development of apparatus for intermittent negative pressure respiration: 1832–1918. Anaesthesia 31:537–547, 1976.]
18. Eisenmenger R: Apparatus for maintaining artificial respiration. Lancet iii:515, 1904.
19. Council on Physical Medicine: Acceptability of the Fairchild-Huxley cuirass respirator. JAMA 143:1157, 1950.
20. Council on Physical Medicine: The Monaghan Portable Respirator acceptance report. JAMA 139:1273, 1949.
21. Newman JH, Wilkins JK: Fabrication of a customized cuirass for patients with severe thoracic asymmetry. Am Rev Respir Dis 137:202–204, 1988.
22. Bach JR, Alba AS: Total ventilatory support by the intermittent abdominal pressure ventilator. Chest 99:630–636, 1991.
23. Spalding JMK, Opie L: Artificial respiration with the Tunnicliffe breathing jacket. Lancet 274:613–615, 1958.
24. Eve FG: Actuation of inert diaphragm by gravity method. Lancet ii:995–997, 1932.
25. Bryce-Smith R, Davis HS: Tidal exchange in respirators. Curr Res Anaesth Analges 33:73–85, 1954.
26. McSweeney CJ: The Bragg-Paul pulsator in treatment of respiratory paralysis. Br Med J 1:1206–1207, 1938.
27. Barach AL: Principles and Practices of Inhalational Therapy. Philadelphia, J.B. Lippincott, 1944.
28. Adamson JP, Lewis L, Stein JD: Application of abdominal pressure for artificial respiration. JAMA 169:153–157, 1959.
29. Abbona H, Navarro R: Mechanical ventilation in Duchenne's disease: A case report. Respir Care 40:734–736, 1995.
30. Dräger B: Technology for Life. Drager Aktiengesellschaft, Lubeck, Germany, 2002.
31. Branson RD: Pioneers in respiratory care: Forrest M. Bird, Ph.D. Am Assoc Respir Care Times 14:50–57, 1990.
32. Levine ER: Effective Inhalation Therapy. Chicago, National Cylinder Gas, 1953, p 8.
33. Peckos T: Respiratory equipment to remember from 20th century. Adv Respir Care Practit July:58, 2000.
34. Trendelenburg F: Beitrage zur den Operationen an den Luftwagen 2. Tamponnade der Trachea. Arch Klin Chir 12:121–233, 1871.
35. MacEwen W: Clinical observations on the introduction of tracheal tubes by the mouth instead of performing tracheotomy or laryngotomy. Br Med J 2:122–124, 1880.
36. Fell GE: Forced respiration. JAMA 16:325–330, 1891.
37. Hochberg LA: Thoracic Surgery Before the 20th Century. New York, Vantage Press, 1960, pp 684–697.
38. Magill IW: Development of endotracheal anesthesia. Proc R Soc Med 22:83–88, 1928.
39. Lassen HCA: The epidemic of poliomyelitis in Copenhagen, 1952. Proc R Soc Med 47:67–71, 1954.
40. Taylor RF: Polio 1953 [monograph]. The Premier's Council on the Status of Persons with Disabilities, Alberta, Canada, 1953.
41. Barach AL, Beck GJ, Bickerman HA, Seanor HE: Physical methods simulating cough mechanisms. JAMA 150:1380–1385, 1952.
42. Bickerman HA, Itkin S: Exsufflation with negative pressure. Arch Intern Med 93:698–704, 1954.
43. The OEM Cof-flator Portable Cough Machine. St. Louis, Shampaine Industries, ca. 1952.
44. Hodes HL: Treatment of respiratory difficulty in poliomyelitis. In Poliomyelitis: Papers and Discussions Presented at the Third International Poliomyelitis Conference. Philadelphia, J.B. Lippincott, 1955, pp 91–113.
45. Barach AL, Beck GJ, Smith WH: Mechanical production of expiratory flow rates surpassing the capacity of human coughing. Am J Med Sci 226:241–248, 1953.
46. Forbes JA: Management of respiratory paralysis using a "mechanical cough" respirator. Br Med J 1:798–802, 1958.
47. Bach JR, Ishikawa Y, Kim H: Prevention of pulmonary morbidity for patients with Duchenne muscular dystrophy. Chest;12:1024–1028, 1997.
48. Bach JR: A comparison of long-term ventilatory support alternatives from the perspective of the patient and care giver. Chest 104;1702–1706, 1993.
49. Alba A, Solomon M, Trainor FS: Management of respiratory insufficiency in spinal cord lesions. In Proceedings of the 17th Veteran's Administration Spinal Cord Injury Conference, 1969. Washington, DC, U.S. Government Printing Office, 1971, pp 200–213 [publication 0-436-398].
50. Aberion G, Alba A, Lee MHM, Solomon M: Pulmonary care of Duchenne type of muscular dystrophy. N Y State J Med 73:1206–1207, 1973.
51. Bach JR, Alba AS, Saporito LR: Intermittent positive pressure ventilation via the mouth as an alternative to tracheostomy for 257 ventilator users. Chest 103:174–182, 1993.
52. Woollam CHM. The development of apparatus for intermittent negative pressure respiration: 1832–1918. Anaesthesia 31:537–547, 1976.
53. Soroka M: Fifty years of progress in respiratory care. Respir Ther 9:21–29, 1979.

54. Bach JR, Alba AS, Bodofsky E, et al: Glossopharyngeal breathing and non-invasive aids in the management of post-polio respiratory insufficiency. Birth Defects 23:99–113, 1987.
55. Bach J, O'Brien J, Krotenberg R, Alba AS: Management of end stage respiratory failure in patients with Duchenne muscular dystrophy. Muscle Nerve 10:177–182, 1987.
56. Curran FJ, Colbert AP: Ventilator management in Duchenne muscular dystrophy and postpoliomyelitis syndrome: Twelve years' experience. Arch Phys Med Rehabil 70:180–185, 1989.
57. Bach JR, Alba AS: Management of chronic alveolar hypoventilation by nasal ventilation. Chest 97:52–57, 1990.
58. Ellis ER, Bye PTP, Bruderer JW, et al: Treatment of respiratory failure during sleep in patients with neuromuscular disease, positive-pressure ventilation through a nose mask. Am Rev Respir Dis 135:148–152, 1987.
59. Hill NS, Eveloff SE, Carlisle CC, et al: Efficacy of nocturnal nasal ventilation in patients with restrictive thoracic disease. Am Rev Respir Dis 145:365–371, 1982.
60. Kerby GR, Mayer LS, Pingleton SK: Nocturnal positive pressure ventilation via nasal mask. Am Rev Respir Dis 135:738–740, 1987.
61. McDermott I, Bach JR, Parker C, Sortor S: Custom-fabricated interfaces for intermittent positive pressure ventilation. Int J Prosthodont 2:224–233, 1989.
62. Round Table Conference on Poliomyelitis Equipment, Roosevelt Hotel, New York City, May 28–29, 1953, National Foundation for Infantile Paralysis–March of Dimes, White Plains, N.Y.
63. Bach J, Alba A, Pilkington LA, Lee M: Long-term rehabilitation in advanced stage of childhood onset, rapidly progressive muscular dystrophy. Arch Phys Med Rehabil 62:328–331, 1981.
64. Delaubier A: Traitement de l'insuffisance respiratoire chronique dans les dystrophies musculaires. In Memoires de certificat d'etudes superieures de reeducation et readaptation fonctionnelles. Paris, Universite R Descarte, 1984, pp 1–124.
65. Rideau Y, Delaubier A: Neuromuscular respiratory deficit: Setting back mortality. Semin Orthop 2:203–210, 1987.
66. Bach JF, Alba A, Mosher R, Delaubier A: Intermittent positive pressure ventilation via nasal access in the management of respiratory insufficiency. Chest 92:168–170, 1987.
67. Sullivan CE, Issa FG, Berton-Jones M, et al: Home treatment of obstructive sleep apnea with continuous positive airway pressure applied through a nose-mask. Bull Eur Physiopatol Respir 20:49–54, 1984.
68. Conference on Respiratory Problems in Poliomyelitis, March 12–14, 1952, Ann Arbor, National Foundation for Infantile Paralysis–March of Dimes, White Plains, N.Y.
68a. Sadoul P: Historique de la réanimation respiratoire. Rev Mal Respir 16:307–312, 1999.
69. Ratzka A: Uberdruckbeatmung durch Mundstuck. In Frehse U (ed): Spatfolgen nach Poliomyelitis: Chronische Unterbeatmung und Moglichkeiten selbstbestimmter Lebensfuhrung Schwerbehinderter, vol. 5. Munchen, Pfennigparade eV, 1989, p 149.
70. Frates RC, Splaingard ML, Smith EO, Harrison GM: Outcome of home mechanical ventilation. J Pediatr 106:850–856, 1985.
71. Kirby NA, Barnerias MJ, Siebens AA: An evaluation of assisted cough in quadriplegic patients. Arch Phys Med Rehabil 47:705–710, 1966.
72. Feigelson CI, Dickinson DG, Talner NS, Wilson JL: Glossopharyngeal breathing as an aid to the coughing mechanism in the patient with chronic poliomyelitis in a respirator. N Engl J Med 254:611–613, 1956.
73. Dail CW. Glossopharyngeal breathing by paralyzed patients. Calif Med 75:217–218, 1951.
74. Dail CW, Affeldt JE: Glossopharyngeal Breathing [video]. Los Angeles, Department of Visual Education, College of Medical Evangelists, 1954.
75. Dempsey CA: 50 Years of Research on Man in Flight. Wright-Patterson AFB, Ohio, U.S. Air Force, Aerospace Medical Research Laboratory.
76. Barach AL, Beck GJ, Bickerman HA, Seanor HE: Mechanical coughing: Studies on physical methods of producing high velocity flow rates during the expiratory cycle. Trans Assoc Am Physicians 64:360–363, 1951.
77. Barach AL, Beck GJ, Bickerman HA, et al: Physical methods simulating mechanisms of the human cough. J Appl Physiol 5:85–91, 1952.
78. Bach JR, Smith WH, Michaels J, et al: Airway secretion clearance by mechanical exsufflation for post-poliomyelitis ventilator assisted individuals. Arch Phys Med Rehabil 74:170–177, 1993.
79. Bach JR: Mechanical exsufflation, noninvasive ventilation and strategies for pulmonary rehabilitation and sleep disordered breathing. Bull N Y Acad Med 68:321–340, 1992.
80. Segal MS, Salomon A, Herschfus JA: Alternating positive-netative pressures in mechanical respiration (the cycling valve device employing air pressures). Dis Chest 25:640–648, 1954.
81. Barach AL, Beck GJ, Smith RH: Mechanical production of expiratory flow rates surpassing the capacity of human coughing. Am J Med Sci 226:241–247, 1953.
82. Bickerman HA: Exsufflation with negative pressure: elimination of radiopaque material and foreign bodies from bronchi of anesthetized dogs. Arch Intern Med 93:698–704, 1954.
83. Beck GJ, Barach AL: Value of mechanical aids in the management of a patient with poliomyelitis. Ann Int Med 40:1081–1094, 1954.

84. Bach JR, Alba AS, Saporito LR: Intermittent positive pressure ventilation via the mouth as an alternative to tracheostomy for 257 ventilator users. Chest 103:174–182, 1993.
85. Bach JR, Alba AS, Bohatiuk G, et al: Mouth intermittent positive pressure ventilation in the management of post-polio respiratory insufficiency. Chest 91:859–864, 1987.
86. Friesen H, Schoemperlen CB: The Cof-flator. Can Inhal Ther 3:11–12, 1967.
87. Beck GJ: Advances in physiologic technics for rehabilitation of asthmatic patient. N Y State J Med 64:993–1000, 1964.
88. Eisenmenger R: Suction and pressure over the belly: Its action and application [in German]. Wien Med Wochenschr 31:807–812, 1939.
89. Beck GJ: Chronic bronchial asthma and emphysema rehabilitation and use of thoracic vibrocompression. Geriatrics 21:139–158, 1966.
90. Chang HK, Harf A: High-frequency ventilation: A review. Respir Physiol 57:135–152, 1984.

4 ——— Noninvasive Ventilation: Mechanisms of Action

MARK W. ELLIOTT, M.D.

BACKGROUND

Interest in the use of noninvasive ventilation has grown rapidly. In this chapter only, the term noninvasive ventilation refers to continuous positive airway pressure (CPAP) as well as to intermittent positive-pressure ventilation (IPPV) and the combination of positive inspiratory pressure and positive end-expiratory pressure (PIP + PEEP). Noninvasive ventilation is used with increasing frequency in the management of acute and chronic respiratory impairment as well as for relatively stable hypercapnic patients. Simonds and Elliott,[1] Leger et al.,[2] and others have reported encouraging long-term benefits of domiciliary nocturnal noninvasive ventilation for patients with a variety of conditions. At least four prospective, randomized, controlled trials have demonstrated benefits of nocturnal noninvasive ventilation[3–6] in managing hypercapnic respiratory failure, mostly due to chronic obstructive pulmonary disease (COPD), and other studies have demonstrated benefit in patients with acute respiratory failure[7] (see Chapters 11 and 12). To understand why assisted ventilation is effective in both acute and chronic respiratory impairment, a basic understanding of pathophysiology is required (see Chapters 1 and 2). This chapter addresses the mechanisms of efficacy of noninvasive ventilation.

To ventilate the lungs effectively, the respiratory muscle pump must have the capacity to sustain ventilation against a given load. It also requires neural drive from the central nervous system (CNS). In other words, there must be a balance between load and capacity, and the system must receive adequate drive. A man attempting to carry a package across the room provides an effective analogy. He may fail for a number of reasons: he may be too weak (i.e., capacity is reduced); the package may be too heavy (i.e., the load is excessive); or he may lack the necessary motivation (i.e., drive is insufficient) (Fig. 1).

ABNORMALITIES OF CAPACITY

Capacity can be reduced because of intrinsic weakness of the respiratory muscles. This weakness may be reversible (when it is due to electrolyte disturbance, hypoxia, hypercapnia, or acidosis) or irreversible (when it is due to neuromuscular disease [NMD]). In addition, muscles of normal strength can work at a mechanical disadvantage—for example, because of hyperinflation[8] or chest wall deformity. Reduced capacity is not an all-or-nothing phenomenon, nor is it static. Instead, it is a continuum that can change minute by minute. When the respiratory muscle pump begins to fail, the pattern of breathing changes with an increase in respiratory rate and a decrease in tidal volume.[9] This pattern of breathing can reduce the demand on the respiratory muscles but at the expense of alveolar ventilation. Hypercapnia and acidosis ensue and further reduce muscle function.[10]

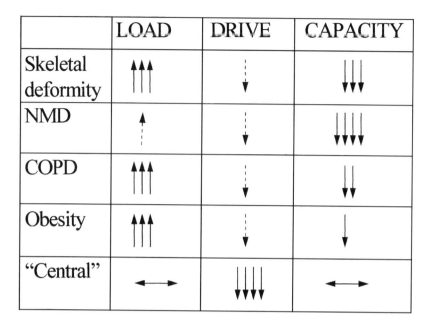

	LOAD	DRIVE	CAPACITY
Skeletal deformity	↑↑↑↑↑↑	↓	↓↓↓↓↓↓
NMD	↑	↓	↓↓↓↓↓↓↓↓
COPD	↑↑↑↑↑↑	↓	↓↓↓↓
Obesity	↑↑↑↑↑↑	↓	↓↓
"Central"	←→	↓↓↓↓↓↓↓↓	←→

FIGURE 1.   The relative contribution of abnormalities of load, drive, and capacity in conditions commonly treated by noninvasive ventilation. Solid lines represent primary abnormalities; dotted lines represent secondary changes.

ABNORMALITIES OF LOAD

Changes in the load against which the respiratory muscle pump is working also may be reversible or irreversible. The load, too, is not constant. Changes can occur either because of disease (e.g., sputum, fluid retention, or increased airflow obstruction) or as part of normal circadian physiologic changes (e.g., during sleep loss of upper airway muscle tone leads to increased upper airway resistance). Load can be excessive because of reduced compliance of the chest wall (e.g., due to scoliosis) or the lungs (e.g., due to atelectasis and diseases of the airways or lung parenchyma). Abnormalities of the pulmonary vasculature, such as occur in COPD and scoliosis, can put an additional load on the respiratory muscles through the need for increased ventilation to maintain adequate gas exchange.

ABNORMALITIES OF DRIVE

Neural drive can be reduced by structural or metabolic abnormalities of the respiratory control center in the brainstem or by sedative drugs. People who develop chronic hypercapnia also can have secondary abnormalities of drive as a consequence of changes during sleep. Ventilation is reduced during sleep in normal people because of the loss of the wakefulness drive to breathe. A rise in carbon dioxide up to 1 kPa is normal. Greater increases in carbon dioxide cause a transient acidosis that results in compensatory renal retention of bicarbonate. As a result, chemosensitivity to carbon dioxide, which is mediated by changes in pH, is reduced. In addition, patients with chronic ventilatory insufficiency often have disturbed sleep. White et al.[11] showed that normal people who were sleep-deprived had abnormal ventilatory responses to both hypoxia and hypercapnia during the day. In the acute setting, worsening hypercapnia, due either to injudicious oxygen therapy or sedatives or to the severity of the primary pathology, can cause narcosis and loss of the central drive to breathe.

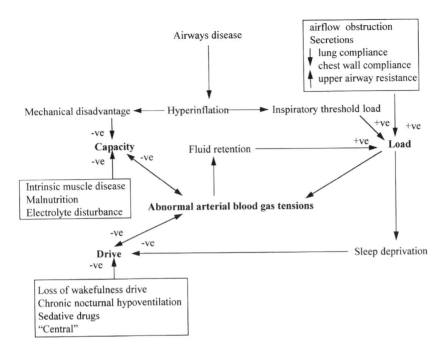

FIGURE 2. A schematic representation of how abnormalities in one system may cause or exacerbate ventilatory failure and how vicious cycles may develop. ve = ventilation. (Adapted from Elliott MW: Long-term ventilation in severe COPD. In Hill NS (ed): Long-Term Mechanical Ventilation. New York, Marcel Dekker, 2001, p 155.)

DEVELOPMENT OF VENTILATORY FAILURE

Severe derangements of load, drive, or capacity or small abnormalities of any combination of these factors can lead to the development of ventilatory failure (Fig. 2). For example, ventilatory failure occurs in a normal person if the respiratory muscle pump is working against an intolerable load, as in severe acute asthma. Similarly, a normal person given large doses of sedative drugs can become apneic even though the lungs and respiratory muscles are normal. By contrast, in a patient with severe NMD the respiratory muscles can be so weak that they may not be able to sustain ventilation even of normal lungs. Combinations of abnormal load, drive, and capacity can result in ventilatory failure even with relatively trivial reductions of a single parameter. For example, the patient with severe weakness of the respiratory muscles may be able to maintain effective ventilation and normal arterial blood gas tensions, but a small reduction in lung compliance or airway mucus accumulation (e.g., during a chest infection) can cause severe decompensation. Similarly, a patient with severe chronic airflow limitation may maintain almost normal blood gas tensions until load is increased during an acute exacerbation or drive is reduced for any reason. An understanding of the contribution of each of these factors to the development of ventilatory failure and the way in which they can change either physiologically or pathologically can help to formulate a logical strategy for both acute and long-term management. A recent study of patients during acute exacerbations of COPD reported that improvements in arterial blood gases during noninvasive ventilation were essentially due to higher alveolar ventilation, not to improvement in ventilation/perfusion relationships. The increase in PaO_2 was explained by a rise in the respiratory exchange ratio due to an increased clearance of body stores of carbon dioxide. The authors suggested that attainment of an efficient breathing pattern rather than high inspiratory pressures should be the primary goal to improve arterial blood gases in such patients.[13] Figure 2 shows how one factor can affect others and culminate in arterial blood gas deterioration.

NONINVASIVE VENTILATION IN CHRONIC RESPIRATORY FAILURE: MECHANISMS OF ACTION

Effect of Noninvasive Ventilation on Capacity

Studies of noninvasive ventilation suggest that it works by resting fatigued respiratory muscles. Most studies have included small numbers of patients with COPD, most often recovering from an acute exacerbation, and have not considered other possible explanations, such as changes in load and drive. Small increases in maximal inspiratory pressures at the mouth have been cited as evidence of improved capacity, although in the absence of a control group, these increases may have been due to learning effects and increased motivation. Others,[13,14] however, have reported improved daytime arterial blood gas tensions in the absence of changes in the indices of respiratory muscle strength. In an attempt to determine whether respiratory muscle fatigue exists in COPD, Shapiro et al.[15] randomized 184 patients to active or sham negative-pressure ventilatory assistance at home, using a poncho wrap ventilator. They found no significant difference between the two groups, but compliance with treatment was much less than anticipated. They compared their primary endpoint, a 6-minute walking test, with the amount of respiratory muscle rest actually delivered and found no correlation. They also found no relationship between baseline characteristics, such as hypercapnia and forced expiratory volume in one second (FEV_1), and benefit. However, subgroup analysis lacked the necessary power to be certain that no relationship existed. The authors concluded that respiratory muscle fatigue did not exist and that little was to be gained by resting the respiratory muscles. However, a 6-minute walking distance is an unconventional measure of respiratory muscle fatigue and can be affected by other factors. Of note, the mean $PaCO_2$ of the patients in the study was only 44 mmHg, and a review of the literature suggests that hypercapnic patients are most likely to benefit from noninvasive ventilation. Because of the problems with the application of negative-pressure ventilation and the use of a crude measure of respiratory muscle fatigue, it is difficult to draw meaningful conclusions from this study other than the following: (1) the failure of patients to comply suggests that they derived no symptomatic relief, or (2) relief was outweighed by the disadvantages associated with using the ventilator.

The question of whether chronic respiratory muscle fatigue exists or whether resting these muscles is beneficial remains unanswered because there are no reliable measures of inspiratory muscle fatigue. The issue is also confused by definition. Fatigue is often defined as a complete failure of force generation.[16,17] The marathon runner provides a helpful analogy: he may feel that he is functioning at his physical limit and can go no faster until confronted by a large menacing dog, in which case he can temporarily increase his speed to escape. Although he has not reached the point of fatigue, his performance would be enhanced by a period of rest. One can argue that the same may be true in chronic ventilatory insufficiency. Patients can increase ventilation temporarily when required to do so, but they may still benefit from a period of rest. Carefully designed studies that control for the effects of motivation and learning on test performance are needed in stable patients.

Effect of Noninvasive Ventilation on Load

There are few data about the effect of noninvasive ventilation on load. Theoretically, atelectatic lung may be recruited and chest wall compliance improved in patients with skeletal deformity by stretching the stiff chest wall with positive-pressure ventilation, particularly with the addition of extrinsic PEEP. Simonds et al.[18] found no change in accessible lung volume by providing large tidal volumes for 10–15 minutes per day. This finding suggests that atelectasis was either not present or irreversible, that lung and chest wall tissue contractures were irreversible, or that the delivered volumes were inadequate, not sufficiently prolonged, or initiated too late (i.e., after too much pulmonary compliance had been lost). However, they noted a sustained improvement in vital capacity and maximal voluntary ventilation, and it was suggested that this improvement may have been due to changes in chest wall compliance. In eight patients with COPD, Elliott et al.[13] found a small reduction in gas trapping and an increase in dynamic compliance and hypothesized that the cause was a reduction in lung water. An elevation in pulmonary artery pressure may increase load because ventilation has to be increased to maintain gas exchange. Schonhofer et al., in a preliminary report,[19] have shown a reduction in mean pulmonary artery pressure from 32.0 ± 0.5 mmHg to 24.1 ± 5.8 mmHg in patients with extrapulmonary restrictive disorders treated with nocturnal noninvasive ventilation for 1 year.

Effect of Noninvasive Ventilation on Drive

If hypercapnia can be prevented, particularly overnight, bicarbonate retention does not occur. Indeed, if the carbon dioxide level is lowered to normal by using noninvasive ventilation and excessive bicarbonate is eliminated, chemosensitivity to carbon dioxide is restored. Berthon-Jones et al.[20] showed a left shift of the ventilatory response curve to progressive hypercapnia in patients with severe obstructive sleep apnea after 90 days of treatment with CPAP. In eight patients with severe COPD who were ventilated noninvasively during sleep for 6 months, Elliott et al.[13] showed a reduction in bicarbonate and base excess and a resetting of the ventilatory response to carbon dioxide at a lower level. Laier-Groenveld et al.[21] showed a lowering of the recruitment threshold in 19 patients with a variety of disorders after intermittent mechanical ventilation, suggesting a resetting of the central controller to a lower level of carbon dioxide.

Effect of Noninvasive Ventilation on Sleep Quality

So far the discussion has focused on the effect of nocturnal noninvasive ventilation on diurnal arterial blood gas tensions. Indeed, an improvement in PaO_2 and $PaCO_2$ is usually taken as an indication of successful assisted ventilation. However, patients receiving domiciliary nocturnal noninvasive ventilation often report an improved sense of well-being, better quality of sleep, and a reduction in the sensation of breathlessness. Large symptomatic improvements can occur with only small changes in arterial blood gas tensions. It is also possible that patients may not show evidence of nocturnal hypoventilation because sleep is so disturbed that they are effectively protected from the deleterious effects of sleep on ventilation. In other words, gas exchange is protected at the expense of sleep quality. A number of studies have reported severe sleep disruption in patients with COPD[22] as well as patients with NMD or chest-wall deformity.[23]

Elliott et al.[24] and Meecham-Jones et al.[25] showed an improvement in SpO_2, transcutaneous carbon dioxide, and various measures of sleep quality in patients with COPD who were ventilated noninvasively during sleep. Barbe et al.[14] showed improved sleep efficiency and sleep architecture in eight patients with NMD who received noninvasive ventilation during sleep for a mean of 18 months. Although the cause of sleep disturbance is different, dramatic improvements in daytime symptoms are also seen in patients with obstructive sleep apnea syndrome who are treated with CPAP.

Long-term nocturnal noninvasive ventilation also may improve gas exchange and sleep quality on subsequent nights when ventilation is not assisted.[26,27] This finding is not surprising given that ventilatory failure is thought to develop insidiously over time.[28] Piper et al.[26] studied 14 patients who had used nocturnal nasal ventilation for at least 6 months. Polysomnography on a night without ventilatory assistance was compared with that of the initial diagnostic study. Spontaneous breathing during sleep after long-term treatment was markedly improved, although still abnormal. During non–rapid-eye-movement (non-REM) sleep without ventilatory assistance, decreases in SpO_2 were significantly less severe compared with the initial study (mean $SpO_2 = 88 \pm 4\%$ vs. $78 \pm 8\%$; $p < 0.001$). Minimum SpO_2 during REM sleep similarly improved from a mean value of $49 \pm 14\%$ during the diagnostic night to $73 \pm 10\%$ at follow-up ($p < 0.001$). In 12 patients, transcutaneous carbon dioxide was measured continuously during sleep on both occasions and demonstrated significantly less carbon dioxide retention during the follow-up studies compared with the initial control studies during both non-REM and REM sleep. How long this benefit is maintained is not known. Hill et al.[29] found a return of symptoms (daytime sleepiness, morning headache, and dyspnea) and worsening nocturnal SpO_2 but no change in diurnal arterial blood gas tensions or maximal mouth pressures when noninvasive nocturnal ventilation was withdrawn for 1 week in six patients with restrictive chest wall disease. Jiminez et al.[30] also showed a deterioration in sleep quality, accompanied by severe derangements in SpO_2, when nocturnal noninvasive ventilation was stopped for 15 days in five patients who had been using it for at least 2 months. It is likely that the rate of deterioration is determined by the severity of the underlying disease. More recently, brief discontinuation of nocturnal noninvasive ventilation was reported to result in deterioration in arterial blood gases for six patients with COPD and five patients with restrictive thoracic disease.[31] Hill et al.[29] concluded that their data suggest that control of nocturnal hypoventilation is more important than resting of inspiratory muscles. However, it is likely that effective control of nocturnal hypoventilation allows at least partial rest of the inspiratory muscles, and changes in maximal inspiratory pressures measured at the mouth are not a good measure of the presence or absence of fatigue.

Schonhofer et al.[27] attempted to elucidate possible mechanisms of improvement in physiologic parameters seen with nocturnal nasal ventilation. In a carefully designed study, patients were allocated to receive noninvasive ventilation either during sleep or during the day for 1 month. In the latter group, patients were prevented from sleeping during ventilator use by having to respond to intermittent prompts by pressing a button when a light came on. Thus, the authors were able to compare the effects of noninvasive ventilation during sleep and wakefulness. There were no differences between the two groups. Each showed improved diurnal blood gas tensions, increased respiratory muscle strength, and a slight reduction in mouth occlusion pressures. Overnight SpO_2 and transcutaneous carbon dioxide tensions also were improved in both groups at the end of the study during spontaneous breathing overnight. Sleep quality was shown to improve in a small subgroup that underwent full polysomnography. The authors concluded that nocturnal derangements of gas exchange alone were not important in the development of ventilatory failure. However, the finding that assisted ventilation was equally effective during wakefulness and sleep does not mean that abnormalities during sleep are not important. By analogy, if a bucket leaks during the night, the abnormality can be corrected by filling it up either during the day or at night. The fact that both achieve the same result does not mean that the leak at night is unimportant. Bicarbonate can be excreted equally by day as $PaCO_2$ levels are improved by noninvasive ventilation. Because of the daytime restoration of central drive, one would then expect better gases during sleep on the following night. This finding, in fact, was seen in the study of Schonhofer et al., which suggests the possibility that the improvements were the consequence of resetting of the central respiratory controller and that nocturnal hypoventilation is fundamental to the development of diurnal ventilatory insufficiency. The finding of a reduction in mouth occlusion pressures and an improvement in respiratory muscle strength, however, suggests that improvement in muscle function rather than restoration of central drive was the important mechanism. Appendini et al.[32] also recorded high mouth occlusion pressures in eight ventilator users with COPD and also suggested that an abnormality of respiratory center output was unlikely in such patients.

There is no doubt that nocturnal assisted ventilation can be effective and is clearly more convenient for the patient than invasive means of ventilatory assistance. In the experience of the author as well as others, properly trained and equipped patients with neuromuscular respiratory muscle impairment rarely find noninvasive ventilation intolerable. For patients with primarily lung disease who do not tolerate noninvasive ventilation during sleep, assisted ventilation by day is as effective in improving blood gas tensions during spontaneous breathing as the use of noninvasive ventilation during sleep.

THERAPEUTIC IMPLICATIONS

An understanding of the pathophysiology of ventilatory failure and of the effects of sleep-disordered breathing is important both in selecting patients who are likely to benefit from noninvasive ventilation and in setting appropriate therapeutic outcome goals. In the early studies of noninvasive ventilation in COPD, benefit was seen in hypercapnic patients but not in eucapnic patients. Because abnormalities of ventilation manifest as hypercapnia, it is not surprising to find little apparent benefit from assisted ventilation when the function of the patient's own "ventilator" can maintain a normal carbon dioxide tension. Ventilation, however, involves more than maintenance of gas exchange. Patients with abnormal breathing during sleep, such as those with severe OSAS, clearly have poor-quality sleep with subsequent daytime symptoms. Even when extreme, however, this pattern may not result in significant changes in overall ventilation, as evidenced by the maintenance of a normal diurnal carbon dioxide tension. In some patients—for example, a subgroup of those with ALS and marked diaphragm weakness—sleep is severely disturbed because of severe orthopnea. Symptoms are much improved by noninvasive ventilation, even in the absence of evidence of abnormal gas exchange during sleep or derangement of daytime blood gas tensions. Thus, sleep-related abnormalities of breathing or severe sleep disturbance, even in the absence of abnormal gas exchange, is an indication for a trial of noninvasive ventilation.

More often, however, the patient presents with evidence of diurnal ventilatory insufficiency and severely disturbed gas exchange. In this situation what should be the therapeutic goal? Should it be to rest the respiratory muscles—in other words, to suppress diaphragm and intercostal EMG activity? If so, how much suppression is adequate? Should we attempt to decrease load by increasing pulmonary compliance by hyperinflating patients with extrapulmonary restrictive disorders? Or should the restoration of central drive by the effective control of nocturnal hypoventilation be the primary aim? Little evidence suggests that frequent hyperinflations to improve chest wall compliance is of benefit for patients with primarily respiratory impairment. Although a number of studies of nocturnal noninvasive ventilation have reported improved respiratory muscle strength, suggesting that improved muscle function may be possible and important, in the absence of control groups it is difficult to exclude the data resulting from a learning effect. In addition, if improvements in muscle strength are real, it is not known whether they are due to the fact that the respiratory muscles have been rested or whether they simply reflect improved arterial blood gas tensions. Because improved respiratory drive and sleep quality also have been reported, it seems unlikely that noninvasive ventilation exerts its benefits exclusively through one mechanism. Therefore, the ventilator should be adjusted to reduce respiratory muscle activity, to lower arterial carbon dioxide, and to improve sleep quality. Fortunately, these goals are not mutually exclusive; indeed, it is difficult to achieve one without the others.

ACUTE RESPIRATORY FAILURE

Many of the mechanisms described above in chronic ventilatory and respiratory insufficiency are also likely to pertain to acute setting use of noninvasive ventilation. Invasive mechanical ventilation often can be avoided or used only briefly while other therapies, such as noninvasive ventilation, bronchodilators, diuretics, antibiotics, and intensive airway secretion clearance, improve the patient's respiratory function. Voltaire said, "The art of medicine lies in keeping the patient alive while nature cures the disease!" This aphorism, however, understates the impact of noninvasive ventilation, which is therapeutic in its own right. In an acute exacerbation of COPD, the primary abnormality is usually an increase in load due to secretion retention or bronchospasm or occasionally to a reduction in drive from injudicious sedative use or over-enthusiastic oxygen supplementation. These problems can lead to a self-perpetuating vicious cycle (see Fig. 2). In such patients, the respiratory muscle pump may be functioning close to its capacity. If load increases, the respiratory muscle pump can no longer maintain ventilation and blood gas tensions deteriorate. This process has a negative effect on respiratory muscle function so that capacity is reduced at a time when load is increased, and the development of respiratory failure accelerates. If carbon dioxide rises further, narcosis may ensue and drive is further compromised. Hypoxia and hypercapnia reduce renal blood flow,[33] and retained fluid can further compromise gas exchange[34] and increase load. Abnormal blood gas tensions also can compromise cardiac function, which has a further untoward effect on gas exchange.

Noninvasive ventilation certainly has a role in accelerating recovery from acute respiratory failure[3–5] and reducing the need for endotracheal intubation[4,5] in selected patients (see Chapter 11). In two studies, the duration of noninvasive ventilation in some patients was less than 1 hour, suggesting that in certain cases this is sufficient time for other therapies to break the cycle of respiratory deterioration. For instance, a slight improvement in arterial blood gas tensions and some off-loading of the respiratory muscles can allow some recovery of respiratory muscle function, which in turn facilitates the return to the patient's previous status. Although this hypothesis is intuitively clear, at present it is confirmed by little direct evidence.

CPAP has theoretical benefits in stabilizing the airway and indirectly aids inspiratory muscles by reducing the inspiratory load due to intrinsic PEEP in patients with COPD. It has been shown to reduce inspiratory muscle activity and alleviate dyspnea in patients with COPD who are being weaned from mechanical ventilation and during acute exacerbations of COPD.[35,36] This finding suggests an unloading of respiratory muscles.[37,38] CPAP also decreases the work of breathing in patients with acute left ventricular failure.[39] Despite its widespread use, few controlled trials support the benefits of CPAP in either acute or chronic respiratory impairment. In patients with restrictive diseases, CPAP may improve gas exchange and reduce the work of breathing by recruiting atelectatic lung and increasing FRC, thereby improving pressure volume relationships. However, maximal insufflations, PIP + PEEP, and assisted coughing are more effective in this regard (see Chapters 6 and 7), and CPAP should not be used as an alternative to noninvasive ventilatory assistance for patients with ventilatory insufficiency.

During use of noninvasive IPPV with or without PEEP a reduction in inspiratory muscle activity has been demonstrated in stable patients[40–42] as well as in patients with acute exacerbations of COPD.[36] A reduction in dyspnea, as measured by a visual analog scale in a randomized, controlled comparison of noninvasive ventilation users with conventionally treated patients,[3] also suggests significant acute unloading of the respiratory muscles. Nava et al. also showed that flow triggering decreases inspiratory work of breathing 15% more than pressure triggering.[43] However, it has not been shown that such unloading is important in recovery. In some patients, acute ventilatory or respiratory failure is the result of reduced drive, usually because of over-enthusiastic oxygen therapy or injudicious use of sedative drugs. In this setting, the reduction in carbon dioxide by noninvasive ventilation can restore alertness and the drive to breathe. Finally, the brisk diuresis that occurs in some patients with the institution of noninvasive ventilation may have a beneficial effect by reducing load.

Noninvasive ventilation may have deleterious or beneficial effects on cardiac function. A slight decrease in mean transmural left and right atrial pressures, suggesting an improvement in cardiac performance, has been demonstrated when CPAP was administered to patients with acute left ventricular failure.[39] In the same study, respiratory muscle activity was reduced without a reduction in cardiac output. Ambrosino et al.[44] demonstrated a small reduction in cardiac output and oxygen delivery with pressure support ventilation via a nasal interface when PEEP was added. In contrast to mechanical ventilation via endotracheal tube, hemodynamic collapse is rarely seen during the use of noninvasive ventilation—probably because anesthetic agents are not needed and positive pressure changes less markedly within the thorax. Noninvasive ventilation probably has only a small effect on cardiac performance, but in some patients this effect may be critical in determining the success or failure of its use.

The mechanisms by which noninvasive ventilation works in both acute and long-term care settings are probably multifactorial, with different factors assuming differing degrees of importance for the individual patient. Because the situation may be unstable in the acute setting and rapid recovery is possible, a small degree of ventilatory assistance may be all that is needed. In any setting, however, the goal of therapy should be an improvement in arterial blood gas tensions, particularly normalization of pH, and unloading of respiratory muscles.

REFERENCES

1. Simonds AK, Elliott MW: Outcome of domiciliary nasal intermittent positive pressure ventilation in restrictive and obstructive disorders. Thorax 50:604–609, 1995.
2. Leger P, Bedicam JM, Cornette A, et al: Nasal intermittent positive pressure ventilation: Long-term follow-up in patients with severe chronic respiratory insufficiency. Chest 105:100–105, 1994.
3. Bott J, Carroll MP, Conway JH, et al: Randomised controlled trial of nasal ventilation in acute ventilatory failure due to chronic obstructive airways disease. Lancet 341:1555–1557, 1993.
4. Brochard L, Mancebo J, Wysocki M, et al: Noninvasive ventilation for acute exacerbations of chronic obstructive pulmonary disease. N Engl J Med 333:817–822, 1995.
5. Kramer N, Meyer TJ, Meharg J, et al: Randomized, prospective trial of noninvasive positive pressure ventilation in acute respiratory failure. Am J Respir Crit Care Med 151:1799–1806, 1995.
6. Barbe F, Togores B, Rubi M, et al: Noninvasive ventilatory support does not facilitate recovery from acute respiratory failure in chronic obstructive pulmonary disease. Eur Respir J 9:1240–1245, 1996.
7. Meduri GU, Turner RE, Abou-Shala N, et al: Noninvasive positive pressure ventilation via face mask: First-line intervention in patients with acute hypercapnic and hypoxemic respiratory failure. Chest 109:179–193, 1996.
8. Macklem PT: Hyperinflation. Am Rev Respir Dis 129:1–2, 1984.
9. Tobin MJ, Perez W, Guenther SM, et al: The pattern of breathing during successful and unsuccessful trials of weaning from mechanical ventilation. Am Rev Respir Dis 134:1111–1118, 1986.
10. Juan G, Calverley P, Talamo C, et al: Effect of carbon dioxide on diaphragmatic function in human beings. N Engl J Med 310:874–879, 1984.
11. White DP, Douglas NJ, Pickett CK, et al: Sleep deprivation and control of ventilation. Am Rev Respir Dis 128:984–986, 1983.
12. Diaz O, Iglesia R, Ferrer M, et al: Effects of noninvasive ventilation on pulmonary gas exchange and hemodynamics during acute hypercapnic exacerbations of chronic obstructive pulmonary disease. Am J Respir Crit Care Med 156:1840–1845, 1997.
13. Elliott MW, Mulvey DA, Moxham J, et al: Domiciliary nocturnal nasal intermittent positive pressure ventilation in COPD: Mechanisms underlying changes in arterial blood gas tensions. Eur Respir J 4:1044–1052, 1991.
14. Barbe F, Quera-Salva MA, de Lattre J, et al: Long-term effects of nasal intermittent positive pressure ventilation on pulmonary function and sleep architecture in patients with neuromuscular diseases. Chest 110:1179–1183, 1996.
15. Shapiro SH, Ernst P, Gray-Donald K, et al: Effect of negative pressure ventilation in severe chronic obstructive pulmonary disease. Lancet 340:1425–1429, 1992.
16. Laroche CM, Moxham J, Green M: Respiratory muscle weaknes and fatigue. Q J Med 265:373–397, 1989.
17. Moxham J: Respiratory muscle fatigue: Mechanisms, evaluation and therapy. Br J Anaesth 65:43–53, 1990.
18. Simonds AK, Parker RA, Branthwaite MA: The effect of intermittent positive-pressure hyperinflation in restrictive chest wall disease. Respiration 55:136–143, 1989.
19. Schonhofer B, Wenzel M, Barchfeld T, Kohler D: Nocturnal mechanical ventilation decreases pulmonary hypertension in chronic respiratory failure. Eur Respir J 10:35s, 1997.
20. Berthon-Jones M, Sullivan CE: Time course of change in ventilatory response to CO_2 with long-term CPAP therapy for obstructive sleep apnea. Am Rev Respir Dis 135:144–147, 1987.

21. Laier-Groeneveld G, Huttemann U, Criee C: The ventilatory recruitment threshold to CO2 can be restored to normal by intermittent mechanical ventilation [abstract]. Am J Respir Crit Care Med 149:A130, 1994.
22. Calverley PMA, Brezinova V, Douglas NJ, et al: The effect of oxygenation on sleep quality in chronic bronchitis and emphysema. Am Rev Respir Dis 126:206–210, 1982.
23. Sawicka EH, Branthwaite MA: Respiration during sleep in kyphoscoliosis. Thorax 42:801–808, 1987.
24. Elliott MW, Simonds AK, Carroll MP, et al: Domiciliary nocturnal nasal intermittent positive pressure ventilation in hypercapnic respiratory failure due to chronic obstructive lung disease: Effects on sleep and quality of life. Thorax 47:342–348, 1992.
25. Meecham Jones DJ, Paul EA, et al: Nasal pressure support ventilation plus oxygen compared with oxygen therapy alone in hypercapnic COPD. Am J Respir Crit Care Med 152:538–544, 1995.
26. Piper AJ, Sullivan CE: Effects of long-term nocturnal nasal ventilation on spontaneous breathing during sleep in neuromuscular and chest wall disorders. Eur Respir J 9:1515–1522, 1996.
27. Schonhofer B, Geibel M, Sonnerborn M, et al: Daytime mechanical ventilation in chronic respiratory insufficiency. Eur Respir J 10:2840–2846, 1997.
28. Guilleminault C, Kurlan G, Winkle R, Miles LE: Severe kyphoscoliosis, breathing and sleep. The Quasimodo syndrome during sleep. Chest 79:626–630, 1981.
29. Hill NS, Eveloff SE, Carlisle CC, Goff SG: Efficacy of nocturnal nasal ventilation in patients with restrictive thoracic disease. Am Rev Respir Dis 145:365–371, 1992.
30. Jiminez JFM, Sanchez de Cos Escuin J, Vicente CD, et al: Nasal intermittent positive pressure ventilation: Analysis of its withdrawal. Chest 107:382–388, 1995.
31. Karakurt S, Fanfulla F, Nava S: Is it safe for patients with chronic hypercapnic respiratory failure undergoing home noninvasive ventilation to discontinue ventilation briefly? Chest 119:1379–1386, 2001.
32. Appendini L, Purro A, Patessio A, et al: Partitioning of inspiratory muscle workload and pressure assistance in ventilator-dependent COPD patients. Am J Respir Crit Care Med 154:1301–1309, 1996.
33. Howes TQ, Deane CR, Levin GE, et al: The effects of oxygen and dopamine on renal and aortic blood flow in chronic obstructive pulmonary disease with hypoxemia and hypercapnia. Am J Respir Crit Care Med 151:378–383, 1995.
34. Noble MIM, Trenchard D, Guz A: The value of diuretics in respiratory failure. Lancet ii:257–260, 1966.
35. Petrof BJ, Legare M, Goldberg P, et al: Continuous positive airway pressure reduces work of breathing and dyspnea during weaning from mechanical ventilation in severe chronic obstructive pulmonary disease. Am Rev Respir Dis 141:281–289, 1990.
36. Appendini L, Patessio A, Zanaboni S, et al: Physiologic effects of positive end-expiratory pressure and mask pressure support during exacerbations of chronic obstructive pulmonary disease. Am J Respir Crit Care Med 149:1069–1076, 1994.
37. Lim TK: Effect of nasal-CPAP on patients with chronic obstructive pulmonary disease. Sing Med J 31:233–237, 1990.
38. de Lucas P, Tarancon C, Puente L, et al: Nasal continuous positive airway pressure in patients with COPD in acute respiratory failure: A study of the immediate effects. Chest 104:1694–1697, 1993.
39. Lenique F, Habis M, Lofaso F, et al: Ventilatory and hemodynamic effects of continuous positive airway pressure in left heart failure. Am J Respir Crit Care Med 155:500–505, 1997.
40. Carrey Z, Gottfried SB, Levy RD: Ventilatory muscle support in respiratory failure with nasal positive pressure ventilation. Chest 97:150–158, 1990.
41. Elliott MW, Mulvey DA, Moxham J, et al: Inspiratory muscle effort during nasal intermittent positive pressure ventilation in patients with chronic obstructive airways disease. Anaesthesia 48:8–13, 1993.
42. Elliott MW, Aquilina R, Green M, et al: A comparison of different modes of noninvasive ventilatory support: effects on ventilation and inspiratory muscle effort. Anaesthesia 49:279–283, 1994.
43. Nava S, Ambrosino N, Confalonieri M, Rampulla C: Physiologic effects of flow and pressure triggering during non-invasive mechanical ventilation in patients affected by chronic obstructive pulmonary disease. Thorax 52:249–254, 1997.
44. Ambrosino N, Nava S, Torbicki A, et al: Haemodynamic effects of pressure support and PEEP ventilation by nasal route in patients with stable chronic obstructive pulmonary disease. Thorax 48:523–528, 1993.

5 —— Noninvasive Ventilation: Mechanisms for Inspiratory Muscle Substitution

JOHN R. BACH, M.D.

> *The test of a first-rate intelligence is the ability to hold two opposed ideas in the mind at the same time, and still retain the ability to function.*
>
> F. Scott Fitzgerald, *The Crack-up*

REST, PULMONARY COMPLIANCE, CHEMOTAXIC SENSITIVITY, AND HEMODYNAMICS

The combination of respiratory muscle weakness and increased elastic load is responsible for a modulation of central respiratory output that results in a shallow breathing pattern or neuroventilatory uncoupling of the ventilatory pump.[1] The shallow breathing pattern avoids inspiratory muscle fatigue[2] but results in hypercapnia and is an indication of limited inspiratory reserve. Excessive positive pressures during inspiration and expiration can increase air trapping and lead to barotrauma in patients with intrinsic lung disease, and blood gas improvements, induced by noninvasive ventilation, in patients with acute exacerbations of chronic obstructive pulmonary disease (COPD) result largely from re-establishing an efficient breathing pattern rather than providing high inspiratory pressures.[3] For patients with primarily ventilatory impairment, however, inspiratory muscle rest and the increased tidal volumes permitted by using noninvasive intermittent positive-pressure ventilation (IPPV) and a high- rather than low-span combination of positive inspiratory pressure and positive end-expiratory pressure (PIP + PEEP) relieve nocturnal hypoventilation and, thus, are important means for improving daytime symptoms and gas exchange.[4,5] Indeed, the improvements in daytime $PaCO_2$ with the use of nocturnal noninvasive IPPV appear to be dose-related because equal improvements have been observed with equivalent duration of noninvasive IPPV during daytime hours.[6,7] In addition, the rest afforded respiratory muscles may result in increased inspiratory muscle strength. Furthermore, with ongoing nocturnal nasal IPPV, decreases in mouth occlusion pressures (PO.1) with carbon dioxide stimulation have been observed. These decreases may be due to an increase in tidal volume, which allows a reduction in respiratory rate.[8]

In awake patients, diaphragm and accessory muscle activity has been shown to decrease with the use of body ventilators[9] or nasal IPPV.[10] Body ventilators and noninvasive IPPV[2] also decrease inspiratory muscle use during sleep. Nasal IPPV, which improves blood gases during sleep,[11] also suppresses phasic respiratory drive via thoracic afferent inhibition and therefore effectively unloads the ventilatory pump and permits a decrease in respiratory muscle activity during sleep.[2] The carbon dioxide threshold is increased in patients with hypercapnic ventilatory failure, probably to minimize the load to the ventilatory muscles. With the increase in inspiratory capacity, the pCO_2 threshold can be restored to normal by intermittent noninvasive or invasive IPPV. By increasing nocturnal lung ventilation and thereby maintaining more normal carbon dioxide tension and blood pH during sleep, nocturnal ventilatory assistance also decreases the tendency to develop or reverses any hypercapnia-associated compensatory metabolic alkalosis. Elevated bicarbonate levels blunt central respiratory sensitivity to carbon dioxide tensions and permit worsening hypercapnia. Annane et al. found that with nocturnal noninvasive IPPV, daytime PaO_2 increases, $PaCO_2$ and bicarbonate decrease, the apnea-hypopnea index and time spent with SpO_2 below 90% during sleep decrease, sleep efficiency and mean SpO_2 increase, and ventilatory response to carbon dioxide increases significantly.[12] Patients can deteriorate rapidly when, with discontinuance of nocturnal nasal IPPV, nocturnal SpO_2 levels decrease each night,[4,13] carbon dioxide levels increase each night, and symptoms return.

Noninvasive IPPV also has been shown to reverse cor pulmonale without concomitant oxygen therapy.[14,15] Eleven patients with edema and recent hypercapnic and hypoxic worsening of chronic ventilatory insufficiency were shown to have normalization of carbon dioxide, improvement in oxygenation, complete relief of edema, decrease in body weight of 4 kg, and decreases in systolic and mean pulmonary arterial pressures.[14,15] They also had a long-term increase in right ventricular ejection fraction (with no change in left ventricular ejection fraction), and normalization of neuroendocrine levels.[14]

In addition, nocturnal nasal ventilation has been reported to increase maximal inspiratory pressures[16] and may transiently increase or stabilize vital capacity in patients with ventilatory insufficiency.[17] Functional residual capacity (FRC) and dynamic lung compliance also may be increased by IPPV.[16,18,19] This effect may reduce the work of breathing and further improve daytime ventilation. Nocturnal nasal IPPV also may improve daytime pulmonary function in some patients.[11,16] Thus, the benefits of nasal IPPV appear to be largely due to some combination of respiratory muscle rest, increasing tidal volumes, alveolar ventilation and blood gases, improved lung compliance and chemotaxic sensitivity, and possibly improved ventilation/perfusion matching by reduction of atelectasis and small airway closure. Noninvasive IPPV can reduce the airway closure caused by the supine position and thus may maintain more advantageous lung volume-pressure relationships.

WHAT CAN BE LEARNED FROM CLOSED-SYSTEM VENTILATION

In 1989, Banzett et al. described chronic hypocapnia in a patient with high-level spinal cord injury (SCI) who received IPPV 24 hours/day via a tracheostomy tube.[20] In 1992 Manning et al. reported severe hypocapnia in five patients with traumatic SCI who were supported by tracheostomy and IPPV and had a vital capacity less than 90 ml.[21] Bach et al. then described chronic hyperventilation in 33 tracheostomized ventilator users with a variety of paralytic/restrictive conditions (Fig. 1).[22] Watt, Oo, and Silva reported hypocapnia in 30 high-level tetraplegic patients supported by tracheostomy and IPPV.[23] Patterson et al. reported similarly severe hypocapnia in a tracheostomized patient with poliomyelitis and less than 30 ml of vital capacity who was supported by an iron lung.[24] Patterson suggested that the patient "was unable to increase the magnitude of the volley of impulses from the stretch receptors of the lung, or the frequency of these volleys (and was therefore) unable to increase by the Hering-Breuer mechanism the inhibition of inspiratory cell discharge in the respiratory center." Wright earlier suggested that loss of such inhibition may play a central role in the production of breathlessness.[25] All of the hypocapnic ventilator users in these reports were unable to trigger the ventilator and had received the same ventilator-delivered volumes for extended periods. Thus, the absence of control over inspiratory effort

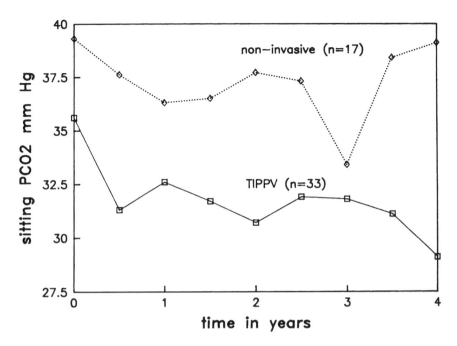

FIGURE 1. Plot of end-tidal partial pressure of carbon dioxide (PCO_2) recorded with the ventilator users in the sitting position and the data summarized in 6-month intervals. The noninvasive IPPV users were significantly less hypocapnic than the tracheostomy IPPV users.

may be related in some way to the increased inspiratory cell activity in the production of breathlessness at hypocapnic levels.

Air satiety is governed by $PaCO_2$.[26] In normal people, any increase in $PaCO_2$ from baseline causes an increase in alveolar ventilation.[27] The hypocapnia of tracheostomized IPPV users greatly hampers breathing tolerance because hypocapnic patients with 500 ml or so of vital capacity cannot autonomously ventilate the lungs sufficiently to maintain the low carbon dioxide needed for acid-base homeostasis in the hyperventilated state. Often breathing tolerance is regained only after the tracheostomy tube is removed, the patient is switched to noninvasive IPPV, and the carbon dioxide levels drift back to normal.[28] In an attempt to reverse chronic hypocapnia without decannulation, tracheostomized IPPV users experienced severe dyspnea when the addition of carbon dioxide to inspired gases led to an 18-mmHg increase in $PaCO_2$ (up to 38 mmHg).[27] In another study of hypocapnic tracheostomized IPPV users, elevations of $PaCO_2$ by only 10 mmHg created air hunger.[20] When IPPV tidal volumes were decreased to reverse hypocapnia, dyspnea began at a $PaCO_2$ of 26 mmHg.[27] When supplemental oxygen was given, breath-holding could be maintained to an increase of 16 mmHg; however, the increased tolerance to $PaCO_2$ depended on continued oxygen supplementation.[29] Gradual reductions in tidal volume also created intolerable air hunger in tracheostomized IPPV users with SCI, whose $PaCO_2$ and PaO_2 were maintained constant by control of the inspired gas mixture concentrations.[21] Severe oxyhemoglobin desaturation immediately follows acute hyperventilation.[30] Discontinuation of noninvasive IPPV, especially nocturnal use, may be accompanied by oxyhemoglobin desaturation, dyspnea, and increases in $PaCO_2$. These facts further imply an untoward effect on resumption of autonomous breathing when lung ventilation is artificially maintained.[30]

As opposed to tracheostomy IPPV with an inflated cuff, which provides a closed system of ventilatory support in which alveolar ventilation is supported passively, carbon dioxide levels also can be maintained within normal limits by patients using the open systems of noninvasive IPPV. As demonstrated in this chapter, successful use of open noninvasive IPPV systems appears to depend largely on the intactness of ventilatory drive. As noninvasive IPPV users sleep, ventilator-delivered (insufflation) volumes leak out of the nose or mouth rather than go entirely into the lungs. Higher ventilator-delivered volumes than those typically used during conventional tracheostomy IPPV compensate in part for variable air delivery leakage (insufflation leakage) during noninvasive IPPV.[31] Pressure-limiting of air delivery with volume-cycled ventilators or use of pressure-cycled ventilators (e.g., BiPAP-ST machines) also can help to compensate for insufflation leakage,[32] although the increase in flows can disturb sleep. As demonstrated below, chemotaxic-mediated reflex muscular activity intermittently decreases or eliminates insufflation leakage to normalize SpO_2 and avert excessive hypoxia and hypoventilation during sleep.[33]

As noted in Chapter 3, it was common knowledge in the 1950s that patients with low vital capacity who used body ventilators overnight could breathe autonomously during daytime hours, but after undergoing tracheotomy they became ventilator-dependent for 24 hours/day with no breathing tolerance. Resort to tracheostomy for IPPV increases airway secretion production,[34] impairs airway secretion clearance mechanisms, deconditions respiratory muscles,[35] and leads to chronic hypocapnia.[28] Many 24-hour tracheostomized IPPV users with Duchenne muscular dystrophy (DMD), amyotrophic lateral sclerosis (ALS), SCI, and other conditions whom we decannulated and switched to noninvasive IPPV progressed from no breathing tolerance to nocturnal-only use of noninvasive IPPV (see Chapter 8).[36–38]

WHY DOES NONINVASIVE IPPV WORK DURING SLEEP FOR PEOPLE WITH NO BREATHING TOLERANCE?

Although most physicians mistakenly think that intubation or tracheostomy is needed when patients have no ability to breathe, open systems of noninvasive IPPV have been used for continuous ventilatory support for over 40 years in patients with little or no measurable vial capacity or breathing tolerance. When mouthpiece IPPV is used during sleep, why does the insufflated air not leak out of the nose to the extent that carbon dioxide levels increase and the patient asphyxiates? Likewise, when a patient with no inspiratory muscle function uses nasal IPPV, why does too much air not leak out of the mouth during sleep? As the author has observed previously, excessive oral leak (insufflation leak) that limits the effectiveness of noninvasive IPPV is surprisingly uncommon in patients with primarily neuromuscular ventilatory failure.[39] This section explores such questions.

The following factors have been described as required for effective long-term use of noninvasive IPPV in patients with little or no breathing tolerance: absence of a history of substance abuse, absence of acute pulmonary or intrinsic lung disease that warrants oxygen therapy, and absence of seizure activity.[39] Narcotics, sedatives,[40] and oxygen administration depress ventilatory drive, leading the sleeping brain of patients with inspiratory muscle dysfunction to permit excessive insufflation leakage and hypercapnia. Seizure activity and postictal central nervous system depression also interfere with ventilatory drive, volitional access to a mouthpiece for noninvasive IPPV, and the movements required to limit insufflation leakage during sleep.[41] Indeed, in the author's experience, the only patients who have had no breathing tolerance and who have died during sleep using noninvasive IPPV either (1) received narcotics, sedatives, or supplemental oxygen or (2) consumed excessive alcohol. All of these nocturnal deaths had in common the suppression of ventilatory drive.

PATTERNS OF INSUFFLATION LEAKAGE

In one report, four patterns of ventilator insufflation air leakage were observed in 36 patients using nocturnal nasal IPPV:

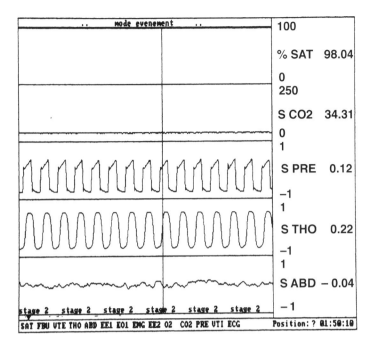

FIGURE 2. Mininal or no leakage pattern during stage 2 sleep. The monitored parameters are oxyhemoglobin saturation (SAT), end-tidal partial pressure of carbon dioxide (CO_2), nasal interface pressure (PRE), and thoracoabdominal movement (THO and ABD). The SAT and CO_2 are normal, the airway pressures increase steadily and smoothly with the air delivered by the ventilator, and thorax movements are full and smooth.

1. Minimal insufflation leakage and no significant oxyhemoglobin desaturation (Fig. 2) when the lips remained closed or were plugged by tongue movement with each breath or when oral leakage was blocked by the passive mechanical effect of nasal IPPV, which seals the soft palate against the tongue. In patients who plug the lip opening with the tip of the tongue with each breath, the floor of the mouth moves upward and outward with each insufflation. This finding may be a passive mechanical effect because the one patient who used nasal IPPV and had EMG monitoring of the genioglossus during sleep demonstrated no increase in electrical activity during this movement.

2. Continual, limited leakage out of the mouth, which creates a snoring effect with vibration of the lips (Fig. 3 and 4). Insufflation pressures drop with resulting periods of mild hypercapnia and oxyhemoglobin desaturation.

3. Intermittent leakage with the mouth open, which leads to oxyhemoglobin desaturation of 4% or more over 20- to 60-second intervals (see Fig. 4). Oropharyngeal movements at the nadir of oxyhemoglobin desaturation diminished insufflation leakage. These movements appeared to be reflexive tongue and pharyngeal movements triggered by the central nervous system. They were usually associated with brief arousals or lightening of sleep stage. As the movements eliminated leakage, the SpO_2 returned to baseline before the next leak episode. These insufflation leakages and the leak elimination movements that they triggered at SpO_2 nadirs resulted in a "sawtooth" pattern of oxyhemoglobin desaturation.

4. Prolonged insufflation leakage. Nocturnal noninvasive IPPV users who are hypercapnic during daytime hours but do not use daytime noninvasive IPPV tend to have more severe nocturnal insufflation leakage, along with prolonged severe episodes of nocturnal oxyhemoglobin desaturation (Fig. 5).[11]

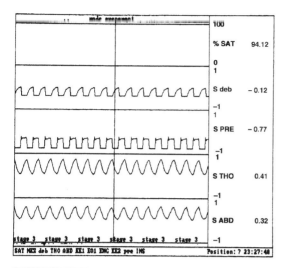

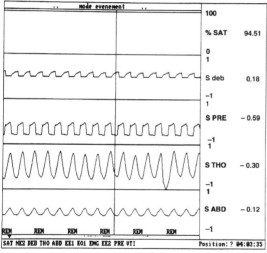

FIGURE 3. Minimal or partial insufflation leakage pattern during stage 3 *(top)* and REM *(bottom)* sleep associated with lip vibration and mild oxyhemoglobin desaturation to 94.1–94.5%. The monitored parameters are oxyhemoglobin saturation (SAT), exhaled air volume through the nose (DEB), nasal interface pressure (PRE), and thoracoabdominal movement (THO and ABD). The airway pressures tend to be flat by comparison with those in Figure 2, but thoracoabdominal movements are still good.

FIGURE 4 *(facing page).* *A,* Capnograph recording of a sleeping patient using mouthpiece IPPV without a lipseal. Although the mouthpiece remains in place, insufflation leakage occurs to the point of oxyhemoglobin desaturation, which triggers the patient to grasp the mouthpiece firmly for several deep insufflations that once again normalize the SpO$_2$ until the next leak episode. *B,* Sawtooth pattern of oxyhemoglobin desaturation common in patients with sleep-disordered breathing as well as during use of nasal ventilation or mouthpiece ventilation without lipseal retention. *C,* Severe desaturations can be eliminated by using lipseal retention for nocturnal IPPV. *D,* The severe desaturations are eliminated in a patient with poliomyelitis by using lipseal retention for nocturnal mouthpiece IPPV. The patient's wife is also applying a tussive thrust to the chest to assist his cough. *E,* Abrupt termination of 147 leaky insufflations by reflex muscle activity during a brief arousal. The exhalation flows (VTE), airway pressure pattern (PRE) and thoracoabdominal movements (THO and ABD) are characteristic of a variable insufflation leakage pattern. Nevertheless, the result is an increase in oxyhemoglobin saturation (SAT) to about 99%. The initial sharp upward inflection of the airway pressure wave form (PRE) of the 5th, 6th, 7th, and 10th breaths indicates an initial obstruction to the ventilator delivered volume of air. The obstruction may be due to passive airway closure related to the pressure or flow wave in the upper airway or to active contraction of the upper airway muscles. A decrease in air delivery to the lungs can be seen in the decreases in air flow exhaled at the nose (VTE) and thoracoabdominal movement (THO and ABD).

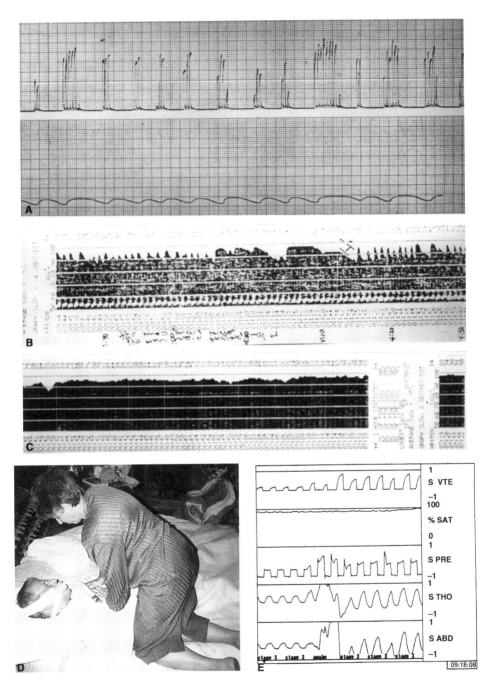

Leak-Limiting Measures and Sleep

Patients who benefit from nocturnal noninvasive ventilation, with or without breathing tolerance and whether using simple mouthpiece IPPV, bite-plates without firm lipseal retention, or nasal IPPV during sleep, usually develop a sawtooth pattern of oxyhemoglobin desaturation and often have a mean nocturnal SpO_2 slightly under 95%.[39,41] When mouthpiece

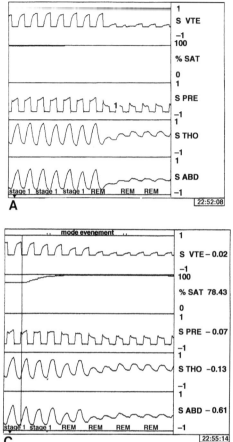

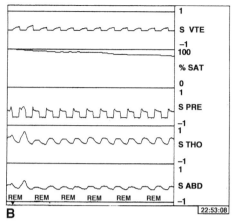

FIGURE 5. A patient who is hypercapnic during the day receives effective assisted insufflations during stage 1 sleep *(A)*, as indicated by high mask pressures (PRE) and expiratory flows recorded at the nose (VTE) and good thoracoabdominal movement (THO, ABD). When the patient enters REM sleep, all parameters indicate massive insufflation leakage. Autonomous ventilation is ineffective because virtually all of the ventilator-delivered air leaks from the mouth and oxyhemoglobin saturation (SAT) decreases to 78% in 3 min *(B)*. On reaching the SAT nadir, he returns to stage 1 sleep and completely terminates insufflation leakage; SAT returns to 98% *(C)*. Insufflation leakage resumed as soon as he entered REM sleep. Once the SAT decreased to 87%, he had a brief arousal of which he was unaware and again returned insufflation parameters and SAT to normal levels.

IPPV users (without lipseals), for example, loosen their grip on the mouthpiece during sleep, it does not fall from the mouth. The result, however, is insufflation air leakage and oxyhemoglobin desaturation. At the nadir of oxygen saturation, the user invariably regrips the mouthpiece with teeth and oral musculature to eliminate leakage until SpO_2 increases to the preleakage baseline. Insufflation leakage is thus stopped or markedly decreased, and SpO_2 is normalized during the oropharyngeal muscular activity associated with (and perhaps triggered by) oxyhemoglobin desaturation or increases in carbon dioxide, changes in airflow sensation, or other factors (see Figs. 5C and 6). Although oxyhemoglobin desaturation (see Fig. 4B) was common, nocturnal mouthpiece IPPV has been used by patients with no breathing tolerance for years[38] before lipseals became available in 1968 or 24-hour nasal IPPV was first described in 1987.

Excessive nocturnal hypercapnia and oxyhemoglobin desaturation are avoided by neurophysiologic mechanisms that include intermittent mechanical sealing of the oropharynx by the soft palate or lip closure during nasal IPPV and sealing off of the nasopharynx by the soft palate during mouthpiece IPPV. Although at times a passive mechanical seal operates to a certain degree, we found that the sawtooth pattern of oxyhemoglobin desaturation manifested by most nasal and simple mouthpiece IPPV users during sleep is reversed by brief arousal in 71% of cases, by lightening of sleep stage or arousal in 76% of cases (see Figs. 4E and 5C), and without apparent sleep-stage change on electroencephalography in

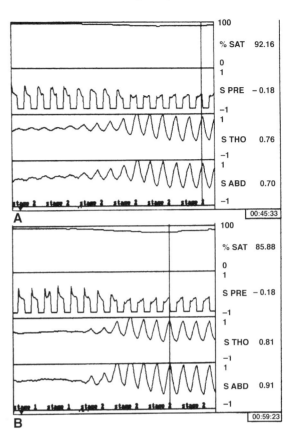

FIGURE 6. Normalization of tidal volumes and oxyhemoglobin saturation with reduction of insufflation leakage without apparent sleep stage change *(A)* and with deepening of sleep to stage 2 *(B)*. The parameters include oxyhemoglobin saturation (SAT), nasal interface pressure (PRE), and thoracoabdominal movement (THO and ABD).

24% of cases[33] (see Fig. 6A). Because brief arousals may not be found during electroencephalography and are sometimes detectable only by monitoring the autonomic nervous system,[42] it is possible that all termination of insufflation leakage is associated with arousals. However, if such were the case, it would be difficult to explain why—after a brief, undetectable arousal that terminates insufflation leakage—the patient returns to the same sleep stage. On rare occasions, oxyhemoglobin desaturation and insufflation leakage were reversed at the point of entering a deeper stage of sleep (see Fig. 6B). The importance of soft palate movements can be seen in the fact that patients who undergo uvulopharyngoplasties experience increased insufflation leakage through the mouth when using nasal CPAP.[43]

The results of increasing ventilatory stimulation of eight normal men during sleep were studied to determine whether arousals would result from increased inspiratory effort. Electroencephalography, electromyography, electro-oculography, minute ventilation, end-tidal carbon dioxide concentration, SpO_2, and esophageal (balloon) pressure were measured while arousal from non-REM sleep was induced by using added resistive loads, progressive hypoxia, and progressive hyperoxic hypercapnia. The extent of increased inspiratory effort was determined by measuring esophageal pressures to estimate pleural pressures. All subjects were eventually aroused by the addition of a 30-cmH$_2$O/L/sec load and during progressive hypercapnia. However, only six of the eight men were aroused when the SpO_2 was reduced to a minimum permissible 70%. For each stimulus, arousal occurred at different levels of ventilation, carbon dioxide concentration, and SpO_2. The ventilatory effort was similar at the point of arousal, regardless of the stimulus.[44] It makes sense that arousals would be induced by increasing inspiratory effort, but it is interesting to speculate about how increased inspiratory effort would be assessed in patients with severe inspiratory muscle weakness or those unable to make any measurable inspiratory effort, such as 24-hour noninvasive IPPV users with no measurable vital capacity. Thus, the question becomes whether arousal is caused by the effect of the added inspiratory muscle effort or some central drive to increase that effort.

With or without sleep-stage changes, all recoveries in SpO_2 were accompanied by changes in the configuration of the pneumotachograph flows or mask pressure patterns that indicated decreased insufflation leakage. This finding can be explained by an adjustment in body position, triggered by oxyhemoglobin desaturation, or initiation of specific oromotor and pharyngeal movements to decrease or eliminate leakage. The former mechanism was not seen and indeed, for many patients, would be impossible. The second mechanism, however, was clearly observed at the nadir of most episodes of oxyhemoglobin desaturation, resulting in the characteristic sawtooth pattern.

In a polysomnography study of six hypercapnic patients with chest wall abnormality or NMD and mean forced expiratory volume in one second (FEV_1) of 1 ± 0.2 L, all of whom were supported by PIP + PEEP, oral insufflation leakage was detected during the majority of the sleep period. Sleep quality was diminished because of poor sleep efficiency and reduced percentages of slow-wave and REM sleep. Oral leakage was associated with frequent arousals during stages 1 and 2 and REM sleep that contributed to sleep fragmentation, but arousals were infrequent during slow-wave sleep despite leakage. Thus, the threshold for arousals seems to increase during slow-wave sleep. Sixty to 99% of arousals occurred toward the end of a period of leakage, bringing about a temporary cessation of leakage. Patients used a combination of passive and active mechanisms to control air leaking. When no leak was detectable, the submental EMG showed absent upper airway muscle activity consistent with a passive-leak control mechanism. Once leaking occurred, patients repositioned the mandible and performed "what appeared to be a swallowing maneuver associated with an increase in submental EMG activity and no other perceptible body movements. Air leaking through the mouth would then cease and assisted breathing would continue without leaking until, after a few minutes, the lips would part again and the cycle would repeat itself."

A study of CPAP use noted similarly absent genioglossus EMG activity with an essentially passive sealing off of the oropharynx until insufflation leakage increased, causing the lips to part and flutter. Eventually the submental EMG activity and swallowing-like motion would temporarily terminate the leakage.[45] The six patients with nasal ventilation in this study[46] demonstrated only a slight drop-off in tidal volumes during insufflation leakage. This finding was possible because the lowest forced vital capacity (FVC) of any of the five successful users was 870 ml. Oxygenation was also well maintained with a mean nocturnal SpO_2 of 94% in all but one patient, whose FVC was only 560 ml This patient, who had restrictive disease secondary to tuberculosis and obesity, also received supplemental oxygen and was the most severely hypercapnic during daytime hours both before and during treatment. He refused an oral-nasal interface and a tracheotomy but was never offered a lipseal or daytime support. He died a few weeks after the sleep study.[46]

The patients who had 4% or less REM sleep had six times more leak-associated arousals/hour than patients with more than 10% REM sleep, despite the same amount of time spent with air leaking in stages 1 and 2 sleep. These patients may have had innately higher arousal thresholds than those with lower REM percentages; alternatively, they may have accommodated to leaks by raising the arousal threshold in a process resembling adaptation of the arousal threshold for noise, which has been demonstrated experimentally.[46] Insufflation leakage, therefore, is associated with frequent arousals during lighter stages of sleep that interfere with progression to REM and deeper stages, thus compromising sleep quality. However, sleep quality is unquestionably better with nasal ventilation than without it. The patients in this study could not sleep without nasal ventilation, and we and others have shown deterioration in sleep quality with withdrawal of nocturnal nasal ventilation.[4,13]

The obese patient with tuberculosis is a special case. For many patients who are hypercapnic during daytime hours and use only nocturnal noninvasive IPPV, nocturnal hypercapnia and oxyhemoglobin desaturation persist and nasal ventilation is less successful. Extending ventilator use into daytime hours reverses the compensatory metabolic alkalosis that suppresses the chemotaxic response to insufflation leakage and oxyhemoglobin desaturation. In one study, 16 patients who had less than 400 ml of supine vital capacity and less than 15 minutes of breathing tolerance were able to maintain normal alveolar ventilation by using noninvasive IPPV up to 24 hours/day and had a mean nocturnal SpO_2 of $95.9 \pm 2.6\%$ with nasal IPPV. Seventeen other patients who were hypercapnic during daytime hours and used only nocturnal nasal IPPV did not normalize nocturnal SpO_2.[47] Thus, nocturnal use of open systems of noninvasive IPPV may not be adequate, and it may be necessary either to close the system by using mouthpiece IPPV with a lipseal and, possibly, nasal plugs or to extend ventilatory assistance into daytime hours.[38] Patients who use daytime as well as nocturnal assisted ventilation are able to maintain intact chemotaxic drive; use of nasal or mouthpiece IPPV during sleep results in few episodes of oxyhemoglobin destauration. On the other hand, patients with daytime hypercapnia have less improvement in nocturnal ventilation with the use of nasal IPPV.[38,41]

No simple passive methods have been reported to be very useful for mechanical prevention of excessive oral air leakage during nocturnal nasal IPPV. Taping the mouth closed (Fig. 7) and stuffing the mouth with a bite-plate (Fig. 8) or other object are rarely effective. Strapping the chin to keep the mouth closed (Fig. 9) can be helpful but does not compensate for suboptimal daytime ventilation or an optimal interface for nocturnal aid. Often, switching from nasal to lipseal IPPV (Fig. 10) is an effective alternative when oral leakage results in severe nocturnal oxyhemoglobin desaturation.

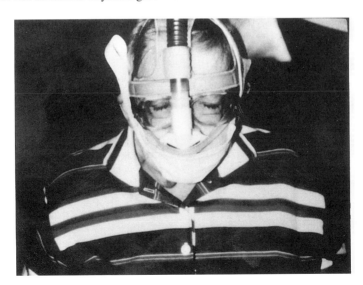

FIGURE 7. Hypercapnic patient with advanced chronic obstructive pulmonary disease receiving continuous supplemental oxygen therapy and nasal ventilation. The clinician attempts to decrease oral insufflation leakage by taping the mouth shut—an effective technique only if one is prepared to replace the tape every 15 minutes.

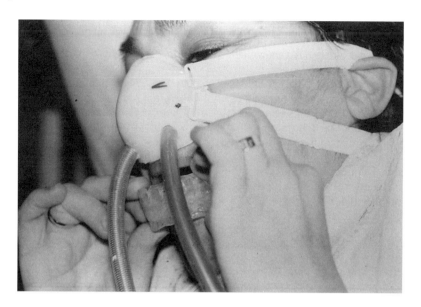

FIGURE 8.   Severely kyphoscoliotic nocturnal nasal IPPV user who remains hypercapnic during daytime hours and attempts to decrease oral insufflation leakage by wearing a bite-plate.

When nasal congestion precludes effective use of nasal IPPV, we routinely switched the patient to lipseal IPPV. Mouthpiece IPPV with lipseal retention passively seals the lips and mouth and, along with an increase in ventilator-delivered volumes, compensates for insufflation leakage from the nose and can change a sawtooth desaturation pattern into a normal pattern (see Fig. 4C). Thus, nocturnal lipseal IPPV can normalize mean nocturnal SpO_2 and probably improve sleep quality because arousals may be unnecessary to normalize

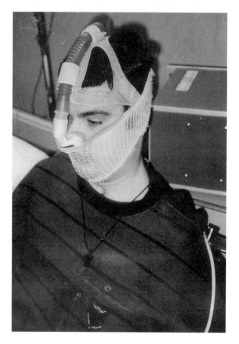

FIGURE 9.   A patient with high-level spinal cord injury was switched from continuous tracheostomy IPPV to daytime mouthpiece and nocturnal nasal IPPV in 1992 and continues to require continuous noninvasive ventilation. He believes that strapping the mouth closed in this fashion helps to decrease oral insufflation leakage during sleep.

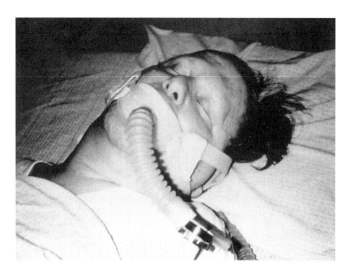

FIGURE 10.   Patient with poliomyelitis who used mouthpiece IPPV with lipseal retention (seen here) 24 hours/day from 1955 until 1995, when he died of leukemia.

SpO_2.[47] In one study of patients using nocturnal mouthpiece IPPV with lipseal retention, expiratory passage of air through the nose occurred during an average of only $33 \pm 27\%$ of total sleep time. Despite the fact that only three of the 27 lipseal IPPV users had sufficient vital capacity for 10 minutes of breathing tolerance in the supine position and only one used supplemental oxygen, all slept in the supine position, 22 (82%) of the nocturnal oximetry studies yielded normal mean SpO_2, and 12 of 15 had maximal end-tidal carbon dioxide levels lower than 45 mmHg. The lowest mean nocturnal SpO_2 for any patient using nocturnal lipseal IPPV was 92%. The smoothing out of the sawtooth pattern of oxyhemoglobin desaturation and the normalization of mean nocturnal SpO_2 imply that lipseal IPPV normalizes nocturnal ventilation by creating at least a partially closed system to ventilate the lungs without as much need for arousal or reflex elimination of insufflation leakage. For 13 nocturnal mouthpiece/lipseal IPPV users undergoing inpatient polysomnography, the time spent in the deeper sleep stages tended to be normal as a percentage of total sleep time.[47] Duration of stage 3 and 4 sleep was normal in 10 patients and increased in three. REM sleep duration, as a percentage of sleep time, was normal in eight patients and decreased in five. Only five patients had numerous episodes of transient oxyhemoglobin desaturation, with a mean SpO_2 less than 95% for 1 hour or more and less than 90% for 6% or more of the recording time. Three of these five used mouthpiece IPPV without a lipseal or with a lipseal with inadequate retention. All three also experienced symptomatic hypoventilation during daytime hours but did not use daytime ventilatory assistance.[47]

Lipseal IPPV can be made into an entirely closed system of ventilatory support by plugging the nostrils or by switching to masks that cover both nose and mouth. These approaches have been shown to normalize nocturnal SpO_2[38] by reducing or eliminating insufflation leakage and, thereby, the need to resort to centrally mediated mechanisms for effective alveolar ventilation. However, covering the nostrils was found to be necessary to maintain adequate alveolar ventilation in only five of 163 nocturnal mouthpiece IPPV users with little or no breathing tolerance.[38]

Just as nocturnal nasal IPPV is ineffective in ventilator users receiving heavy sedation or narcotics, evidence also indicates that nasal IPPV is less effective in the acute setting for ventilator users requiring high oxygen supplementation, particularly during sleep.[38,48] We speculate that this finding can be explained in large part by failure of centrally mediated activity to decrease insufflation leakage when SpO_2 is maintained by excessive oxygen supplementation.

Periods of insufflation leakage and oxyhemoglobin desaturation alternate with effective insufflations during all sleep stages. In nasal IPPV users with DMD, leakage can occur in association with downward movements of the soft palate and tongue that narrow the pharynx during REM sleep and apparently result in episodes of oxyhemoglobin desaturation.[49] Indeed, the SpO_2 pattern can oscillate between 94% and 95% (Fig. 11). Perhaps the most interesting pattern is alternation of effective assisted ventilation and insufflation leakage with every breath (Fig. 12). This pattern also may represent activation of central neural mechanisms. The highest percentage of desaturation episodes per unit of time occur during REM sleep despite the fact that effective insufflation patterns are often maintained during REM sleep for prolonged periods (Fig. 13). As for patients with obstructive sleep apnea syndrome,[50] episodes of oxyhemoglobin desaturation and arousal are less frequent in the deeper stages than in stages 1, 2, and REM sleep.

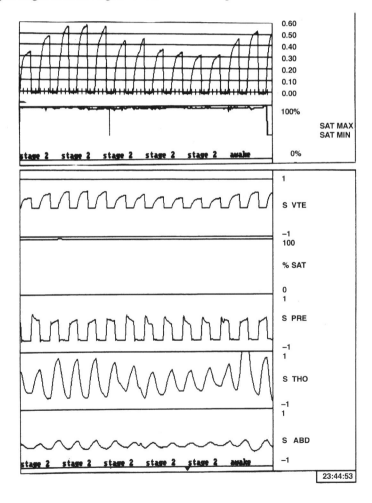

FIGURE 11. Alternating optimal insufflations with variable insufflation leakage as oxyhemoglobin saturation oscillates in eight breath cycles between 94% and 95% in stage 2 sleep. This scenario may represent intermittent activation of central neural mechanisms. Parameters include expired flow (VTE), oxyhemoglobin saturation (SAT), nasal mask pressure (PRE), and thoracoabdominal movement (THO and ABD).

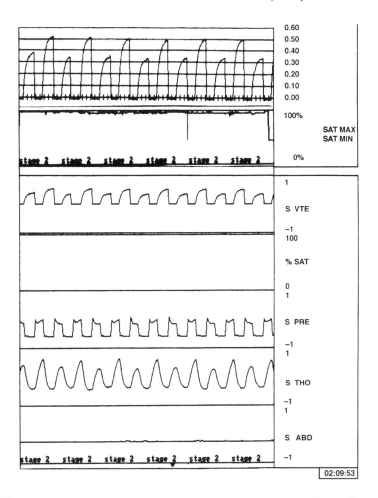

FIGURE 12. Another example of alternating optimal insufflations with variable insufflation leakage as oxyhemoglobin saturation oscillates between 94% and 95% in stage 2 sleep. In this case, however, the cycles consist of two breaths. Parameters include expired flow (VTE), oxyhemoglobin saturation (SAT), nasal mask pressure (PRE), and thoracoabdominal movement (THO and ABD).

When mouthpiece IPPV is used without a lipseal, the central nervous system, probably through chemotaxic sensitivity, reflexively triggers the muscular activity needed to prevent potentially life-threatening air leakage and oxyhemoglobin desaturation. This finding is not surprising because it is unlikely that open systems of ventilatory support, such as nasal or simple mouthpiece IPPV, could sustain patients with little or no vital capacity 24 hours/day by postural or passive mechanisms alone. The centrally triggered activity occurs at the nadir of oxyhemoglobin desaturation or possibly at nadirs of PaO_2, with differing sensitivity to oxygen saturation in all stages of sleep. The improvements in nocturnal SpO_2 are in large part due to the deeper lung insufflations that are fostered by arousal-triggered oromotor movements to decrease insufflation leakage. Respiratory muscle recruitment cannot explain the maintenance of nocturnal ventilation for patients who use noninvasive IPPV and have no measurable vital capacity.[38,41,51] Such patients could not have tolerated 147 severe leaky insufflations, as seen in Figure 4E, before eliminating excessive leaking. The fact that patients with little or no measurable vital capacity

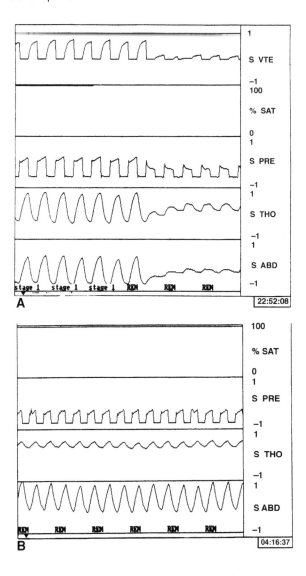

FIGURE 13. *A,* Assisted insufflations in stage 1 sleep indicated by high mask pressures (PRE) and expiratory flows (VTE) and good thoracoabdominal movement (THO and ABD). With change into rapid eye movement sleep, all parameters indicate massive insufflation leakage. Once the oxyhemoglobin saturation (SAT) decreased to 87%, the patient had a brief arousal of which he was unaware. The arousal returned insufflation parameters and SpO$_2$ to normal levels. (From Bach JR, Robert D, Leger P, Langevin B: Sleep fragmentation in kyphoscoliotic individuals with alveolar hypoventilation treated by nasal IPPV. Chest 107:1552–1558, 1995; with permission of the American College of Chest Physicians.) *B,* Maintenance of effective ventilation during REM sleep. The monitored parameters are oxyhemoglobin saturation (SAT), nasal interface pressure (PRE), and thoracoabdominal movement (THO and ABD).

can often tolerate periods of limited insufflation leakage without significant changes in SpO$_2$ during all sleep stages implies that passive mechanisms such as lip plugging by the tongue or apposition of the tongue and soft palate are also likely to be at work to prevent excessive insufflation leakage.[41,51]

UPPER AIRWAY MOVEMENTS TO OBSTRUCT AIR DELIVERY

Figure 4E demonstrates inspiratory cycle obstruction to ventilator-delivered volumes initially during an arousal after a long period of insufflation leakage and later during stage 3 sleep. Glottic movements and the compliance of the upper airways modulate ventilator-delivered volumes entering the lungs. Obstructions to airflow can increase insufflation leakage and may be centrally triggered events to prevent hyperventilation. Jounieux et al. found that the glottic aperture narrows and delivered tidal volumes fall during lighter stages of sleep, but the aperture widens, permitting more ventilation, during the deeper stages. If minute ventilation is increased excessively, the aperture narrows, correlating with reduction in carbon dioxide.[52] Parreira et al. reported that these changes occur more often with control mode-assisted ventilation than with PIP + PEEP in the spontaneous mode.[53,54] Delguste et al. observed apnea for up to 1 minute in association with hypocapnia caused by passive nasal IPPV in three of four patients during sleep.[55] The apneas seemed to be caused by complete upper airways obstruction. This finding also suggests that active glottic closure occurred to avoid excessive hypocapnia during nocturnal noninvasive IPPV.

In addition to narrowing or obstructing the airway to prevent hyperventilation during nocturnal noninvasive ventilation, obstructive apneas can result in frequent arousals and disturbed sleep architecture during use of noninvasive IPPV and may cause severe episodes of oxyhemoglobin desaturation, as they do for patients with sleep-disordered breathing.[42] Obstruction can be due to pharyngeal wall instability and collapse. Indeed, airway muscles are normally activated during both inspiration and expiration to preserve an open upper airway.[56] Patients with neuromuscular weakness or obstructive sleep apnea syndrome (OSAS) may have excessive upper-airway collapsibility, which, when observed and measured by applying negative pressure to the airway in awake patients, predicts airway collapsibility during sleep.[57] Pharyngeal collapse occurred in response to pressures of -17 to -40 cmH$_2$O and may be due to loss of protective reflexes and decreased dilator muscle activation as well as the pressure gradient. Inspiratory resistive loading correlated with negative-pressure pulses in predicting airway collapse. This correlation explains in large part the high incidence of OSAS in obese patients. Likewise, pharyngeal collapsibility can be so severe in patients with neuromuscular disease, especially in those with bulbar ALS, that it not only reduces assisted peak cough flows to unmeasurably low levels but also results in stridor during both inspiration and expiration.

Obstructions can decrease with extension of the head and neck, use of a collar, and modification of ventilator settings to improve patient coordination with the ventilator. As for obstructive sleep apneas that may cause and, at times, be caused by arousals and continuous activation of the sympathetic nervous system,[42] as seen in Figure 4E, obstruction can appear at the end of a period of massive insufflation leakage as well as during brief arousals during which SpO$_2$ recovers. Thus, sleep stage, bulbar muscle function, and the amount of ventilatory assistance influence the glottic and upper airway aperture, an important determinant of the efficacy of noninvasive ventilation.

LUNG AND CHEST-WALL RANGE OF MOTION

The lungs and chest walls of infants with neuromuscular weakness do not grow normally because of inability to take deep breaths. The results are severely restricted pulmonary volumes, decreased pulmonary compliance, and undergrowth of the thoracic cage (see Chapter 2). Likewise, as the vital capacity of adults with NMD diminishes, they, too, lose the ability to attain predicted inspiratory capacities. There are similarities in the development of extremity joint contractures, rib cage contractures, and loss of maximal insufflation capacity (MIC).[35,58] The use of air-stacking and maximal insufflations via oral, nasal, or oral-nasal interfaces can provide respiratory muscle and rib cage range of motion (ROM)in pediatric and adult patients with NMD to maintain or increase MIC in much the same way that passive ROM exercises benefit the ROM of skeletal articulations (see Chapter 7).[58]

The only studies that have explored the effects of regimens of deep insufflations on static pulmonary compliance were instituted only after patients had developed severe pulmonary restriction (vital capacity < 50% of predicted normal), involved the use of insufflation pressures that were less than 30 cmH$_2$O and thus grossly inadequate to expand fully even normally compliant lungs, and called for the use of insufflations for only minutes each day. No evidence indicates that static pulmonary compliance was maintained or improved by such regimens,[59] On the other hand, it has been shown that the MIC can be increased with the use of regimens designed to expand the lungs.[60,61]

CONCLUSION

Inability to take in adequate tidal volumes autonomously can affect both alveolar ventilation and airway secretion management. Diminished inspiratory muscle function results in depressed mucociliary clearance, which appears to be caused by the reduced mechanical movement of the lungs and a concomitant reduction in airflows.[62] Thus, mechanisms by which nasal or mouthpiece/lipseal IPPV can improve the clinical picture include resting respiratory muscles and decreasing metabolic demand; increasing tidal volumes and relieving hypercapnia; resetting chemoreceptors; opening atelectatic airways; maintaining airway patency; improving ventilation/perfusion matching; maintaining lung and chest-wall range of motion and possibly compliance; improving mucociliary clearance; and, of greatest importance, assisting, supporting, and substituting for inspiratory muscle function. Assisted lung ventilation and normal SpO_2 can be maintained indefinitely during sleep as well as during daytime hours for patients with little or no vital capacity by using noninvasive IPPV.[32,38,41]

Es menester que andemos por el mundo, como en aprobación, buscando aventuras.
(It is necessary that we go through the world, as if on approval, looking for adventures.)

Miguel de Cervantes, *Don Quijote de La Mancha*

REFERENCES

1. Rochester DF: Respiratory muscle weakness, pattern of breathing, and CO2 retention in chronic obstructive pulmonary disease. Am Rev Respir Dis 143:901–903, 1991.
2. Laier-Groeneveld G, Schucher B, Criee CP: The etiology of chronic hypercapnia. Med Klin 92(Suppl 1):33–38, 1997.
3. Diaz O, Iglesia R, Ferrer M, et al: Effects of noninvasive ventilation on pulmonary gas exchange and hemodynamics during acute hypercapnic exacerbations of chronic obstructive pulmonary disease. Am J Respir Crit Care Med 156:1840–1845, 1997.
4. Hill NS, Eveloff SE, Carlisle CC, Goff SG: Efficacy of nocturnal nasal ventilation in patients with restrictive thoracic disease. Am Rev Respir Dis 145:365–371, 1992.
5. Pankow W, Hijjeh N, Schuttler F, et al: Influence of noninvasive positive pressure ventilation on inspiratory muscle activity in obese subjects. Eur Respir J 10:2847–2852, 1997.
6. Schonhofer B, Geibel M, Haidl P, Kohler D: Daytime mechanical ventilation in chronic ventilatory insufficiency [in German]. Med Klin 94:9–12, 1999.
7. Servera E, Perez M, Marin J, et al: Noninvasive nasal mask ventilation beyond the ICU for an exacerbation of chronic respiratory insufficiency. Chest 108:1572–1576, 1995.
8. Feldmeyer F, Randerath W, Ruhle KH: Time course of ventilatory drive in patients with kyphoscoliosis before and during intermittent ventilation [in German]. Pneumologie 1999;53:S93–S94.
9. Rochester DF, Braun NMT, Laine S: Diaphragmatic energy expenditure in chronic respiratory failure: The effect of assisted ventilation with body respirators. Am J Med 63:223–232, 1977.
10. Carrey Z, Gottfried SB, Levy RD: Ventilatory muscle support in respiratory failure with nasal positive pressure ventilation. Chest 93:150–158, 1990.
11. Bach JR, Alba AS: Management of chronic alveolar hypoventilation by nasal ventilation. Chest 97:52–57, 1990.
12. Annane D, Quera-Salva MA, Lofaso F, et al: Mechanisms underlying effects of nocturnal ventilation on daytime blood gases in neuromuscular diseases. Eur Respir J 13:157–162, 1999.
13. Jimenez JFM, Sanchez de Cos Escuin J, Vicente CD, et al: Nasal intermittent positive pressure ventilation: Analysis of its withdrawal. Chest 107:382–388, 1995.
14. Thorens JB, Ritz M, Reynard C, et al: Haemodynamic and endocrinological effects of noninvasive mechanical ventilation in respiratory failure. Eur Respir J 11:2553–2559, 1997.

15. Schlenker E, Feldmeyer F, Hoster M, Ruhle KH: Effect of noninvasive ventilation on pulmonary artery pressure in patients with severe kyphoscoliosis. Med Klin 92(Suppl 1):40–44, 1997.
16. Goldstein RS, DeRosie JA, Avendano MA, Dolmage TE: Influence of noninvasive positive pressure ventilation on inspiratory muscles. Chest 99:408–415, 1991
17. Vianello A, Bevilacqua M, Salvador V, et al: Long-term nasal intermittent positive pressure ventilation in advanced Duchenne's muscular dystrophy. Chest 105:445–448, 1994.
18. Sinha R, Bergofsky EG: Prolonged alteration of lung mechanics in kyphoscoliosis by positive hyperinflation. Am Rev Respir Dis 106:47–57, 1972.
19. Hoeppner VH, Cockcroft DW, Dosman JA, Cotton DJ: Nighttime ventilation improves respiratory failure in secondary kyphoscoliosis. Am Rev Respir Dis 129:240–243, 1984.
20. Banzett RN, Lansing RW, Reid MB, et al: Air hunger arising from increased PCO2 in mechanically ventilated quadriplegics. Respir Physiol l76:53–68, 1989.
21. Manning HL, Shea SA, Schwartzstein RM, et al: Reduced tidal volume increases air hunger at fixed pCO_2 in ventilated quadriplegics. Respir Physiol 90:9–30, 1992.
22. Bach JR, Haber II, Wang TG, Alba AS: Alveolar ventilation as a function of ventilatory support method. Eur J Phys Med Rehabil 5:80–84, 1995.
23. Watt JWH, Oo T, Salva P: Biochemical profile and long-term hyperventilation in high tetraplegia. Eighth Journées Internationales de Ventilation à Domicile, abstract 128, March 7, 2001, Hôpital de la Croix-Rousse, Lyon, France.
24. Patterson JL, Mullinax PF, Bain T, et al: Carbon dioxide-induced dyspnea in a patient with respiratory muscle paralysis. Am J Med 32:811–816, 1962.
25. Wright GW, Branscomb BV: The origin of the sensations of dyspnea. Trans Am Climat Clin 66:116–125, 1954.
26. Fowler WS: Breaking point of breath holding. J Appl Physiol 6:539–545, 1954.
27. Opie LH, Smith AC, Spalding JM: Conscious appreciation of the effects produced by independent changes of ventilation volume and of end-tidal pCO2 in paralyzed patients. J Physiol 149:494–499, 1959.
28. Haber II, Bach JR: Normalization of blood carbon dioxide levels by transition from conventional ventilatory support to noninvasive inspiratory aids. Arch Phys Med Rehabil 75:1145–1150, 1994.
29. Rahn H, Bahnson HT, Muxworthy JF, Hagen JM: Adaptation to high altitude: Changes in breath-holding time. J Appl Physiol 6:154–157, 1953.
30. Ohi M, Chin K, Hirai M, et al: Oxygen desaturation following voluntary hyperventialtion in normal subjects. Am J Respir Crit Care Med 149:731–738, 1994.
31. Tzeng AC, Bach JR: Prevention of pulmonary morbidity for patients with neuromuscular disease. Chest 118:1390–1396, 2000.
32. Leger P, Jennequin J, Gerard M, Robert D: Home positive pressure ventilation via nasal mask for patients with neuromuscular weakness or restrictive lung or chest-wall disease. Respir Care 34:73–77, 1989.
33. Bach JR, Robert D, Leger P, Langevin B: Sleep fragmentation in kyphoscoliotic individuals with alveolar hypoventilation treated by nasal IPPV. Chest 107:1552–1558, 1995.
34. Bach JR, Rajaraman R, Ballanger F, et al: Neuromuscular ventilatory insufficiency: The effect of home mechanical ventilator use vs. oxygen therapy on pneumonia and hospitalization rates. Am J Phys Med Rehabil 77:8–19, 1998.
35. Le Bourdelles G, Viires N, Boczkowski J, et al: Effects of mechanical ventilation on diaphragmatic contractile properties in rats. Am J Respir Crit Care Med 149:1539–1544, 1994.
36. Bach JR, Alba AS: Noninvasive options for ventilatory support of the traumatic high level quadriplegic. Chest 98:613–619, 1990.
37. Bach JR: New approaches in the rehabilitation of the traumatic high level quadriplegic. Am J Phys Med Rehabil 70:13–20, 1991.
38. Bach JR, Alba AS, Saporito LR: Intermittent positive pressure ventilation via the mouth as an alternative to tracheostomy for 257 ventilator users. Chest 103:174–182, 1993.
39. Bach JR: Alternative methods of ventilatory support for the patient with ventilatory failure due to spinal cord injury. J Am Parapleg Soc 14:158–174, 1991.
40. Berggren L, Eriksson I, Mollenholt P, Sunzel M: Changes in respiratory pattern after repeated doses of diazepam and midazolam in healthy subjects. Acta Anaesthesiol Scand 31:667–672, 1987.
41. Bach JR, Alba AS: Management of chronic alveolar hypoventilation by nasal ventilation. Chest 97:52–57, 1990.
42. Kohler D, Schonhofer B: How important is the differentiation between apnea and hypopnea? Respiration 64(Suppl):15–21, 1997.
43. Mortimore IL, Bradley PA, Murray JAM, Douglas NH: Uvulopalatopharyngoplasty may compromise nasal CPAP therapy in sleep apnea syndrome. Am J Respir Crit Care Med 154:1759–1762, 1996.
44. Gleeson K, Zwillich CW, White DP: The influence of increasing ventilatory effort on arousal from sleep. Am Rev Respir Dis 142:295–300, 1990.
45. Strohl KP, Redline S: Nasal CPAP therapy, upper airway activation, and obstructive sleep apnea. Am Rev Respir Dis 134:555–558, 1986.

46. Meyer TJ, Pressman MR, Benditt J, et al: Air leaking through the mouth during nocturnal nasal ventilation: Effect on sleep quality. Sleep 20:561–569, 1997.
47. Bach JR, Alba AS: Sleep and nocturnal mouthpiece IPPV efficiency in post-poliomyelitis ventilator users. Chest 106:1705–1710, 1994.
48. Wysocki M, Tric L, Wolff MA, et al: Noninvasive pressure support ventilation in patients with acute respiratory failure. Chest 103:907–913, 1993.
49. Nakayama T, Saito Y, Yatabe K, et al: The usefulness of tracheostomy in Duchenne muscular dystrophy ventilated by a chest respirator [in Japanese]. Rinsho Shinkeigaku 39:606–609, 1999.
50. Takasaki Y, Kamio K, Okamoto M, et al: Altered arousability in non-REM sleep during sleep progression in patients with moderate to severe obstructive sleep apnea. Am Rev Resp Dis 147:A513, 1993.
51. Bach JR, Alba AS, Mosher R, Delaubier A: Intermittent positive pressure ventilation via nasal access in the management of respiratory insufficiency. Chest 92:168–170, 1987.
52. Jounieaux V, Parreira VF, Delguste P, et al: Nasal mask pressure waveform and inspiratory muscle rest during nasal assisted ventilation. Am J Respir Crit Care Med 155:2096–2101, 1997.
53. Parreira VF, Delguste P, Jounieaux V, et al: Effectiveness of controlled and spontaneous modes in nasal two-level positive pressure ventilation in awake and sleep normal subjects. Chest 112:1267–1277, 1997.
54. Parriera VF, Delguste P, Jounieaux V, et al: Glottic aperature and effective minute ventilation during nasal two-level positive pressure ventilation in spontaneous mode. Am J Respir Crit Care Med 154:1857–1863, 1996.
55. Delguste P, Aubert-Tulkens G, Rodenstein DO: Upper airway obstruction during nasal intermittent positive pressure ventilation in sleep. Lancet 338:1295–1297, 1991.
56. Sanna A, Veriter C, Stanescu D: Expiratory supraglottic obstruction during muscle relaxation. Chest 108:143–149, 1995.
57. Malhotra A, Pillar G, Fogel R, et al: Upper-airway collapsibility: Measurements and sleep effects. Chest 120:156–161, 2001.
58. Bach JR, Kang SW: Disorders of ventilation: weakness, stiffness, and mobilization. Chest 117:301–303, 2000.
59. McCool FD, Mayewski RF, Shayne DS, et al: Intermittent positive pressure breathing in patients with respiratory muscle weakness: Alterations in total respiratory system compliance. Chest 90:546–552, 1986.
60. Kang SW, Bach JR: Maximum insufflation capacity. Chest 118:61–65, 2000.
61. Huldtgren AC, Fugl-Meyer AR, Jonasson E, Bake B: Ventilatory dysfunction and respiratory rehabilitation in post-traumatic quadriplegia. Eur J Respir Dis 61:347–356, 1980.
62. Mier A, Laroche C, Agnew JE, et al: Tracheobronchial clearance in patients with bilateral diaphragmatic weakness. Am Rev Respir Dis 142:545–548, 1990.

6 —— Home Mechanical Ventilation for Neuromuscular Ventilatory Failure: Conventional Approaches and Their Outcomes

JOHN R. BACH, M.D.

Tradition nicht anders sei als Schlamperei. (Tradition is nothing other than negligence.)

Gustav Mahler

CONVENTIONAL STRATEGIES

Conventional respiratory management strategies for patients with neuromuscular conditions are invasive and reactive rather than noninvasive and proactive. They essentially ignore the problem until the inevitable occurrence of respiratory failure, at which point the patient seeks help in a local emergency department or dies before getting there. Current strategies for managing progressive respiratory muscle insufficiency include the following:

1. Treating ventilatory insufficiency with narcotics, sedatives, and supplemental oxygen to lighten and hasten the pathway to the grave while obtaining a "living will" or "informed consent" that prohibits the use of "heroic measures," generally intubation or tracheotomy, or simply mandates no treatment at all.

2. Treating ventilatory insufficiency and episodes of acute ventilatory failure as though they were respiratory insufficiency with some combination of oxygen, medications, chest physical therapy, airway suctioning, and, ultimately, intubation and tracheostomy.

3. "Prophylactic" tracheostomy.

4. Using nocturnal positive inspiratory pressure and positive end-expiratory pressure (PIP + PEEP) at low pressure spans that are ultimately inadequate to prevent ventilatory failure.

Easing and Hastening Death: Not-so-benign Neglect

Prescribing oxygen therapy with or without morphine is an especially popular approach with clinicians who lack knowledge of noninvasive respiratory aids and preach "therapeutic nihilism."[1] This approach decreases dyspnea while hastening death.[2,3] Often, without consulting the patient, the physician judges the patient's quality of life to be unacceptable and the disease terminal, ignores options that prevent respiratory complications, and biases the family against ventilator use, which the physician associates with tracheostomy.[4] This approach emphasizes "palliation" but results in hopelessness and thus augments mental anguish. Either patients die from carbon dioxide narcosis, or an intercurrent chest cold results in pneumonia and acute respiratory failure.[5,6] When patients are desperately short of breath, despite having a living will, they often agree to be intubated and ultimately undergo tracheotomy.

Treating Ventilatory Insufficiency Like Respiratory Insufficiency

If the only tool one knows is a hammer, everything is treated like a nail.

Conventional approaches to managing ventilatory insufficiency are identical to those for respiratory insufficiency and include medical therapy typical for patients with chronic obstructive pulmonary disease (COPD). The goals of medical therapy can be to increase diaphragm contractility, dilate the airways and facilitate airway secretion clearance, improve ventilatory drive, and improve oxygenation without exacerbating hypercapnia. Unfortunately, no medical therapy has been shown to be effective and safe for any of these goals in patients with neuromuscular disease (NMD). In a review of 25 studies of patients with musculoskeletal and neuromuscular respiratory insufficiency, methylxanthine administration was not found to alleviate diaphragm fatigue.[7] Indeed, in the presence of hypercapnia and hypoxia, theophylline appeared to increase or delay recovery from diaphragm fatigue, and side effects were common.[8] I have observed two patients who suffered generalized seizures due to long-term methylxanthine therapy, from which they had derived no benefit. Bronchodilators, too, are often used on a long-term basis with no subjective or objective benefits. Bronchodilators often cause anxiety and by increasing heart rate can exacerbate cardiac dysfunction for patients with NMD, who often have severe cardiomyopathies. Bronchodilators can even increase airway secretion production.

Low-flow oxygen in combination with protriptyline[9] or clomipramine[10] has been used to treat sleep hypoxia in this patient population. However, these medications appear to decrease hypoxia by suppressing rapid-eye-movement (REM) sleep.[9] Any resulting increase in fatigue may increase the risk of pulmonary complications. Furthermore, the anticholinergic effects of protriptyline preclude regular use and may be hazardous for patients with cardiomyopathy, who often have decreased cardiac reserve and cardiac conduction abnormalities. Other medications such as doxapram hydrochloride, acetazolamide, medroxyprogesterone, and almitrine have not been shown to benefit patients with NMD.[11,12]

Although first used to treat lung disease in 1924,[13] oxygen therapy became widely accepted for treating hypoxia only in the mid-1960s. Subsequently, oxygen therapy has been shown to improve significantly the prognoses of patients who suffer primarily from severe respiratory impairment. This success and general familiarity with oxygen therapy have led to its use for treating hypoxia due to ventilatory impairment. However, considering the pathophysiology of ventilatory impairment (see Chapter 2), such patients fare poorly because hypercapnia is exacerbated. Oxygen supplementation results in a significantly higher incidence of pneumonias and hospitalizations and prolonged length of stay compared with untreated patients or patients treated with respiratory muscle aids.[5] In addition, because of its relatively high pressure gradient for absorption in comparison with nitrogen, supplemental oxygen can cause and help to maintain atelectasis.[14] Most patients with neuromuscular weakness who become comatose from carbon dioxide narcosis do so while receiving oxygen supplementation. Although most conventionally managed patients avoid carbon dioxide narcosis, they inevitably undergo tracheotomy or die from airway secretion retention during chest infections because of failure to teach and equip them to use mechanically assisted coughing (MAC).[15] Attempts to suction patients' airways via the nose or mouth are rarely effective and extremely uncomfortable and may further impair already severely impaired breathing. There is even less chance to enter the left mainstem bronchus in this manner than when suctioning via a tube. Lung suctioning via the upper airway should rarely if ever be required or used as an alternative to mechanically assisted coughing.

Prophylactic Tracheotomy

Because a higher rate of complications is associated with emergency than elective tracheotomy and because respiratory failure is inevitable for conventionally managed patients, physicians unfamiliar with respiratory muscle aids or the indications for tracheostomy[16] (see Chapter 7) may recommend it prophylactically.[17] Most patients, however, appropriately refuse this option. In general, prophylactic tracheotomy may be appropriate only for patients with severe bulbar amyotrophic lateral sclerosis (ALS)and the rare adult patient with maximally assisted peak cough flows less than 160 L/min and SpO_2 persistently less than 95% (see Chapter 7).

Low-Span PIP + PEEP (Bilevel Positive Airway Pressure)

Modern therapy with continuous positive airway pressure (CPAP) was described in 1976.[18] As the widespread prevalence of obstructive sleep apnea syndrome (OSAS) became appreciated in the 1980s, CPAP was used to maintain upper airway patency. CPAP pneumatically splints open the airway and increases functional residual capacity (FRC). CPAP, however, is ineffective for patients whose hypercapnia is based on absolute or relative inspiratory muscle weakness because it does not directly assist inspiratory muscle function. Although this point may appear to be obvious, it was confirmed by a recent study of pressure support ventilation vs. CPAP.[19]

In pressure support ventilation, the ventilator delivers a preset inspiratory pressure to assist spontaneous breathing efforts. Most ventilators permit patient triggering with a set back-up rate. With pressure control ventilation, preset time-cycled inspiratory and expiratory pressures are delivered at a controlled rate with adjustable inspiratory-to-expiratory ratios. Ventilators can cycle to expiration when they sense a fall in inspiratory flow below a threshold value or at a pre-set time. Flow triggering appears to be more sensitive than pressure triggering.[20]

The BiPAP machine (Respironics, Inc., Murrysville, PA) is a pressure-cycled ventilator. It was developed because of the frequent ineffectiveness of CPAP and the difficulties of tolerating high CPAP levels. The quick acceptance and widespread use of the BiPAP device were due to its light weight, inspiratory pressures greater than 20 cmH_2O, PEEP (equivalent to expiratory positive airway pressure [EPAP]) capabilities, similarity to CPAP (CPAP plus inspiratory positive airway pressure [IPAP]), and its relatively low cost compared with volume-cycled ventilators.

The BiPAP-ST, Synchrony, and BiPAP Harmony (Respironics, Murrysville, PA); the PB335 Respiratory Support System and the Quantom (Mallincrodt, Pleasanton, CA); the ResMed VPAP-STII (ResMed, San Diego, CA); and other similar units are essentially pressure-limited blowers with pressures up to 22–40 cmH_2O and plateauing of delivered volumes at the higher pressures. The IPAP and EPAP are adjusted manually, and the ventilator delivers air flows to achieve the set pressures.

The failure of all of the ventilator-delivered air to enter the lungs (i.e., insufflation leakage) is due to both mask leakage and leakage from the nose for mouthpiece ventilation or from the mouth for nasal ventilation. Increased airway resistance (e.g., due to mucus plugging) results in a decrease in delivered volumes. The inspiratory pressure minus the PEEP (IPAP-EPAP difference) or pressure span is essentially the amount of inspiratory muscle assistance that the patient receives. Excessive mask leakage can impair the expiratory trigger cycling mechanism and result in prolonged duration of the inspiratory phase, auto-PEEP, and patient-ventilator dyssynchrony. In the presence of air leaks, time-cycled expiratory triggers facilitate patient-machine synchrony more effectively than flow-cycled expiratory triggers.[21]

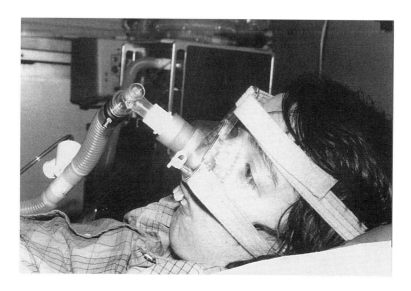

FIGURE 1.   A woman with spinal muscular atrophy and chronic respiratory muscle insufficiency who was born in 1959. She used nasal IPPV via a standard CPAP mask for nocturnal ventilatory assistance from 1971 until March of 1988, when she underwent tracheotomy during hospitalization for a respiratory tract infection. She died of pneumonia in April of 1990.

Nocturnal-only delivery of PIP + PEEP at low spans (IPAP minus EPAP less than 10 cmH_2O) using commonly available, inexpensive, generic CPAP masks as patient-ventilator interfaces provides a small pressure boost to assist inspiratory effort (Fig. 1). This approach is widely used even in the absence of diurnal hypercapnia or symptoms of ventilatory insufficiency. Although it can be helpful early on, low spans of typically 5–7 cmH_2O allow inadequate rest of respiratory muscles and insufficient assistance to inspiratory muscle function to sustain patients as inspiratory muscle weakness progresses.

Increasing the EPAP without increasing the IPAP decreases the span. EPAP is conventionally used even though it does not benefit patients with predominantly inspiratory muscle impairment. The greater the level of EPAP that is used, the greater the level of IPAP that must be used to provide the same level of inspiratory assistance and the greater the resulting intrathoracic pressure. It has been shown that increases in intrathoracic pressure cause dose-dependent decreases in cardiac stroke volume and cardiac output.[22] This scenario can be hazardous for ventilator users with cardiomyopathies.

Even the maximal spans of most commonly used machines generally deliver less than 1200-ml volumes to patients with normal lung impedance. These volumes do not permit the cough volumes or flows needed to clear airway secretions or optimally raise voice volumes. When lung impedance is increased, even adequate ventilation may not be achieved. Thus, the fact that pressure-cycled ventilators are widely used at suboptimal spans plays a large role in the development of ventilatory or respiratory failure during intercurrent chest infections in patients with neuromuscular weakness.[23]

Nocturnal low-span PIP + PEEP has become part of the conventional management of patients with NMD. A recent survey of MDA clinic directors indicated that nocturnal PIP + PEEP was used in about 80% of clinics. Unfortunately, physicians confuse the nocturnal use of low-span PIP + PEEP with the use of "noninvasive ventilation."[2,24,25]

In many centers, patients with weak respiratory muscles and possible symptoms of chronic alveolar hypoventilation are sent for polysomnography. The polysomnogram interprets the problem as one of central or obstructive sleep apneas instead of hypercapnia due to inspiratory muscle weakness.[26] CPAP is thought to be the primary treatment for sleep-disordered breathing, and patients are treated with CPAP or low-span PIP + PEEP. Inappropriately low spans are used because of confusion in the interpretation of polysomnography results, failure to appreciate the need for respiratory muscle rest, unjustified fear of barotrauma (see Chapter 7), and physicians' much greater familiarity with CPAP, OSAS, and lung disease than with neuromuscular weakness in patients with otherwise normal lung tissues.

NOCTURNAL-ONLY NASAL VENTILATION

Patients with symptoms of ventilatory insufficiency and hypoxia can benefit from nocturnal nasal ventilation whether it be provided as PIP + PEEP or as IPPV.[5] Nasal ventilation typically relieves fatigue and other symptoms of which patients may have been unaware. When such patients feel better the day after using nocturnal nasal ventilation, they do not need to be prompted to continue use.

Ventilatory insufficiency progresses insidiously. A consensus conference in 1991 suggested the following indications and considerations for instituting nocturnal nasal ventilation in stable patients with Duchenne muscular dystrophy (DMD): rapid speed of disease progression, presence of hypercapnia or end-tidal carbon dioxide exceeding 50 mmHg during sleep, mean nocturnal SpO_2 less than 95%, and symptoms of ventilatory insufficiency. In addition, it was agreed that in the absence of symptoms, nocturnal nasal ventilation is indicated for patients with DMD when $PaCO_2$ exceeds 45 mmHg and/or PaO_2 is less than 60 mmHg in blood gas samples taken early in the morning, late in the day, or during periods of oxyhemoglobin desaturation.[27] Another consensus conference in 1999 decided that for patients with NMD and chest wall deformities the indications for nocturnal nasal ventilation were symptomatic hypoventilation, $PaCO_2$ greater than 45 mmHg, nocturnal SpO_2 less than 89% for at least five consecutive minutes, or maximal inspiratory pressures less than 60 cmH_2O or forced vital capacity less than 50% of predicted.[28] For patients with COPD, indications were listed as symptoms plus one of the following: $PaCO_2$ greater than 55 mmHg, $PaCO_2$ of 50–54 mmHg, nocturnal SpO_2 less than 89% for at least five continuous minutes while the patient is receiving oxygen therapy of 2 L/m or more, or $PaCO_2$ of 50–54 mmHg and hospitalizations related to recurrent episodes of hypercapnic respiratory failure.[28] Some of these indications (e.g., speed of progression) are irrelevant, and others are draconian. The only true indication is relief of symptoms, although before treatment an increase from normal in episodes of nocturnal oxyhemoglobin desaturation is usually present.[29]

Patients tend to be symptomatic when diurnal hypercapnia causes the SpO_2 to decrease below 95%. However, even when untreated, many patients can tolerate hypercapnia for years—or until they have an intercurrent chest cold—when diurnal SpO_2 is normal. Although nocturnal low-span PIP + PEEP can benefit mildly affected patients, clinicians too often prescribe oxygen or recommend tracheotomy instead of increasing the spans or switching to the use of volume-cycled ventilators for daytime IPPV via a mouthpiece when low-span pressure assistance is no longer adequate.[27,30] Once the patient is intubated or a tracheostomy tube is placed, he or she receives appropriate tidal volumes at adequate peak inspiratory pressures (usually 20–25 cmH_2O) to maintain normal lung ventilation and facilitate coughing. Ironically, if these pressures had been provided noninvasively, the patient would not have needed invasive management.

Along with suboptimal PIP + PEEP spans, conventional management includes medical interventions, chest physical therapy, and occasionally IPPB, used for inadequate periods and at inadequate pressures, to expand fully the lungs and chest walls or to support or rest inspiratory muscles. Chest physical therapy, including chest percussion and postural drainage, can facilitate the proximal migration of airway secretions but at the cost of acute increases in metabolic rate, oxygen consumption (by 40–50%), heart rate, blood pressure, and plasma catecholamine concentrations.[31] These therapeutic measures do not address the fundamental need to support inspiratory muscles and increase cough flows. Patients receiving chest physical therapy who are able to increase minute ventilation do so by about 35%, and those not able to increase minute ventilation require ventilatory assistance to the same extent.[31] Failure to assist the cough must inevitably result in respiratory failure for patients with NMD. Even now airway mucus accumulation tends to be considered a "complication" of the use of noninvasive ventilation rather than the failure of the clinician to institute insufflation therapy and MAC.[32]

A recent review of nocturnal nasal ventilation inadvertently provided a good example of common misunderstandings related to the use of noninvasive IPPV. The review notes that "patients with severe neuromuscular weakness, prominent pulmonary secretions, or significant bulbar dysfunction" may require tracheostomy. This review ignored the fact that patients with no measurable vital capacity successfully use noninvasive IPPV; it failed to consider assisted coughing to clear secretions; and it failed to quantitate bulbar muscle dysfunction (see Chapter 7). The review arbitrarily recommended normalizing end-tidal carbon dioxide by "no more than 15 mmHg." It advised that ventilatory assistance be initiated in a monitored environment, even though we have instituted noninvasive IPPV for hundreds of patients, many of whom eventually became 24-hour users, in the outpatient clinic and home settings. The review notes that polysomnography and supplemental oxygen are required when PIP + PEEP does not increase SpO_2 to greater than 90%.[33] Both suggestions are harmful and dangerous for patients with primarily ventilatory impairment.

VOLUME-CYCLED VENTILATORS

The expiratory volume alarm of intensive care volume ventilators makes them impractical for the delivery of noninvasive IPPV, and they are usually not sufficiently portable for home use. Nasal ventilation has been most frequently described using portable volume-cycled ventilators.[34–36] Portable volume-cycled ventilators, however, are most often conventionally used for providing long-term tracheostomy rather than noninvasive IPPV.

Volume-cycled ventilators—such as the PLV-100 (Respironics, Inc., Murrysville, PA), the Achieva, LP-10, and LP-20 (Mallincrodt, Pleasanton, CA), and LTV-900, a volume- or pressure-cycled machine (Pulmonetic Systems Inc., Colton, CA)—can generally deliver volumes up to 2500 ml. Typically, control, assist-control, and synchronized intermittent mandatory ventilation (SIMV) modes can be used. The most commonly used mode for home noninvasive ventilation is assist-control, which delivers set volumes of air are delivered, triggered by the patient's inspiratory effort. A back-up rate provides for air delivery in the absence of effort. For volume-cycled ventilators, the volume to be delivered to the ventilator circuit—once set—remains constant regardless of the insufflation leakage, pulmonary compliance, and airway resistance. However, because insufflation leakage can change from breath to breath, the volumes delivered to the lungs change from breath to breath. The volumes delivered to the lungs correlate with ventilator gauge pressures. Thus, the pressures indicated on the volume ventilator pressure gauge vary, depending on ventilator-delivered volumes, insufflation leakage, and lung impedance. Volume-cycled ventilators also have low- and high-pressure alarms, sensitivity controls that permit the patient to trigger ventilator-delivered breaths, and flow-rate adjustments. They can be pressure-limited, like pressure-cycled ventilators, by increasing the delivered volumes and lowering the high-pressure alarm.

VOLUME-CYCLED VS. PRESSURE-CYCLED VENTILATORS

A number of studies have attempted to compare the efficacy of ventilatory assistance using PIP + PEEP vs. noninvasive IPPV using volume-cycled ventilators in both acute and long-term settings and for both daytime and overnight use. In a review of these studies, no clear advantage could be appreciated using either system. Hill concluded that "the choice between the two comes down to clinician preference and a consideration of the particular advantages and disadvantages."[37]

Advantages and disadvantages of using volume-cycled and pressure-cycled ventilators are listed in Table 1. Because the currently available pressure-cycled units are limited to pressures of less than 40 cmH_2O, they can be inadequate for managing conditions characterized by poor pulmonary compliance or high work of breathing, as in patients with severe scoliosis or obesity. On the other hand, PIP + PEEP can be useful for managing COPD and sleep-disordered breathing. Even low-span PIP + PEEP can effectively assist inspiratory muscle function for emphysematous patients with hypercompliant lungs. The positive pressures also can stabilize the airway in the event of concurrent obstructive sleep

---

TABLE 1. Pressure Assist Vs. Portable Volume Ventilators

Advantages of volume ventilators
1. Can deliver higher volumes and at potentially higher pressures, as needed, for patients with poor lung compliance
2. Can adjust flow rates for comfort
3. Uses 3–8 times less electricity for comparable air delivery, permitting greater patient mobility for the same battery capacity
4. Operates more quietly
5. Less mean thoracic pressures create less untoward hemodynamic effects on cardiac preload; particularly hazardous for patients with cardiomyopathies
6. Permits air-stacking to obtain maximal insufflations for increasing dynamic pulmonary compliance as well as for raising voice volume and increasing cough flows
7. Can be used to operate intermittent abdominal pressure ventilators as well as for noninvasive IPPV
8. Has alarm systems that can facilitate effective use of nocturnal noninvasive IPPV

Disadvantages of volume ventilators
1. Heavier
2. Annoying alarms (low-pressure alarm can be eliminated by setting alarm to minimum and using flexed mouthpiece, bacterial filter, or a regenerative humidifier to create sufficient back pressure)
3. Needlessly complicated; ventilators with fewer modes should be available

Advantages of BiPAP
1. No annoying alarms
2. Light weight
3. Lower cost
4. Can compensate to some extent for small insufflation leaks

Disadvantages of PIP + PEEP
1. Inability to air stack
2. Fixed, high initial flow rates can cause mouth drying and gagging, especially with insufflation leakage, and arousals from sleep
3. High power utilization limits patient mobility
4. Inadequate pressure generation capabilities for some patients
5. Discomfort and increased thoracic pressures due to unnecessary expiratory positive airway pressure
6. The gauge of pressure-cycled devices is less useful for feedback about insufflation leakages
7. No alarms to facilitate effective nocturnal IPPV for some patients
8. Noisier
9. EPAP unnecessary for most patients
10. Ventilatory assistance at higher mean intrathoracic pressures than with the use of volume-cycled ventilators
11. Significant carbon dioxide rebreathing occurs; can be corrected by using a nonrebreathing valve at the cost of greater expiratory resistance[147]
12. EPAP can make eating difficult or hazardous for 24-hour ventilator users

BiPAP = biphasic positive airway pressure, PIP = positive inspiratory pressure, PEEP = positive end-expiratory pressure, IPPV = intermittent positive-pressure ventilation, EPAP = expiratory positive airway pressure.

apneas or bulbar muscle dysfunction with airway collapse. The PEEP can decrease the work of breathing by relieving the effort required to reverse the expiratory flows associated with air trapping, thus countering the auto-PEEP effect. In general, depending on settings, the work of breathing can be equally decreased during pressure-cycled and volume-cycled mechanical ventilation.[38] Because patients cannot air-stack when using pressure-cycled ventilators, their long-term use in patients with NMD is suboptimal unless the patient is equipped with the means to expand the lungs and assist the cough.

Currently available pressure-cycled ventilators can weigh as little as 5.5 lb. They are becoming lighter, smaller, and more quiet. The Harmony, for example, weighs only 2.5 kg, operates quietly, and can provide IPAP up to 30 cmH$_2$O. It uses only 10% more amperage than typical portable volume-cycled ventilators and can operate most of the day on a fully charged external battery. The ResMed VPAP-STII is 1 kg heavier but provides IPAP up to 40 cmH$_2$O and therefore may be more useful for deep insufflation therapy in patients who do not have Cough Assist devices or volume-cycled ventilators and who are unable to air-stack via a manual resuscitator. These machines are useful for air delivery without high- and low-pressure alarms. This feature can be an advantage or a disadvantage, depending on the particular patient. Such devices do not have internal batteries, use more electricity than volume-cycled ventilators, and, therefore, run for shorter periods on an external battery source when they are equipped to do so.

The LTV-900 is a 12-pound, versatile, lap-top sized ventilator. Air flows are created by turbine, and the ventilator can be volume- or pressure-cycled. The LTV-900, however, is noisier than other volume-cycled ventilators, it is the most expensive portable ventilator on the market, and frequent technical glitches have been reported. This and other small units, however, may be ideal for patients who are able to walk despite ventilator dependence (see Chapter 15) as well as for others who need small, light units to optimize mobility.[39]

Air-stacking to facilitate coughing, to increase voice volume, and to expand the lungs optimally is not possible with pressure-cycled ventilators. Depending on the unit and lung impedance characteristics, most patients cannot obtain the minimal 1.5 L insufflation volumes generally needed for an effective assisted cough.[40] In addition, despite increases in minute ventilation and reductions in respiratory effort, PIP + PEEP does not always reduce PaCO$_2$—perhaps because of the carbon dioxide rebreathing inherent with the standard exhalation device (Whisper-Swivel, Respironics, Inc., Murrysville, PA). With the fixed-resistance exhalation Whisper-Swivel, the patient rebreathes air exhaled into the ventilator tubing, as dead-space ventilation is increased.[41] Elimination of rebreathing would require a completely unacceptable EPAP level of 8 cmH$_2$O. The problem can be solved by using nonrebreather valves and exhalation plateau valves. However, nonbreather valves can malfunction if valve materials stiffen or secretions become impacted within it, and exhalation plateau valves are not yet commercially available. A generally better alternative is to switch to volume-cycled ventilation at appropriate settings. The use of PIP + PEEP by clinicians with little experience in noninvasive aids almost invariably leads to failure to intervene appropriately during intercurrent chest infections.

CONVENTIONAL EXTUBATION

Like any emergency department patient presenting with respiratory distress, intubated patients using ventilatory support typically receive supplemental oxygen along with bronchodilators, mucolytics, chest physical therapy, and, possibly, sedation. Ventilator-weaning attempts are made with some combination of assist-control ventilation, SIMV, pressure support, PEEP, and supplemental oxygen. Occasionally, periods of ventilator-free breathing are tried with the patient receiving CPAP or oxygen and humidification by T-piece. With these approaches, "weaning schedules" are imposed on the patient. This approach usually involves one of two problems: either it causes anxiety because the patient is not ready to breathe autonomously, or the schedule is too conservative, delaying respiratory muscle reconditioning. Furthermore, the use of pulse oximetry, which can signal the presence of airway mucus encumberment as well as its elimination with treatment, is lost with oxygen administration. The supplemental oxygen therapy becomes tantamount to putting a "Bandaid on a cancer," with the "cancer" being some combination of hypoventilation and airway mucus.

Because SpO_2 from 90–95% is considered acceptable for most patients with lung disease, patients with neuromuscular weakness are often extubated without concern for their ability to maintain normal SpO_2 on room air. However, when the SpO_2 in ambient air is not greater than 94%, it is invariably because of hypoventilation, airway mucus, or residual lung disease. Thus, when such patients are extubated without normal SpO_2 in ambient air, they are expected to be ventilator-weaned despite some combination of hypercapnia, airway mucus encumberment, and residual lung disease. Furthermore, they are often extubated to CPAP, inappropriately low-span PIP + PEEP, or simply breathing on their own, without cough aids. This approach effectively puts them in a "sink-or-swim" situation and often results in reintubation.

Intubated ventilator-supported patients can develop hypo- or hypercapnia, decreases in pulmonary function due to airway mucus, and inspiratory muscle deconditioning. A study of normal rats demonstrated a daily decrease in diaphragm weight, contractile properties, and enzymatic profile after just 48 hours of mechanical ventilation.[42] These factors, along with laryngeal edema or airway damage, can make post-extubation peak cough flow ineffective. In addition, the patients' mucociliary elevators are impaired by intubation. Thus, mucus accumulation can greatly hamper ventilator weaning and the ability to remain extubated and is the main reason that patients require intubation and reintubation.[16] These effects are exacerbated by the tendency of intubated patients to develop malnutrition, often due in part to the presence of the tube (see Chapter 6). Thus, it is not surprising that conventional extubation is significantly less often successful in comparison with extubation using respiratory muscle aids (see Chapter 10).

COMPLICATIONS OF INVASIVE MANAGEMENT

Once the patient undergoes tracheotomy, the tube cuff is conventionally left inflated and verbal communication is lost (see Case 9 in Chapter 15)—even though prolonged cuff inflation is virtually never necessary for stable patients who suffer primarily from ventilation impairment.[43] Patients then experience the inevitably greater morbidity, swallowing difficulties (see Chapter 6), and higher mortality risk associated with tracheostomy and prolonged cuff inflation.[5] The tube and cuff also disrupt mucociliary transport.[44] Four hours of tracheostomy cuff inflation was shown to affect ciliary appearance and function for 3 days.[45] Cuff pressure causes tracheal wall ischemia, necrosis, and ulceration that scars and leads to stenosis or malacia and tracheal collapse during inspiration or expiration. Tracheobronchomalacia has been defined as a greater than a 50% narrowing of the distal trachea and mainstem bronchi on expiration during spontaneous breathing.[46]

Whether performed under emergency or elective circumstances—and despite the proliferation of ventilation modes that include proportional assist, pressure support, jet, SIMV, and assist-control ventilation as well as PEEP and the availability of precise oxygen delivery systems—the hospital survival rates of intubated and tracheostomy IPPV users have not improved over the past 20 years.[47] Numerous complications of invasive support have been described,[48] including infection and destruction of airway cilia[49–52] associated with pathogenic bacterial colonization of the airway.[52] Chronic purulent bronchitis, granuloma formation, and sepsis from paranasal sinusitis are associated with pathogenic bacterial colonization.[53,54] Sudden death is common as a result of mucus plugging,[55–57] cardiac arrhythmias,[58–60] accidental disconnections, and other causes related to the presence of an indwelling tube.[61,62]

Other complications include tracheomalacia and tracheal perforation, innominate artery hemorrhage, an 8%[63] to 65%[64] incidence of tracheal stenosis,[65] tracheoesophageal fistula,[66,67] painful hemorrhagic tube changes, aspiration of upper airway secretions and food,[68] and psychosocial difficulties. Vocal cord paralysis, laryngeal strictures, hypopharyngeal muscle dysfunction, and airway collapse also can result from invasive ventilation.[69,70] Tracheotomy was shown to exacerbate endotracheal tube-associated laryngeal damage and to increase the risk of laryngeal stenosis.[71] In fact, because of the higher incidence of laryngotracheal stenosis in intubated patients who undergo tracheostomy than in patients intubated for several weeks or patients undergoing tracheotomy without prior intubation, it appears preferable to maintain intubation longer in the hope of successful extubation than to resort to tracheotomy.[72] The airway obstruction of laryngeal stenosis decreases cough flows and, thus, can ultimately prevent tracheostomy tube removal.[73]

In addition, patients receiving tracheostomy rather than noninvasive IPPV tend to become dependent on more ventilatory support per day because of deconditioning of the inspiratory muscles.[42] Often, hypercapnic patients who never before used ventilatory assistance and patients who use nocturnal-only noninvasive IPPV become 24-hour ventilator dependent immediately after tracheostomy (see Chapter 5).[74]

Pulmonary function (vital capacity) also decreases because of the long-term presence of airway mucus and impaired mucociliary clearance caused by the tube. Adequate expiratory flows cannot be generated by coughing or assisted coughing methods because of leakage from or around the walls of the tube. The presence of the tube, suctioning, and bacterial colonization result in loss of physiologic coughing, chronic inflammation, denuding, ulceration, and scarring of the mucociliary elevator,[75-77] especially when suction catheters are inserted until resistance is met.[78,79] Deep suctioning, in general, is associated with greater necrosis and inflammation and greater loss of cilia and increased mucus than shallow suctioning.[80] Thus, physiologic and assisted airway secretion elimination methods are incapacitated by intubation or tracheostomy.

Although indications for airway suctioning have not been determined, patients with tracheostomy tubes are routinely suctioned an average of 8 times per day—and 30 or more times per day when they have chest infections.[5] In a survey of ICU nurse managers, the indications for suctioning, in order of decreasing frequency, were time from last suctioning, coughing, rhonchi, increased work of breathing, visible mucus in the tube, dyspnea, patient request, extubation, increased peak inspiratory pressures, decreased breath sounds, and drawing of blood gases.[81] At best, suctioning can clear only superficial airway secretions. Suctioning misses mucus adherent between the tube and the tracheal wall, and routine suctioning misses the left mainstem bronchus in up to 92% of cases.[82] The results are a high incidence of left-lung pneumonias,[82] potentially fatal mucus plugging, and perceived need for bronchoscopies. Airway suctioning also is often accompanied by severe hypoxia.[83]

An indwelling tracheostomy tube necessitates regular cleaning of the site and tube, tubing changes, and supplemental humidification. Appetite is decreased. The chronic hypocapnia often associated with long-term tracheostomy IPPV also may result in bone decalcification.[84,85] In addition, in many states tracheostomy is considered an "open wound." This classification can prevent community living without prohibitively expensive nursing care for suctioning and stomal care and can restrict access to schools, places of employment, and recreational facilities such as swimming sites.

OUTCOMES WITH CONVENTIONAL MANAGEMENT

Spinal Cord Injury

It is estimated that there are about 3000 ventilator users with spinal cord injury (SCI) at any one time in the United States.[86] In a study of 435 patients with SCI and a mean age at injury of 39.6 ± 22.6 years between 1973 and 1992, who either used a ventilator at discharge from rehabilitation or died before discharge while still using a ventilator daily, the overall survival rates were 25.4% at 1 year and 16.8% at 15 years. Tracheostomy tube cuff status was not reported. For patients who survived the first year after injury, the cumulative survival rate over the next 14 years was 61.4%. For patients who survived the first two years after injury, the cumulative survival rate over the next 13 years was 70.7 ± 6.0%. Among the 1-year survivors, the subsequent mortality rate was reduced by 39% for people injured between 1980 and 1985 and by 91% for people injured since 1986 compared with those injured between 1973 and 1979.[87] By comparison with the general population, the annual death rate after the initial 2-year period was 20.86 times greater for 1- to 30-year-old patients, 8.87 times greater for 31- to 60-year-old patients, and 2.38 times greater for patients older than 61 years. For example, the life expectancy for 15 ventilator users with SCI who were injured at 10 years of age and survived the first two years after injury was 43.2 years.[87] The mean survival for ventilator users with SCI at age 30 who survived one and two years after injury was another 15.9 and 23.6 years, respectively.

Although the overall mortality rate after SCI has been declining, one of the three most common causes of serious morbidity and mortality, both in the acute period and over the long term, is respiratory complications.[87] In one study, respiratory complications accounted for 45.8% of deaths and contributed to the 24.6% mortality rate attributed to probable heart disease.[87] Fifty-one percent of the deaths attributed to probable heart disease were noted as sudden cardiac arrest, a condition with which sudden death from mucus plugging is often confused. An additional 16.7% of deaths were attributed to unknown causes. Unexplained deaths often are due to bronchial mucus plugging and cardiac arrhythmias associated with hypoxia or perhaps to the presence of the tube. The common potentially fatal complications of pneumonia, mucus plugging, asphyxia from accidental tracheostomy tube disconnection, and cardiac arrhythmias are directly associated with failure of conventional management approaches.

Electrophrenic pacing has been used for over 900 patients, mostly those with SCI. It can improve outcomes when it is sufficiently successful to permit tracheostomy tube removal for use of glossopharyngeal breathing (GPB) and noninvasive ventilation as backup. Pacing is discussed in Chapter 7.

Guillain-Barré Syndrome

Of 79 patients with acute Guillain-Barré syndrome, 21 were admitted to a respiratory intensive care unit for 58 ± 26 days. Thirteen underwent nasotracheal intubation followed by tracheostomy and IPPV. The tracheostomy remained in place for a mean of 50 ± 27 days. Two of the 13 patients receiving ventilatory support died. Four patients had complications of tracheostomy, one of which was innominate artery hemorrhage and fatal sepsis.[88]

The duration of mechanical ventilation in patients with Guillain-Barré syndrome is usually 8–12 weeks. Although there are no reports of need for permanent ventilatory support after disease onset, we had one patient who remained dependent on 24-hour tracheostomy IPPV for 14 years with no measurable vital capacity until she was disconnected from the ventilator. In this case bulbar muscle weakness precluded the use of noninvasive ventilation.

Duchenne Muscular Dystrophy

Fifty-five percent[89,90] to 90%[91–93] of conventionally managed patients with DMD die from pulmonary complications between 16.2 and 19 years of age; death from pulmonary complications is uncommon after age 25.[92,94] Most of the remaining patients succumb to dilated cardiomyopathy. A number of studies have reported outcomes of tracheostomy IPPV for patients who undergo prophylactic tracheostomy or who survive an initial episode of respiratory failure and subsequently undergo tracheostomy. Gatin reported eight such patients. Two died 36 and 30 days after tracheostomy, one from accidental decannulation and the other from massive tracheal hemorrhage.[17] The other six patients survived at least 38 months. None required more than 16 hours per day of IPPV. They experienced a total of four episodes of pneumonia and two near-respiratory arrests due to tracheobronchial mucus plugging as well as tracheal stenosis, granulation, and pseudopolyp formation.[17] Splaingard et al. reported three patients with DMD who survived 3, 5, and 2 years, respectively, with tracheostomy tubes. At least the last patient apparently died from respiratory complications.[61] Baydur et al. reported seven patients with DMD who received full-time tracheostomy IPPV for 18.2, 4.2, 3, 4.2, 6.3, 3.5, and 3.2 years, respectively, from the mean age of 22.3 ± 6.5 (range: 17–36) to 28.5 ± 8.1 (range: 20.5–42.3) years. Two of the seven patients died from pneumonia, and five of the seven patients were reported as having had pneumonia or recurrent pneumonias.[95] Fukunaga et al. reported three patients with DMD who received tracheostomy IPPV for 0.6, 1.5, and 2.5 years after using a chest-shell ventilator overnight for 3.5 4.5, and 2 years, respectively.[96] Complications were not reported. Soudon reported a mean survival of 3.6 years for 23 tracheostomy IPPV users, most of whom had DMD.[97] Eagle et al. reported survival periods of 200 patients with DMD as 19.5 years for those untreated and 24.8 years for those receiving tracheostomy IPPV.[98] Cardiomyopathy was the cause of death in 7.4% of untreated patients and 36.8% of ventilator users. Bach et al. reported seven patients who received tracheostomy IPPV for a mean of 7.1 years; age ranged from 21.1 ± 3.8 to 28.1 ± 4.5 years. Two of the seven patients were still alive.[99] Complications were not reported. The Baydur and Bach patients who had survived long enough after episodes of acute respiratory failure to be referred to rehabilitation centers had mean prolongations of survival of 6.2 and a bit more than 7.1 years, respectively, with tracheostomy IPPV.

Noninvasive IPPV, along with mini-tracheostomy, has been reported to successfully avert intubation for patients with NMD in acute hypercapnic failure.[100] This finding is not surprising because this approach both assists alveolar ventilation and clears airway secretion. Of course, if these patients had used noninvasive IPPV and cough aids properly at home, they would not have developed hypercapnic failure in the first place.

Use of the 4.5-mm mini-tracheostomies by patients with DMD is consistent with the paradigm that a tracheostomy tube is needed for ventilatory support and airway secretion management, and it ultimately condemns patients with NMD to use of normal-sized tubes of 5 mm or more. Along with the usual tracheostomy sizes, mini-tracheostomy necessitates hospitalization for surgery. The tubes block the upper airway and, even when capped, diminish the generation of thoracoabdominal pressures needed for effective coughing. Mini-tracheostomy also can prevent glossopharyngeal breathing for breathing tolerance. In one center, the misguided patients with mini-tracheostomy used nocturnal-only, low-span PIP + PEEP and were thereby unable to air-stack deep volumes to facilitate coughing.[101] They were ventilated at inadequate volumes, both by nasal interface and by mini-tracheostomy. As a result of suboptimal assisted ventilation and secretion elimination, 6 of 10 patients with DMD received oxygen therapy; at least one patient died within 1 year, and the others died shortly thereafter. The patients were never introduced to mouthpiece interfaces for daytime IPPV, nor were they trained in maximal insufflations or manual or mechanical cough assistance methods. With such limitations it is not surprising that the outcomes were so poor. More recently, the 5-year survival rate was reported to be only 50% for 89 patients with muscular dystrophy, including 51 with DMD at the same center.[102]

Tonoyama National Hospital in Osaka reported its experience from 1984 to 1998.[103] Nocturnal nasal IPPV was used for 61 patients with NMD, of whom 46 had DMD. The indications were arbitrarily set at pCO_2 greater than 60 mmHg, regardless of symptoms, for all patients with NMD except those with ALS, for whom the pCO_2 had to be only greater than 50 mmHg because "ALS is more rapidly progressive." Eight patients underwent tracheostomy after 39.9 (range: 8.5–73) months of nocturnal-only nasal IPPV because "they wanted to be tracheostomized." Thirteen used low-span PIP + PEEP, and the others used volume-cycled ventilators at the low volumes associated with equally poor assisted ventilation. Eight patients who never underwent tracheotomy died after an average of 46.8 months—three from pneumonia, two from presumed congestive heart failure (circumstances not given), and three from "suffocation." Sixty-two patients with NMD underwent tracheotomy without being introduced to noninvasive IPPV. Twenty-seven died. This number included 19 of the 25 patients with DMD after use of tracheostomy IPPV for an undisclosed period. Causes of death were not reported. Nineteen additional patients with DMD who, instead of using ventilatory assistance received supplemental oxygen, had pCO_2 greater than 60 mmHg and died at age 20 after a mean of 6 months (range: up to 1.5 years) of oxygen therapy.

In 1994 during a visit to Tonoyama Hospital, the author observed patients with ALS and DMD. Most of the patients with DMD had severe scoliosis from failure to intervene surgically, and many were confined to their beds. All had indwelling cuffless tracheostomy tubes and were severely hypercapnic. Ventilator-delivered volumes were typically 250 ml. Despite the cuffless tubes, they had inadequate air delivery for speech. When I increased the delivered volumes for one patient from 250 to 350 ml, he complained of chest pain. This pain was most likely due to intercostal muscle stretching on the ipsilateral side of the scoliotic convexity. Patients received no "sighs," nor had their tidal volumes varied for years in many cases. Perhaps a more humane approach to limit the duration of suffocation would be simply to hang the patients once the pCO_2 reaches 70 mmHg! Unfortunately, the Tonoyama approach is not atypical for conventional management elsewhere.

In 80% of NMD clinics in the U.S., with and sometimes without any sleep-related or hypoventilation symptoms, patients are offered nocturnal-only low-span PIP + PEEP on the basis of polysomnograms.[104] Many of these patients are found to have nocturnal desaturations and frequent hypopneas.[104] The hypopneas tend to be associated with reduced chest wall movement or chest wall paradox, suggesting a noncentral origin, that is, inspiratory muscle weakness. The use of low-span PIP + PEEP has been shown to prolong tracheostomy-free survival by a matter of only months; respiratory failure is ultimately inevitable (Table 2).

In a curious letter to the editor, Yasuma et al. reported that 27 nasal IPPV users lived to 30.4 years of age, whereas 65 untreated patients with DMD died at 20.1 years of age. The authors did not report causes of death or whether daytime aid or assisted coughing was used.[105] Their report makes no sense because patients with DMD cannot possibly survive for 10 years using nocturnal-only nasal IPPV. For example, Simonds et al. began nocturnal-only nasal ventilation in 23 patients with DMD. The mean age was 20.3 ± 3.4 years, and the mean vital capacity was 306 ± 146 ml. The 1-year survival rate was 85%; the 2-year survival rate, 73%; and the 5-year survival rate, less than 40%, with at least five deaths due to respiratory failure.[106] Another example, in which 70 patients with DMD were limited to nocturnal-only nasal ventilation and demonstrated no benefit, is discussed in Chapter 9.[107] Many other examples of poor outcomes are listed in Table 2. Indeed, conventional management can be so inadequate that patients "asphyxiate" or even "ask to undergo tracheotomy"![103]

At several centers in the U.S. and at least one in Europe, more than nocturnal nasal ventilation is used, but important aspects of providing respiratory muscle aids are lacking. For example, Soudon reported the use of mechanical ventilation by 86 patients with NMD. Of these, 44 used nasal IPPV; 23 used tracheostomy IPPV; and one used lipseal IPPV. One patient progressed to daytime IAPV use along with nocturnal nasal IPPV, but when the other patients needed aid more than 16 hours per day, they underwent tracheostomy instead of being offered continuous noninvasive IPPV. The patients also had access to manually but not mechanically assisted means of coughing, and oximeters were not mentioned. No meaningful outcome measures were reported.[97]

TABLE 2. Nocturnal Nasal Ventilation: Results in Neuromuscular Ventilatory Impairment*

Year	1st Author	Ventilator[a]	Users	Diagnoses[b]	Results[c]
1987	Kerby[36]	Volume	5	NMD	> 3 months
1987	DiMarco[148]	Pressure	1	Scoliosis	NR[g]
1988	Ellis[149]	Volume	5	Scoliosis	> 3 months
1988	Carroll[150]	Volume	6	Various	> 3–9 months
1989	Guille[151]	Volume	1	OSAS	NR[g]
1990	Heckmatt[152]	Volume	14	NMD	2–34 months
1991	Goldstein[153]	Volume	6	NMD/scoliosis	> 14 months
1991	Gay[154]	Volume	21	NMD	Up to 39 months
1991	Laier[155]	Volume	23	Restrictive[d]	Up to 33 months
1991	Thommi[156]	Pressure	1	OSAS	NR[g]
1992	Hill[157]	Pressure	6	Scoliosis/DMD[e]	> 12.7 months
1992	Waldhorn[158]	Pressure	8	Restrictive	> 3 months
1993	Paulus[159]	Volume	34	NMD	> 3.0 years
1993	Delguste[160]	Volume	9	NMD	NR[G]
1993	Barois[161]	Volume	46	NMD	See h
1993	Chetty[162]	Pressure	1	Phrenic neuropathy	NR[g]
1993	Sekino[163]	Volume	6	Ventilation-impaired	NR[g]
1994	van Kesteren[164]	Pressure	64	NMD, polio, scoliosis	NR[g]
1994	Vianello[165]	Volume	5	DMD	> 2 years
1994	Leger[166]	Volume	279	See f	> 2 years[i]
1994	Piper[167]	Volume	13	OSAS	NR[g]
1994	Raphael[107]	Volume	70	DMD	No benefit
1994	Robertson1[68]	Pressure	2	LGMD	NR[g]
1995	Pinto[134]	Pressure	10	ALS	Up to 36 mos
1996	Piper[164]	Volume/pressure	14	NMD	NR[g]
1996	Yasuma[105]	Unknown	27	DMD	10.3 years
1997	Aboussouan[135]	Volume/pressure	39	ALS	13 months
1998	Simonds[106]	Volume/pressure	23	DMD	< 40% 5 year survival rate
1998	Escarrabill[169]	Pressure	6	NMD	NR[g]
1998	Schlamp[170]		24	ALS	17/24NR[g]
1998	Guilleminault[171]	Pressure	20	NMD	NR[g]
1999	Polkey[2]	Unknown	25	ALS	None
1999	Jardine[172]	Unknown	103	78% NMD	NR[g]
1999	Kleopa[25]	Pressure	38	ALS	7–11 months
1999	Annane[173]	Pressure	20	NMD	None
1999	Schucher[174]	Volume	87	Ventilation-impaired	NR[g]
1999	Bullemer[175]	Volume/pressure	277	Scoliosis/NMD	NR[g]
2000	Kang[103]	Pressure	13	DMD	8 died/2 years
2000	Hukins[176]	Unknown	19	DMD	None
2000	Ohi177	Unknown	51	Hypercapnia	None
2000	Baydur[146]		73/79	Various	See text
2001	Masa[142]	Unknown	36	Scoliosis/obesity	NR[g]

Note: Settings were not noted in 15 studies; other studies used PIP+PEEP at low spans or set to titrate improvements in carbon dioxide or AHI. In general, in the studies in which volume-cycled ventilators were used, the settings were more appropriate to rest inspiratory muscles.

* In these studies, the indications for nocturnal nasal IPPV included symptomatic alveolar hypoventilation. Symptoms were alleviated, and arterial blood gases improved with treatment.

[a] Volume = volume-cycled; pressure = bilevel positive airway pressure or other pressure-cycled ventilator.

[b] NMD= neuromuscular diseases/weakness, OSAS = obstructive sleep apnea syndrome, DMD = Duchenne muscular dystrophy, ALS = amyotrophic lateral sclerosis, scoliosis = kyphoscoliosis.

[c] Time in years of clinical improvement and delay in resort to tracheostomy or death.

[d] Restrictive pulmonary syndromes include 3 patients with OSAS.

[e] 4 with kyphoscoliosis and 2 with muscular dystrophy.

[f] Diagnoses included scoliosis, 56; tuberculosis, 52; DMD, 75; COPD, 49; and bronchiectasis, 49.

[g] Successful for ameliorating symptoms and arterial blood gases but duration of benefit not reported

[h] In this study of patients with congenital myopathies, congenital muscular dystrophy, and spinal muscular atrophy, at least 14 patients underwent tracheostomy after periods of nocturnal nasal IPPV for up to greater than 3 years, and several patients died from cardiomyopathies.

[i] Tracheostomy was delayed for greater than 2 years for 183 patients, and 54 patients underwent tracheostomy or died in less than 2 years. The treatment populations included 155 patients with intrinsic lung diseases.

Non-Duchenne Myopathies

Robert et al. reported that of 18 patients with muscular dystrophy (including DMD) who used tracheostomy IPPV in the home setting, 77% survived for 1 year and 62% for 5 years. Ten-year survival was not reported.[108]

Acute episodes of ventilatory failure were reported in at least six patients with mitochondrial myopathies. One 31-year-old woman was intubated and ultimately weaned from ventilatory support in 12 days. One 65-year-old woman had a history of multiple episodes of pneumonia, the last of which necessitated mechanical ventilation, for which an indwelling tracheostomy tube was placed. Two months later she died of another episode of pneumonia and sepsis. A 37-year-old woman had had at least one episode of pneumonia per year for 12 years before presenting with atelectasis and a $PaCO_2$ of 89 mmHg. She underwent intubation and bronchoscopy and required ventilatory support for 7 days. Five months later, despite a vital capacity of 2.1 L, she presented with a $PaCO_2$ of 68 mmHg and underwent tracheotomy. A patient with mitochondrial myopathy who developed nocturnal ventilatory insufficiency at 55 years of age underwent tracheostomy for nocturnal ventilatory support but died 2 months later.[109] A 56-year-old patient developed ventilatory failure and was intubated for 5 months but died one week after extubation. This patient nicely demonstrated the conventional approach of weaning at the cost of hypercapnia or "weaning to death." A 70-year-old patient developed pneumonia and acute respiratory failure and required intubation for 6 weeks but was extubated successfully and without further episodes of respiratory failure for at least 1 year.[110]

Two patients with nemaline myopathies had episodes of ventilatory failure. The first presented at age 9 with a $PaCO_2$ of 56 mmHg when awake and 67 mmHg when asleep. Oxygen therapy progressively exacerbated the hypercapnia. Three months later, with severe ventilatory insufficiency, he underwent tracheotomy for nocturnal IPPV. The second patient became symptomatic for ventilatory insufficiency at 6.5 years of age, developed hypercapnic coma, and underwent tracheotomy. She continued to require nocturnal ventilatory support 4 years after the initial admission.[111]

A 64-year-old patient with acid maltase deficiency presented with symptoms of hypersomnolence. He was treated with nocturnal oxygen administration and CPAP at 9 cmH_2O with "marked symptomatic relief." On the following day, however, the patient developed confusion and cyanosis: "The lone preintubation blood gas measurement revealed a PaO_2 of 74 mmHg, $PaCO_2$ of 102 mmHg, and a pH of 7.29 on 2 L nasal oxygen. Nasotracheal intubation was performed and mechanical ventilation was instituted. Further pulmonary deterioration ensued, and the patient died on October 7, 1991."[112] No surprise here either!

These anecdotal cases typify the conventional approach of failing to assist or support weak respiratory muscles or, even worse, treating ventilatory insufficiency with supplemental oxygen until hypercapnic coma, pneumonia, or other complications provoke acute ventilatory or respiratory failure.

Spinal Muscular Atrophy

Gilgoff et al. reported 15 patients with spinal muscular atrophy (SMA) who received tracheostomy IPPV for an average of 8 years and 10 months (range: 5 months to 23 years 10 months) from the average age of 12 years 5 months (range: 5 months to 18 years 10 months).[113] Three patients required 24-hour support after undergoing tracheotomy. The other 12 used nocturnal-only assistance for an average of 8 years 7 months. All patients had a vital capacity under 20% of predicted normal when using IPPV. Six patients underwent tracheotomy to clear airway secretions before requiring continuous ventilator use, and most patients had multiple episodes of pneumonias before and after tracheostomies. All patients had uncuffed tracheostomy tubes and were able to speak. Two patients died after 5 and 14 years of support, respectively; one was weaned; and 9 were still using nocturnal support at the time of the report. One patient was institutionalized. Of the 10 patients over 18 years of age, three had college degrees, two were college students, three graduated from high school, and two completed eleventh grade. One patient is the mother of a healthy child. Two patients are employed, and two others do volunteer work.

In another study, six patients with SMA survived for a mean of 11.7 ± 17.7 years using IPPV continuously via indwelling tracheostomy tubes despite frequent episodes of mucus plugging and pneumonia.[114] Four of the patients also received all nutrition via indwelling gastrostomy tubes because of bulbar muscle weakness. Four patients used tracheostomy IPPV with the tracheostomy cuffs deflated and were able to communicate verbally. Five of the six patients remained institutionalized from the onset of ventilator use. Two patients survived for 15 and 4 years, respectively, despite need for ventilatory support since infancy. All four ventilator users who could communicate remained socially active, and one was gainfully employed.

These patient series do not take into account patients with SMA who died suddenly during initial episodes of respiratory failure, and the reports tend to ignore the more severe forms of infantile SMA that are considered in Chapter 10. Clearly, however, as for patients with other NMDs, the survival of many patients with SMA, with or without severe bulbar muscle involvement, can be prolonged by ventilatory support via indwelling tracheostomy tubes. Of interest, however, although bulbar muscle dysfunction was not so severe as to necessitate enteral nutrition or preclude verbal communication for most patients, the incidence of pneumonia and bronchial mucus plugging was high in tracheostomy IPPV users compared with the incidence in noninvasive IPPV users in a large national survey.[5]

Amyotrophic Lateral Sclerosis/Motor Neuron Disease

Pulmonary complications and respiratory failure account for at least 84% of mortality due to ALS.[115,116] After establishment of the diagnosis, vital capacity typically remains normal for several years. However, ventilatory failure and death occasionally occur as soon as 2 months after onset of symptoms and can occur at the time of initial presentation.[117] The mean survival time after onset of symptoms without the use of ventilatory support has been reported as 2.4,[118] 3.1,[119] and 4.1 years and from 2.5 to 5.9 years, depending on age at onset.[120] Jablecki et al., on the other hand, reported that about 20% of 194 patients survived 10 years without ventilatory support.[119]

In the U.S. fewer than 10% of patients with ALS undergo tracheotomy.[121] However, 80–97% of patients with ALS who use tracheostomy continuous IPPV are satisfied with the choice of mechanical ventilation and with their lives and would choose mechanical ventilation again if it were needed.[121–124] Only about 8% seriously consider discontinuation of ventilatory support.[124] Yet many physicians inappropriately judge the "lack of quality" of patients' lives to justify withholding mechanical ventilation, even during episodes of acute respiratory failure.

Reviewing the outcomes of programs offering ventilatory support, from the point of undergoing tracheotomy, a mortality rate of 76% was reported by 12 months in 24 IPPV users.[125] For other tracheostomy IPPV user groups, mean survival was reported as 20 months for 18 users,[126] 15 months (range: 3–48 months) for 12 users,[127] 26.6 months for four users,[123] 2.3 years for three users,[128] and 7 months for three users.[129] In another study, 89 ventilator users with ALS survived using 24-hour assistance for a mean of 4.4 ± 3.9 years (range: 1 month to 26.5 years); 37 of the patients were still alive at the time of the report. Thirteen of the 89 patients had used only noninvasive methods of ventilatory support. The 76 ventilator users who ultimately received tracheostomy IPPV survived using ventilatory support for a mean of 4.5 ± 4.0 years (range: 1 month to 26.3 years). Six patients survived using tracheostomy IPPV for over 10 years, including three who survived for over 14 years (Fig. 2). The 52 deceased patients used ventilatory support for a mean of 3.8 ± 2.9 years (range: 3 months to 14.5 years), including 4.1 ± 2.9 years (range: 1 month to 14.5 years) of tracheostomy IPPV for the 45 deceased patients who ultimately underwent

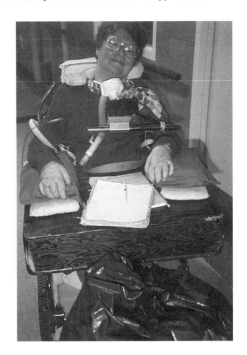

FIGURE 2. Eighty-one-year-old woman with onset of motor neuron disease at age 23 who has been wheelchair-dependent since age 27 and is a 24-hour ventilator user with no residual upper extremity function since age 47. She continues to sell clothing (in the dark sack below her lap tray) and, with assistance, to keep her accounts (open account book on her lap tray).

tracheotomy. In this study of 89 patients with ALS, 74 with rapidly progressive disease and 15 with a slower form, 42 with the rapidly progressive form (57%) and 11 with a slower form (73%) were managed predominantly in the community.[130] In another study of 362 patients with ALS, 194 were managed without respiratory intervention, 84 with noninvasive IPPV, and 84 with tracheostomy IPPV. Postdiagnosis survival was 19.4 months for the untreated group, 42.9 months for the noninvasive IPPV users, and 87.9 months for the tracheostomy IPPV users.[131] Thus, tracheostomy at times can prolong survival by 10 years or more. However, deterioration in physical functioning and in the ability to communicate,[130] limited family resources, and, most importantly, lack of a national policy for personal attendant care often make it impractical to manage patients with ALS in the community. In addition, many of the sudden deaths after tracheotomy may be due to airway mucus plugging or autonomic dysfunction.[132]

In a recent survey, 1.2% of 2357 patients with ALS from 48 centers were using CPAP, 49% were currently under do-not-resuscitate orders or refusing "mechanical ventilation," 1.5% were using IPPB, 15% (360) were using low-span PIP + PEEP, and 2.8% had tracheostomies.[133] Thus, although only a small percentage of patients with ALS undergo tracheotomy, many more now receive nocturnal PIP + PEEP. The following goals were suggested: detection of early respiratory failure, early intervention if it develops, prevention of complications, avoidance of tracheostomy ventilation, standardization of respiratory care, and improvement in survival and quality of life. Unfortunately, supporting respiratory muscle function was not a goal.

Indications for instituting nocturnal noninvasive ventilation continue to be debatable for patients with ALS as for patients with others NMDs. Institution of PIP + PEEP has been recommended once the patient is symptomatic or the FVC falls below 50%. Although symptomatic nocturnal hypoventilation is a valid indication, patients do not always realize that they are symptomatic until they have a treatment trial. Third-party payors often demand quantifiable indications, including criteria for maximal inspiratory pressures, FVC, carbon dioxide levels, and SpO_2. In one study, however, symptomatic hypoventilation occurred at greatly varying levels for these parameters, such as normal SpO_2 and FVC ranging from 16% to 111% of normal. Of interest, 23 of 29 patients with at least two symptoms of hypoventilation had a total of only 1 minute or more of SpO_2 below 90% during sleep.[29]

Many studies have reported statistical prolongation of survival by 2–13 months with the use of generally low-span PIP + PEEP for ventilatory assistance during sleep (see Table 2).[24,25,134–136] At times, control groups consisted of similar patients with ALS who were treated with supplemental oxygen. Thus, some of the apparently positive outcomes from ventilatory assistance were probably due to the untoward effects of oxygen therapy on alveolar ventilation and airway secretion management in the controls.[134] Most studies did not take the extent of bulbar muscle involvement into account when considering the benefits to patients with ALS who tolerated the use of PIP + PEEP.[25] Regardless of the minimal benefits for survival, however, many studies have demonstrated improvements in quality of life by reversing the symptoms of sleep-disordered breathing with nocturnal ventilatory assistance.[137] It is not surprising that minimal ventilatory assistance minimally benefits patients with mild-to-moderate inspiratory muscle weakness who have not yet developed respiratory failure due to airway secretion encumberment, but the difference between outcomes in these studies and patients who benefit from respiratory muscle aids is striking.[138]

About 10–30% of patients with ALS who use tracheostomy IPPV over the long term eventually lose the ability to blink and therefore become blind and cannot operate augmentative communication systems.[131] Communication also can be lost when patients are placed into nursing facilities where their communication systems may not be set up or may be ignored. Institutionalization can result in severe isolation and the loss of any meaningful interaction with the environment. Understanding the family's commitment to the patient, therefore, is essential before tracheotomy is considered.

Kyphoscoliosis and Obesity-Hypoventilation

Use of nocturnal-only noninvasive IPPV has been shown to improve daytime blood gases, to relieve symptoms of sleep-disordered breathing and hypoventilation, and to avert tracheostomy for patients with scoliosis and thoracic wall deformity as well as patients with obesity-hypoventilation (see Table 2).[139–142] Patients with extreme morbid obesity or severe scoliosis can deteriorate to the point of requiring continuous ventilatory assistance. They conventionally undergo tracheotomy.

NON–DIAGNOSIS-SPECIFIC OUTCOMES OF LONG-TERM PARTIAL NONINVASIVE VENTILATORY ASSISTANCE

Nocturnal-only ventilatory assistance of any kind,[143,107] especially low-span PIP + PEEP, must eventually fail for patients with progressive disease, as observed in all of the studies cited in Table 2. Failure of nocturnal-only nasal IPPV and the need for resort to tracheotomy have been defined as occurring when symptoms and signs of hypoventilation persist or recur or when use of nasal IPPV becomes necessary for more than 15 hours a day.[27,144,145] In reality, failure occurs when the contraindications for using noninvasive IPPV are not respected, when insufficient effort is made to find or fabricate comfortable IPPV interfaces, when only low-pressure spans are used, when inadequate attention is made to clearing airway secretions, and when mouthpiece IPPV is not used for air-stacking or daytime aid. Thus, nocturnal-only nasal ventilation can prolong life or delay respiratory failure for patients with NMD only to marginal degrees.[107]

A recent study summarized the authors' "46-year experience" with noninvasive ventilation in 73 (of 79) patients who suffered primarily from ventilatory impairment. Included were 45 patients with polio, 15 ventilator users with DMD, 48 patients who used mouthpiece or nasal ventilation, and 31 patients who used body ventilators. Fourteen of 25 patients with polio used body ventilators, 10 of 15 patients with DMD used noninvasive

IPPV, and five other patients with NMD underwent tracheotomies "because of progressive disease and hypercarbia which could not be controlled by noninvasive ventilation." The nine other tracheostomies were placed "because of bulbar dysfunction." Despite these figures, the authors reported that "the difference in the number of patients eventually receiving tracheostomies between the body ventilator and positive-pressure ventilation groups was fairly high (56% versus 5%, p < 0.001)." Certainly, however, most of the tracheotomies could have been safely avoided. Examples of suboptimal noninvasive management were the fact that 56% of the body ventilator users, mostly post-polio patients with more than adequate bulbar muscle function, underwent tracheotomy instead of being switched to more effective noninvasive IPPV and assisted coughing strategies, whereas the patients with DMD underwent tracheotomies with mean FVCs of 530 ml and daytime hypercapnia.[146] Thus, the tracheostomy tubes must have been placed as a result of episodes of respiratory failure triggered by chest infection, as is the case in 90% of patients.[5] Indeed, most of our patients with DMD (as well as most patients of other physicians[106]) with a vital capacity at this level do not require nightly ventilatory assistance between chest colds. The authors also reported that "[o]ne patient [with DMD] whose FVC declined to an unmeasurable value over five years was adamantly opposed to a tracheostomy and was able to sustain himself using a face mask/IPPV device 24 hours a day." This unfortunate patient had to be "adamantly opposed" to the clinicians' efforts to pressure him into undergoing tracheotomy, whereas, if he had been born in northern New Jersey, tracheostomy would not have needed to be a consideration. Thus, instead of being trained and equipped to maintain normal daytime ventilation and, more importantly, to maintain normal SpO_2 during intercurrent chest infections, these patients were counseled to undergo tracheotomy.

. . . la prudencia requiere que lo que se puede hacer por las buenas, no se haga por las malas.
(. . . prudence requires that what can be done for good effects should not be done for bad effects.)

Miguel de Cervantes, *Don Quijote de La Mancha*

REFERENCES

1. Dubowitz V: Management of muscular dystrophy in 1977. Isr J Med Sci 235–238, 1977.
2. Polkey MI, Lyall RA, Davidson AC, et al: Ethical and clinical issues in the use of home non-invasive mechanical ventilation for the palliation of breathlessness in motor neuron disease. Thorax 54:367–371, 1999.
3. Sykes NP: People with MND/ALS using noninvasive positive pressure ventilation: How do they die? In Proceedings of the 11th International Symposium on Amyotrophic Lateral Sclerosis and Other Motor Neuron Disorders. London, World Federation of Neurology, ALS Foundation, 2000, p 40.
4. Bach JR: Ventilator use by muscular dystrophy association patients: An update. Arch Phys Med Rehabil 73:179–183, 1992.
5. Bach JR, Rajaraman R, Ballanger F, et al: Neuromuscular ventilatory insufficiency: The effect of home mechanical ventilator use vs. oxygen therapy on pneumonia and hospitalization rates. Am J Phys Med Rehabil 77:8–19, 1998.
6. Poponick JM, Jacobs I, Supiski G, DiMarco AF: Effect of upper respiratory tract infection in patients with neuromuscular disease. Am J Respir Crit Care Med 156:659–664, 1997.
7. Moxham J: Aminophylline and the respiratory muscles: An alternative view. Clin Chest Med 9:325–336, 1988.
8. Esau SA: The effect of theophylline on hypoxic, hypercapnic hamster diaphragm muscle in vitro. Am Rev Respir Dis 143:954–959, 1991.
9. Smith PEM, Edwards RHT, Calverley PMA: Protriptyline treatment of sleep hypoxaemia in Duchenne muscular dystrophy. Thorax 44:1002–1005, 1989.
10. Nakayama T, Saito Y, Yatabe K, et al: The usefulness of trachostomy in Duchenne muscular dystrophy ventilated by a chest shell respirator. Rinsho Shinkeigaku 39:606–609, 1999.

11. George CF, Kryger MH: Sleep in restrictive lung disease. Sleep 10:409–418, 1987.
12. Ohi M, Nakashima M, Heki S, et al: Doxapram hydrochloride in the treatment of acute exacerbation of chronic respiratory failure: A patient with four episodes treated without use of a respirator. Chest 74:453–454, 1978.
13. Elliott LS: Steps toward effective pulmonary therapy: Alvan L. Barach, MD. Respir Ther 9:13–18, 1979.
14. Stark P: Atelectasis: Types and pathogenesis. Up-to-Date CD-ROM, 2001.
15. Bach JR, Ishikawa Y, Kim H: Prevention of pulmonary morbidity for patients with Duchenne muscular dystrophy. Chest 112:1024–1028, 1997.
16. Bach JR, Saporito LR: Criteria for extubation and tracheostomy tube removal for patients with ventilatory failure: A different approach to weaning. Chest 110:1566–1571, 1996.
17. Gatin G: Intêret de la ventilation assistée dans les dystrophies musculaires. Ann Réadapt Med Phys 26:111–128, 1983.
18. Greenbaum DM, Miller JE, Eross B, et al: Continuous positive airway pressure without tracheal intubation in spontaneously-breathing patients. Chest 69:615–619, 1976.
19. Brimacombe J, Keller C, Hormann C: Pressure support ventilation versus continuous positive airway pressure with the laryngeal mask airway: A randomized crossover study of anesthetized adult patients. Anesthesiology 92:1621–1623, 2000.
20. Aslanian P, El Atrous S, Isabey D, et al: Effects of flow triggering on breathing effort during partial ventilatory support. Am J Respir Crit Care Med 57:135–143, 1998.
21. Calderini E, Confalonieri M, Puccio PG, et al: Patient-ventilator asynchrony during noninvasive ventilation: the role of expiratory trigger. Intens Care Med 25:662–667, 1999.
22. Montner PK, Greene ER, Murata GH, et al: Hemodynamic effects of nasal and face mask continuous positive airway pressure. 149:1614–1618, 1994.
23. Bach JR, Chaudhry SS: Management approaches in muscular dystrophy association clinics in 1997. Am J Phys Med Rehabil 79:193–196, 2000.
24. Pinto AC, Evangelista T, Carvalho M, et al: Respiratory assistance with a non-invasive ventilator in MND/ALS patients: Survival rates in a controlled trial. J Neurol Sci 129(Suppl):19–26, 1995.
25. Kleopa KA, Sherman M, Neal B, et al: Bi-PAP improves survival and rate of pulmonary function decline in patients with ALS. J Neurol Sci 164:82–88, 1999.
26. Ferguson KA, Strong MJ, Ahmad D, George CFP: Sleep-disordered breathing in amyotrophic lateral sclerosis. Chest 110:664–669, 1996.
27. Robert D, Willig TN, Paulus J, Leger P: Long-term nasal ventilation in neuromuscular disorders: report of a consensus conference. Eur Respir J 6:599–606, 1993.
28. Clinical indications for noninvasive positive pressure ventilation in chronic respiratory failure due to restrictive lung disease, COPD, and nocturnal hypoventilation: A consensus conference report. Chest 116:521–534, 1999.
29. Gelinas D: Nocturnal oximetry as an early indicator of respiratory involvement in ALS: Correlation with FVC plus symptoms and response to NIPPV therapy. ALS Other Motor Neuron Disord 1:38–39, 2000.
30. Estournet-Mathiaud B: La ventilation non invasive domicile dans les maladies neuromusculaires. Arch Pediatr 7(Suppl 2):210–212, 2000.
31. Harding J, Kemper M, Weissman C: Pressure support ventilation attenuates the cardiopulmonary response to an acute increase in oxygen demand. Chest 107:1665–1672, 1995.
32. Wood KE, Flaten AL, Backes WJ: Inspissated secretions: A life-threatening complication of prolonged noninvasive ventilation. Respir Care 45:491–493, 2000.
33. Claman DM, Piper A, Sanders MH, et al: Nocturnal noninavsive positive pressure ventilatory assistance. Chest 110:1581–1588, 1996.
34. Bach JR, Alba AS, Mosher R, Delaubier A: Intermittent positive pressure ventilation via nasal access in the management of respiratory insufficiency. Chest 92:168–170, 1987.
35. Ellis ER, Bye PTP, Bruderer JW, Sullivan CE: Treatment of respiratory failure during sleep in patients with neuromuscular disease, positive-pressure ventilation through a nose mask. Am Rev Respir Dis 135:148–152, 1987.
36. Kerby GR, Mayer LS, Pingleton SK: Nocturnal positive pressure ventilation via nasal mask. Am Rev Respir Dis 135:738–740, 1987.
37. Mehta S, Hill NS: Noninvasive ventilation. Am J Respir Crit Care Med 163:540–577, 2001.
38. Kreit JW, Capper MW, Eschenbacher WL: Patient work of breathing during pressure support and volume-cycled mechanical ventilation. Am J Respir Crit Care Med 149:1085–1091, 1994.
39. Kirshblum SC, Bach JR: Walker modification for ventilator assisted individuals. Am J Phys Med Rehabil 71:304–306, 1992.
40. Bach JR: Mechanical insufflation-exsufflation: comparison of peak expiratory flows with manually assisted and unassisted coughing techniques. Chest 104:1553–1562, 1993.
41. Ferguson GT, Gilmartin M: CO_2 rebreathing during BiPAP ventilatory assistance. Am J Respir Crit Care Med 151:1126–1135, 1995.

42. Le Bourdelles G, Viires N, Boczkowski J, et al: Effects of mechanical ventilation on diaphragmatic contractile properties in rats. Am J Respir Crit Care Med 149:1539–1544, 1994.
43. Bach JR, Alba AS: Tracheostomy ventilation: A study of efficacy with deflated cuffs and cuffless tubes. Chest 97:679–683, 1990.
44. Konrad F, Schreiber T, Brecht-Kraus D, Georgieff M: Mucociliary transport in ICU patients. Chest 105:237–241, 1994.
45. Sanada Y, Kohima Y, Fonkalsrud EW: Injury of cilia induced by tracheal tube cuffs. Surg Gynecol Obstet 154:648–652, 1982.
46. Newth CJL, Lipton JJ, Gould RG, Stretton M: Varying tracheal cross-sectional area during respiration in infants and children with suspected upper airway obstruction by computed cineotomagraphy scanning. Pediatr Pulmonol 9:224–232, 1990.
47. Vasilyev S, Schaap RN, Mortensen JD: Hospital survival rates of patients with acute respiratory failure in modern respiratory intensive care units: an international, multicenter, prospective survey. Chest 107:1083–1088, 1995.
48. Bellamy R, Pitts FW, Stauffer S: Respiratory complications in traumatic quadriplegia. J Neurosurg 39:596–600, 1973.
49. Craven DE, Kunches LM, Kilinsky V, et al: Risk factors for pneumonia and fatality in patients receiving continuous mechanical ventilation. Am Rev Respir Dis 133:792–396, 1986.
50. Johanson WG, Pierce AK, Sanford JP, Thomas GD: Nosocomial respiratory infections with gram-negative bacilli: The significance of colonization of the respiratory tract. Ann Intern Med 77:701–706, 1972.
51. Johanson WG, Seidenfeld JJ, Gomez P, et al: Bacteriologic diagnosis of nosocomial pneumonia following prolonged mechanical ventilation. Am Rev Respir Dis 137:259–264, 1988.
52. Niederman MS, Ferranti RD, Ziegler A, et al: Respiratory infection complicating long-term tracheostomy: The implication of persistent gram-negative tracheobronchial colonization. Chest 85:39–44, 1984.
53. Deutschman CS, Wilton P, Sinow J, et al: Paranasal sinusitis associated with nasotracheal intubation: A frequently unrecognized and treatable source of sepsis. Crit Care Med 14:111–114, 1986.
54. Moar JJ, Lello GE, Miller SD: Stomal sepsis and fatal haemorrhage following tracheostomy. Int J Oral Maxillofac Surg 15:339–341, 1986.
55. Dee PM, Suratt PM, Bray ST, Rose CE: Mucous plugging simulating pulmonary embolism in patients with quadriplegia. Chest 85:363–366, 1984.
56. Cohn JR, Steiner RM, Posuniak E, Northrup BE: Obstructive emphysema due to mucus plugging in quadriplegia. Arch Phys Med Rehabil 68:315–317, 1987.
57. de Groot REB, Dik H, Groot HGW, Bakker W: A nearly fatal tracheal obstruction resulting from a transtracheal oxygen catheter. Chest 104:1634–1635, 1993.
58. Berk JL, Levy MN: Profound reflex bradycardia produced by transient hypoxia or hypercapnia in man. Eur Surg Res 9:75–84, 1977.
59. Mathias CJ: Bradycardia and cardiac arrest during tracheal suction: Mechanisms in tetraplegic patients. Eur J Intens Care Med 2:147–156, 1976.
60. Welply NC, Mathias CJ, Frankel HL: Circulatory reflexes in tetraplegics during artificial ventilation and general anesthesia. Paraplegia 13:172–182, 1975.
61. Splaingard ML, Frates RC, Harrison GM, et al: Home positive-pressure ventilation: Twenty years' experience. Chest 4:376–382, 1984.
62. Carter RE, Donovan WH, Halstead L, Wilkerson MA: Comparative study of electrophrenic nerve stimulation and mechanical ventilatory support in traumatic spinal cord injury. Paraplegia 25:86–91, 1987.
63. Bach JR: A comparison of long-term ventilatory support alternatives from the perspective of the patient and care giver. Chest 104:1702–1706, 1993.
64. Pingleton SK: Complications of acute respiratory failure. Am Rev Respir Dis 37:1463–1493, 1988.
65. Korber W, Laier-Groeneveld G, Criee CP: Endotracheal complications after long-term ventilation: noninvasive ventilation in chronic thoracic diseases as an alternative to tracheostomy. Med Klin 94:45–50, 1999.
66. Hedden M, Ersoz C, Safar P: Tracheoesophageal fistulas following prolonged artificial ventilation via cuffed tracheostomy tubes. Anesthesiology 31:281–289.1969.
67. Malingue S, Prunier F, Egreteau JP: Four cases of tracheoesophageal fistula associated with prolonged ventilation [in French]. Ann Anesthesiol Fr 119:539–544, 1978.
68. Elpern EH, Scott MG, Petro L, Ries M: Pulmonary aspiration in mechanically ventilated adults with tracheostomies [abstract]. Am Rev Respir Dis 147:A409, 1993.
69. Colice GL: Resolution of laryngeal injury following translaryngeal intubation. Am Rev Respir Dis 145:361–364, 1992.
70. Heffner JE: Timing of tracheotomy in mechanically ventilated patients. Am Rev Respir Dis 147:768–771, 1993.
71. Castella X, Gilbert J, Torner F: Letter to the editor. Chest 98:776–777, 1990.
72. Richard I, Giraud M, Perrouin-Verbe B, et al: Laryngotracheal stenosis after intubation or tracheostomy in patients with neurological disease. Arch Phys Med Rehabil 77:493–496, 1996.

73. Bach JR, Saporito LS: Indications and criteria for decannulation and transition from invasive to noninvasive long-term ventilatory support. Respir Care 39:515–531, 1994.

74. Haber II, Bach JR: Normalization of blood carbon dioxide levels by transition from conventional ventilatory support to noninvasive inspiratory aids. Arch Phys Med Rehabil 75:1145–1150, 1994.

75. Todd DA, John E, Osborn RA: Epithelial damage beyond the tip of the endotracheal tube. Early Hum Dev 24:187–200, 1990.

76. Czarnik RE, Stone KS, Everhart CC Jr, Preusser BA: Differential effects of continuous versus intermittent suction on tracheal tissue. Heart Lung 20:144–151, 1991.

77. Clini E: Patient ventilator interfaces: Practical aspects in the chronic situation. Monaldi Arch Chest Dis 52:76–79, 1997.

78. Kleiber C, Krutzfield N, Rose EF: Acute histologic changes in the tracheobronchial tree associated with different suction catheter insertion techniques. Heart Lung 17:10–14, 1988.

79. Brodsky L, Reidy M, Stanievich JF: The effects of suctioning techniques on the distal tracheal mucosa in intubated low birth weight infants. Int J Pediatr Otorhinolaryngol 14:1–14, 1987.

80. Bailey C, Kattwinkel J, Teja K, Buckley T: Shallow versus deep endotracheal suctioning in young rabbits: Pathologic effects on the tracheobronchial wall. Pediatrics 82:746–751, 1988.

81. Thompson CL, Wiggins W, Sheppard L, Sims K: Criteria for tracheal suction of ventilated intensive care adults [abstract]. Am Rev Respir Dis 147:A410, 1993.

82. Fishburn MJ, Marino RJ, Ditunno JF: Atelectasis and pneumonia in acute spinal cord injury. Arch Phys Med Rehabil 71:197–200, 1990.

83. Bach JR, Sortor S, Sipski M: Sleep blood gas monitoring of high cervical quadriplegic patients with respiratory insufficiency by non-invasive techniques [abstract]. Abstracts Digest, 14th Annual Scientific Meeting of the American Spinal Cord Injury Association, 1988, p 102. Available from L. H. Johnson, 2020 Peachtree Road, NW, Atlanta, GA.

84. Bach JR, Haber II, Wang TG, Alba AS: Alveolar ventilation as a function of ventilatory support method. Eur J Phys Med Rehabil 5:80–84, 1995.

85. Watt JWH, Oo T, Salva P: Biochemical profile and long-term hyperventilation in high tetraplegia. Eighth Journées Internationales de Ventilation à Domicile, abstract 128, March 7, 2001, Hôpital de la Croix-Rousse, Lyon, France.

86. Bach JR: Alternative methods of ventilatory support for the patient with ventilatory failure due to spinal cord injury. J Am Parapleg Soc 14:158–174, 1991.

87. DeVivo MJ, Ivie CS: Life expectancy of ventilator-dependent persons with spinal cord injuries. Chest 108:226–232, 1995.

88. Gracy DR, McMichan JC, Divertie MB, Howard FM Jr: Respiratory failure in Guillain-Barré Syndrome: A 6-year experience. Mayo Clin Proc 57:742–746, 1982.

89. Brooke MH, Fenichel GM, Griggs RC, et al: Duchenne muscular dystrophy: patterns of clinical progression and effects of supportive therapy. Neurol 39:475–480, 1989.

90. Mukoyama M, Kondo K, Hizawa K, Nishitani H, and the DMDR Group: Life spans of Duchenne muscular dystrophy patients in the hospital care program in Japan. J Neurol Sci 81:155–158, 1987.

91. Inkley SR, Oldenburg FC, Vignos PJ Jr: Pulmonary function in Duchenne muscular dystrophy related to stage of disease. Am J Med 56:297–306, 1974.

92. Rideau Y, Gatin G, Bach J, Gines G: Prolongation of life in Duchenne muscular dystrophy. Acta Neurol 5:118–124, 1983.

93. Vignos PJ: Respiratory function and pulmonary infection in Duchenne muscular dystrophy. Isr J Med Sci 13:207–214, 1977.

94. Emery AEH: Duchenne muscular dystrophy: Genetic aspects, carrier detection and antenatal diagnosis. Br Med Bull 36:117–122, 1980.

95. Baydur A, Gilgoff I, Prentice W, et al: Decline in respiratory function and experience with long-term assisted ventilation in advanced Duchenne's muscular dystrophy. Chest 97:884–889, 1990.

96. Fukunaga H, Okubo R, Moritoyo T, et al: Long-term follow-up of patients with Duchenne muscular dystrophy receiving ventilatory support. Muscle Nerve 16:554–558, 1993.

97. Soudon P: Tracheal versus noninvasive mechanical ventilation in neuromuscular patients: experience and evaluation. Monaldi Arch Chest Dis 50:228–231, 1995.

98. Eagle M, Chandler C, Giddings D, et al: Survival and cause of death in Duchenne muscular dystrophy. Eighth Journées Internationales de Ventilation à Domicile, abstract 121, March 7, 2001, Hôpital de la Croix-Rousse, Lyon, France.

99. Bach JR, O'Brien J, Krotenberg R, Alba A: Management of end stage respiratory failure in Duchenne muscular dystrophy. Muscle Nerve 10:177–182, 1987.

100. Vianello A, Bevilacqua M, Arcaro G, et al: Non-invasive ventilatory approach to treatment of acute respiratory failure in neuromuscular disorders: A comparison with endotracheal intubation. Int Care Med 26:384–390, 2000.

101. Nomori H, Ishihara T. Pressure controlled ventilation via a mini-tracheostomy tube for neuromuscular disease patients. Neurology12:698–702, 2000.

102. Ishihara T: Management of respiratory failure in patients with muscular dystrophy: Long-term results with nasal IPPV and new aspects at the National Center of Neurology and Psychiatry, Tokyo. Res Nerv Ment Disord [in press].
103. Kang J: Widespread application of NPPV in respiratory failure associated with neuromuscular diseases [in Japanese]. Kokyo To Jyunkan (Respiration and Circulation) 48:11–16, 2000.
104. Smith PEM, Calverley PMA, Edwards RHT: Hypoxemia during sleep in Duchenne muscular dystrophy. Am Rev Respir Dis 137:884–888, 1988.
105. Yasuma F, Sakai M, Matsuoka Y: Effects of noninvasive ventilation on survival in patients with Duchenne's muscular dystrophy [letter]. Chest 109:590, 1996.
106. Simonds AK, Muntoni F, Heather S, Fielding S: Impact of nasal ventilation on survival in hypercapnic Duchenne muscular dystrophy. Thorax 53:949–952, 1998.
107. Raphael J-C, Chevret S, Chastang C, Bouvet F: Randomised trial of preventive nasal ventilation in Duchenne muscular dystrophy. Lancet 343:1600–1604, 1994.
108. Robert D, Laier-Groeneveld G, Leger P: Mechanical assistance. Prax Klin Pneumol 42;846–849, 1988.
109. Byrne E, Dennett X, Trounce I, Burdon J: Mitochondrial myoneuropathy with respiratory failure and myoclonic epilepsy: A case report with biochemical studies. J Neurol Sci 71:273–281, 1985.
110. Cros D, Palliyath S, DiMauro S, et al: Respiratory failure revealing mitochondrial myopathy in adults. Chest 101:824–828, 1992.
111. Maayan C, Springer C, Armon Y, et al: Nemaline myopathy as a cause of sleep hypoventilation. Pediatrics 77:390–395, 1986.
112. Margolis ML, Howlett P, Goldberg R, et al: Obstructive sleep apnea syndrome in acid maltase deficiency. Chest 105:947–949, 1994.
113. Gilgoff IS, Kahlstrom E, MacLaughlin E, Keens TG: Long-term ventilatory support in spinal muscular atrophy. J Pediatr 115:904–909, 1989.
114. Wang TG, Bach JR, Avilez C, et al: Survival of individuals with spinal muscular atrophy on ventilatory support. Am J Phys Med Rehabil 73:207–211, 1994.
115. Mulder DW, Howard FM: Patient resistance and prognosis in amyotrophic lateral sclerosis. Mayo Clin Proc 51:537–541, 1976.
116. Bowman K, Meurman T: Prognosis of amyotrophic lateral sclerosis. Acta Neurol Scand 43:489–498, 1967.
117. Bradley MD, Orrell RW, Williams AJ, et al: Motor neuron disease presenting with acute respiratory failure. ALS Other Motor Neuron Disord 1:21–22, 2000.
118. Strong MJ, Ferguson KA, Ahmad D: The pulmonary function testing as a predictor of survival in amyotrophic lateral sclerosis [abstract]. Chest 102:180S, 1992.
119. Jablecki CK, Berry C, Leach J: Survival prediction in amyotrophic lateral sclerosis. Muscle Nerve 12:833–841, 1989.
120. Norris F, Shepherd R, Denys E, et al: Natural history and outcome in idiopathic adult motor neuron disease. J Neurol Sci 118:48–55, 1993.
121. Moss AH, Casey P, Stocking CB, et al: Home ventilation for amyotrophic lateral sclerosis patients: Outcomes, costs, and patient, family, and physician attitudes. Neurology 43:438–443, 1993.
122. Bach JR: Amyotrophic lateral sclerosis: Predictors for prolongation of life by noninvasive respiratory aids. Arch Phys Med Rehabil 76:828–832, 1995.
123. Oppenheimer EA, Baldwin-Myers A, Tanquary P: Ventilator use by patients with amyotrophic lateral sclerosis. In Proceedings of the International Conference on Pulmonary Rehabilitation and Home Ventilation. Denver, National Jewish Center, 1991, p 49.
124. Moss AH, Oppenheimer EA, Casey P, et al: Patients with amyotrophic lateral sclerosis receiving long-term mechanical ventilation: Advance care planning and outcomes. Chest 110:249–255, 1996.
125. Salamand J, Robert D, Leger P, et al: Definitive mechanical ventilation via tracheostomy in end stage amyotrophic lateral sclerosis. In Proceedings of the International Conference on Pulmonary Rehabilitation and Home Ventilation, Denver, National Jewish Center, 1991, p 51.
126. Gabinski CL, Barthe A, Castaing Y, Favarel-Garrigues JC: Sclérose latérale amyotrophique et réanimation. Concours Med 105:249–252, 1983.
127. Goulon M, Goulon-Goeau C: Sclérose latérale amyotrophique et assistance respiratoire. Rev Neurol (Paris) 145:293–298, 1989.
128. Iwata M: Clinico-pathological studies of long survival ALS cases maintained by active life support. Adv Exper Med Biol 209:223–225, 1987.
129. Sivak ED, Gipson WT, Hanson MR: Long-term management of respiratory failure in amyotrophic lateral sclerosis. Ann Neurol 12:18–23, 1982.
130. Bach JR: Amyotrophic lateral sclerosis: Communication status and survival with ventilatory support. Am J Phys Med Rehabil 72:343–349, 1993.
131. Cazzolli PA: The use of noninvasive and tracheostomy positive pressure ventilation in amyotrophic lateral sclerosis survival, long-term outcomes, factors for success and failure, and quality of life. Eighth Journées Internationales de Ventilation à Domicile, abstract 120, March 7, 2001, Hôpital de la Croix-Rousse, Lyon, France.

132. Shimizu T, Hayashi H, Kato S, et al: Circulatory collapse and sudden death in respirator-dependent amyotrophic lateral sclerosis. J Neurol Sci 124:43–33, 1994.

133. Melo J, Homma A, Iturriaga E, et al: Pulmonary evaluation and prevalence of noninvasive ventilation in patients with amyotrophic lateral sclerosis: A multicenter survey and proposal of a pulmonary protocol. J Neurol Sci 169:114–117, 1999.

134. Pinto AC, Evangelista T, Carvalho M, et al: Respiratory assistance with a non-invasive ventilator (Bipap) in MND/ALS patients: Survival rates in a controlled trial. J Neurol Sci 129(Suppl):19–26, 1995.

135. Aboussouan LS, Khan SU, Mecker DP, et al: Effect of noninvasive positive-pressure ventilation on survival in amyotrophic lateral sclerosis. Ann Intern Med 127:450–453, 1997.

136. Sherman MS, Paz HL: Review of respiratory care of the patient with amyotrophic lateral sclerosis. Respiration 61:61–67, 1994.

137. Lyall RA, Donaldson N, Fleming T, et al: A prospective study of quality of life in ALS patients treated with non-invasive ventilation. Neurology 124:2000–2013, 2001.

138. Bach JR, Li Li, Santos R: Amyotrophic lateral sclerosis: Prolongation of life by noninvasive respiratory aids. Chest [in press].

139. Bach JR, Robert D, Leger P, Langevin B: Sleep fragmentation in kyphoscoliotic individuals with alveolar hypoventilation treated by nasal IPPV. Chest 107:1552–1558, 1995.

140. Bach JR, Alba AS: Management of chronic alveolar hypoventilation by nasal ventilation. Chest 97:52–57, 1990.

141. Bach JR, Alba AS, Saporito LR: Intermittent positive pressure ventilation via the mouth as an alternative to tracheostomy for 257 ventilator users. Chest 103:174–182, 1993.

142. Masa JF, Celli BR, Riesco JA, et al: The obesity hypoventilation syndrome can be treated with noninvasive mechanical ventilation. Chest 119:1102–1107, 2001.

143. Mohn CH, Hill NS: Long-term follow-up of nocturnal ventilatory assistance in patients with respiratory failure due to Duchenne-type muscular dystrophy. Chest 97:91–96, 1990.

144. Leger P, Langevin B, Guez A, et al: What to do when nasal ventilation fails for neuromuscular patients. Eur Respir Rev 3:279–283, 1993.

145. Neri M, Donner CF, Grandi M, Robert D: Timing of tracheostomy in neuromuscular patients with chronic respiratory failure. Monaldi Arch Chest Dis 50:220–222, 1995.

146. Baydur A, Layne E, Aral H, et al: Long-term non-invasive ventilation in the community for patients with musculoskeletal disorders: 46 year experience and review. Thorax 55:4–11, 2000.

147. Lofaso F, Brochard L, Touchard D, et al: Evaluation of carbon dioxide rebreathing during pressure support ventilation with airway management system devices. Chest 108:772–778, 1995.

148. DiMarco AF, Connors AF, Altose MD: Management of chronic alveolar hypoventilation with nasal positive pressure breathing. Chest 92:952–954, 1987.

149. Ellis ER, Grunstein RR, Chan RR, et al: Noninvasive ventilatory support during sleep improves respiratory failure in kyphoscoliosis. Chest 94:811–815, 1988.

150. Carroll N, Branthwaite MA: Control of nocturnal hypoventilation by nasal intermittent positive pressure ventilation. Thorax 43:349–353, 1988.

151. Guilleminault C, Stoohs R, Schneider H, et al: Central alveolar hypoventilation and sleep: Treatment by intermittent positive pressure ventilation through nasal mask in an adult. Chest 96:1210–1212, 1989.

152. Heckmatt JZ, Loh L, Dubowitz V: Night-time nasal ventilation in neuromuscular disease. Lancet 335:579–582, 1990.

153. Goldstein RS, DeRosie JA, Avendano MA, Dolmage TE: Influence of noninvasive positive pressure ventilation on inspiratory muscles. Chest 99:408–415, 1991.

154. Gay PC, Patel AM, Viggiano RW, Hubmayr RD: Nocturnal nasal ventilation for treatment of patients with hypercapnic respiratory failure. Mayo Clin Proc 66:695–703, 1991.

155. Laier-Groeneveld G, Huttemann V, Criee C-P: Nasal ventilation can reverse chronic ventilatory failure in both chest wall diseases and COPD. Proceedings of the International Conference on Pulmonary Rehabilitation and Home Ventilation. National Jewish Center for Immunology and Respiratory Medicine, Denver, 1991, p 104.

156. Thommi G, Nugent K, Bell GM, Liu J: Termination of central sleep apnea episodes by upper airway stimulation using intermittent positive pressure ventilation. Chest 99:1527–1529, 1991.

157. Hill NS, Eveloff SE, Carlisle CC, Goff SG: Efficacy of nocturnal nasal ventilation in patients with restrictive thoracic disease. Am Rev Respir Dis 145:365–371, 1992.

158. Waldhorn RE: Nocturnal nasal intermittent positive pressure ventilation with bi-level positive airway pressure in respiratory failure. Chest 101:516–521, 1992.

159. Paulus J, Willig T-N: Nasal ventilation in neuromuscular disorders: respiratory management and patients' experience. Eur Respir Rev 3:245–249, 1993.

160. Delguste P, Rodenstein T: Implementation and monitoring of mechanical ventilation via nasal access. Eur Respir Rev 3:266–269, 1993.

161. Barois A, Estournet-Mathiaud B: Nasal ventilation in congenital myopathies and spinal muscular atrophies. Eur Respir Rev 3:275–278, 1993.

162. Chetty KG, McDonald RL, Berry RB, Mahutte CK: Chronic respiratory failure due to bilateral vocal cord paralysis managed with nocturnal nasal positive pressure ventilation. Chest 103:1270–1271, 1993.
163. Sekino H, Ohi M, Chin K, et al: Long-term artificial ventilation by nasal intermittent positive pressure ventilation: 6 cases of domiciliary assisted ventilation. Nihon Kyobu Shikkan Gakkai Zasshi 31:1377–1384, 1993.
164. van Kesteren RG, Kampelmacher MJ, Dullemond-Westland AC, et al: Favorable results of nocturnal nasal positive-pressure ventilation in 64 patients with neuromuscular disorders: 5-year experience [in Dutch]. Ned Tijdschr Geneeskd 138:1864–1868, 1994.
165. Vianello A, Bevilacqua M, Salvador V, et al: Long-term nasal intermittent positive pressure ventilation in advanced Duchenne's muscular dystrophy. Chest 105:445–448, 1994.
166. Leger P, Bedicam JM, Cornette A, et al: Nasal intermittent positive pressure ventilation: Long-term follow-up in patients with severe chronic respiratory insufficiency. Chest 105:100–105, 1994.
167. Piper AM, Sullivan CE: Effects of short-term NIPPV in the treatment of patients with severe obstructive sleep apnea and hypercapnia. Chest 105:434–440, 1994.
168. Robertson PL, Roloff DW: Chronic respiratory failure in limb-girdle muscular dystrophy: Successful long-term therapy with nasal bilevel positive airway pressure. Pediatr Neurol 10:328–331, 1994.
169. Escarrabill J, Estopa R, Farrero E, et al: Long-term mechanical ventilation in amyotrophic lateral sclerosis. Respir Med 92:438–441, 1998.
170. Schlamp V, Karg O, Abel A, et al: Noninvasive intermittent self-ventilation as a palliative measure in amyotrophic lateral sclerosis. Nervenarzt 69:1074–1082, 1998.
171. Guilleminault C, Philip P, Robinson A: Sleep and neuromuscular disease: Bilevel positive airway pressure by nasal mask as a treatment for sleep disordered breathing in patients with neuromuscular disease. J Neurol Neurosurg Psychiatry 65:225–232, 1998.
172. Jardine E, O'Toole M, Paton JY, Wallis C: Current status of long term ventilation of children in the United Kingdom: Questionnaire survey. Br Med J 318:295–298, 1999.
173. Annane D, Quera-Salva MA, Lofaso F, et al: Mechanisms underlying effects of nocturnal ventilation on daytime blood gases in neuromuscular diseases. Eur Respir J 13:157–162, 1999.
174. Raffenberg M, Geerdes-Fenge H, Muller-Pawlowski H, et al: Invasive and noninvasive home ventilation: Changes between 1982 and 1996 [in German]. Med Klin 94:18–21, 1999.
175. Pahnke J, Bullemer F, Heindl S, et al: Long-term breathing via traceostoma [in German]. Med Klin 94:40–42, 1999.
176. Hukins CA, Hillman DR: Daytime predictors of sleep hypoventilation in Duchenne muscular dystrophy. Am J Respir Crit Care Med 161:166–170, 2000.
177. Ohi M, Kuno K: Effectiveness of domiciliary noninvasive positive pressure ventilation in improving blood gas levels and the performance of daily activities. NIPPV Study Group. Nihon Kokyuki Gakkai Zasshi 38:166–173, 2000.

7 —— Noninvasive Respiratory Muscle Aids and Intervention Goals

JOHN R. BACH, M.D.
Collation of noninvasive interfaces by Barbara Rogers, B.A.

> *What people say you cannot do, you try and find that you can.*
> Henry David Thoreau

WHAT ARE PHYSICAL MEDICINE RESPIRATORY MUSCLE AIDS?

Inspiratory and expiratory muscle aids are devices and techniques that involve the manual or mechanical application of forces to the body or intermittent pressure changes to the airway to assist inspiratory or expiratory muscle function. The devices that act on the body include the negative-pressure body ventilators (NPBVs) and oscillators that create atmospheric pressure changes around the thorax and abdomen and body ventilators and exsufflation devices that apply force directly to the body for mechanical displacement of respiratory muscles. Negative pressure applied to the airway during expiration or coughing assists the expiratory muscles as forced exsufflation, just as positive pressure applied to the airway during inhalation (noninvasive ventilation) assists the inspiratory muscles.

Certain positive-pressure ventilators or blowers have the capacity to deliver continuous positive airway pressure (CPAP). Likewise, certain negative-pressure generators or ventilators used to power NPBVs can create continuous negative expiratory pressure (CNEP). CPAP and CNEP, both first described in the 1870s,[1] act as pneumatic splints to help maintain airway and alveolar patency and to increase functional residual capacity (FRC). They do not directly assist respiratory muscle activity, are rarely useful for patients who suffer primarily from ventilatory muscle weakness, and are not considered examples of noninvasive ventilation.

INTERVENTION OBJECTIVES

The goals of intervention are to maintain lung and chest-wall elasticity; to promote normal lung and chest wall growth in children by the use of lung and chest-wall mobilization (range of motion [ROM]); to maintain normal alveolar ventilation around the clock; and to maximize cough flows. The long-term goals are to avert episodes of acute respiratory failure during intercurrent chest infections, to avoid hospitalizations, and to prolong survival without resort to tracheotomy. All goals can be attained by evaluating, training, and equipping patients in the outpatient setting and at home.

Goal One: Maintenance of Pulmonary Compliance, Lung Growth, and Chest-Wall Mobility

The reasons for loss of pulmonary compliance are discussed in Chapter 2. As vital capacity decreases markedly, the largest breath that the patient can take can expand only a small portion of the lungs. Use of incentive spirometry or deep breathing cannot expand the lungs beyond vital capacity. Although possibly useful, manual chest-wall stretching and rocking the pelvis onto the chest to decrease costovertebral tightness[2] have not been shown to increase lung volumes. Like limb articulations and other soft tissues, the lungs and chest wall require regular ROM mobilization to prevent chest-wall contractures and lung restriction. As recognized since at least 1952, this goal can be achieved only by providing regular deep insufflations or nocturnal noninvasive ventilation.[2]

Maximal insufflation capacity (MIC) is determined by giving the patient the largest volume of air that he or she can hold with a closed glottis, usually from a volume-cycled ventilator or Cough Assist, or by teaching the patient to stack volumes of air consecutively delivered from a manual resuscitator or volume-cycled ventilator. The patient holds the stacked volumes with a closed glottis until the lungs are expanded as much as possible and no more air can be held. Patients who learn glossopharyngeal breathing (GPB) can often air-stack consecutive GPB gulps to or beyond the MIC without mechanical assistance. This phenomenon is called the glossopharyngeal breathing maximal single breath capacity (GPmaxSBC). The extent to which MIC or GPmaxSBC is greater than vital capacity predicts the patient's capacity to be maintained by noninvasive rather than tracheostomy ventilatory support.[3] The difference between MIC and vital capacity, like the extent of assisted peak cough flow (PCF), is a function of bulbar muscle function.

The primary objectives in using air stacking or providing maximal insufflations as lung and chest wall ROM are to increase MIC (Fig. 1), to maximize PCF (Fig. 2), to maintain or improve pulmonary compliance, to prevent or eliminate atelectasis, and to master

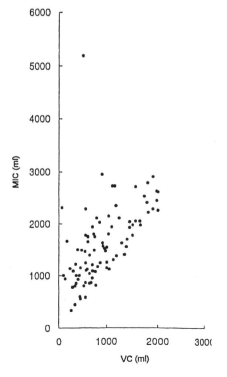

FIGURE 1. Relationship between vital capacity (VC) and maximal insufflation capacity (MIC) in patients with neuromuscular disease. (From Kang SW, Bach JR: Maximum insufflation capacity: The relationships with vital capacity and cough flows for patients with neuromuscular disease. Am J Phys Med Rehabil 79: 222–227, 2000, with permission.)

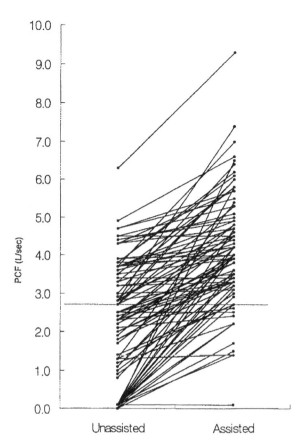

FIGURE 2. Relationship between unassisted and assisted peak cough flows for patients with neuromuscular disease. (From Kang SW, Bach JR: Maximum insufflation capacity: The relationships with vital capacity and cough flows for patients with neuromuscular disease. Am J Phys Med Rehabil 79:222–227, 2000, with permission.)

noninvasive intermittent positive-pressure ventilation (IPPV). Air-stacking not only may help to maintain static lung compliance but also—at least temporarily—improves dynamic pulmonary compliance.[4] In 278 spirometry evaluations of patients with neuromuscular disease (NMD) who were old enough and able to air-stack, we found a mean vital capacity in the sitting position of 1190.5 ml and in the supine position of 974.9 ml, whereas MIC was 1820.7 ml. The higher volumes increase both unassisted and manually assisted PCF and permit the patient to raise voice volume as desired.

Lung ROM, as described above, also can promote lung growth in children (see Chapters 5 and 10). Positioning of the patient to reduce pulmonary stress, avoidance of prolonged singular positioning, and using optimal trunk support during sitting also have been reported to be beneficial in improving chest-wall structure and reducing pectus excavatum.[5]

Any patient who can air-stack also can use noninvasive IPPV. If such a patient is intubated for respiratory failure, he or she can be extubated directly to continuous noninvasive IPPV, regardless of whether any breathing intolerance has been regained (see Chapter 8). This approach is extremely important for eliminating the need to resort to tracheostomy because such patients are extubated without ventilator weaning. Extubation of a patient who has little or no breathing tolerance and has not been trained to receive noninvasive IPPV results in panic, massive insufflation leakage, glottic closure, ventilator dyssyncrony, asphyxia, and possible reintubation.

Before vital capacity decreases to 70% of predicted normal, patients are instructed to air-stack or to receive maximal insufflations 10–15 times at least two or three times daily. Thus, the first respiratory equipment prescribed for patients with ventilatory impairment is a manual resuscitator. In general, because of the importance of air-stacking, patients without air-trapping who have a vital capacity less than 2000 ml use volume-cycled ventilators rather than pressure-cycled ventilators unless the pressure-cycled ventilator can attain the 50–80 cmH_2O pressures required to attain the MIC.

Infants cannot air-stack or cooperate to receive maximal insufflations. All infants with type 1 or type 2 spinal muscular atrophy (SMA) and infants with other NMDs who have paradoxical chest-wall movement require nocturnal high-span positive inspiratory pressure and positive end-expiratory pressure (PIP + PEEP) to prevent pectus excavatum and to promote lung growth (see Chapter 10). In addition to nocturnal aid, deep insufflations can be provided via oral-nasal interface for children over 1 year of age, along with concomitant abdominal compression to prevent abdominal expansion while directing the air into the upper thorax. These insufflations need to be timed to the child's inspirations. Children can become cooperative with deep insufflation therapy by 14–30 months of age.

Goal Two: Continuous Maintenance of Normal Alveolar Ventilation with Inspiratory Muscle Assistance As Needed

Nocturnal Inspiratory Muscle Aids

Negative-pressure Body Ventilators and the Rocking Bed. An NPBV assists inspiratory muscles by applying force or pressure changes to the body. It is practical only during sleep. Currently available NPBVs include the iron lung (see Fig. 8 in Chapter 3), the Porta-Lung (Fig. 3), chest-shell ventilator (Fig. 4), and various wrap-style ventilators. Many previously manufactured iron lungs and wrap-style ventilators are also still available and in use.

The large tank ventilators were discussed in Chapter 3. Unlike the heavy iron lung, the Porta-Lung (Respironics, Inc., Murrysville, PA) weighs 110 lb; its negative pressure generator, which is separate from the main cylinder, weighs another 45 lb. It is more practical and much lighter than the iron lung that is driven by a motor-operated bellows (see Fig. 3).

The chest-shell and wrap-style ventilators (see Fig. 11 of Chapter 2) are more portable than tank ventilators. Negative pressure is created under the shell or wrap to expand the chest and ventilate the lungs. The shells and wraps are made in various styles and of various materials. A wrap with the caudal end sealed over the lower abdomen or pelvis has the advantage of easier patient access for perineal care and permits greater lower extremity mobility, but it has a tendency to slip up and under the grid. This slippage decreases comfort

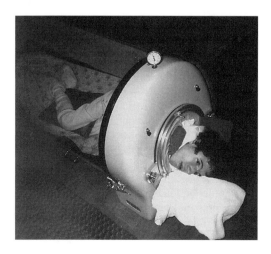

FIGURE 3. The Porta-Lung, a "portable" iron lung (Respironics, Inc., Murrysville, PA), was used by a patient with Duchenne muscular dystrophy during a cold when his nose was too congested to use nasal IPPV and his lips too weak for mouthpiece IPPV.

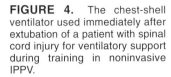

FIGURE 4. The chest-shell ventilator used immediately after extubation of a patient with spinal cord injury for ventilatory support during training in noninvasive IPPV.

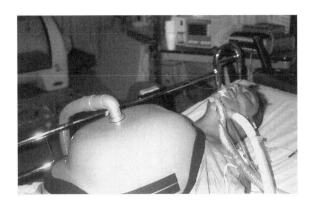

and causes leak, especially at pressures exceeding – 45 cmH$_2$O. Wraps that extend down the legs and are sealed at the thighs or ankles are easier to seal in an air-tight manner, but some patients complain that the fabric squeezes the legs during use. The Pulmobag (formerly from Respironics, Inc., Murrysville, PA) and Pneumobag (J. H. Emerson Company, Cambridge, MA) are essentially full-length wrap ventilators that completely seal the lower extremities. They decrease leakage and facilitate donning, but the dorsiflexion of the feet and the "squeezing" of the legs that occurs during use can be uncomfortable.

Gore-tex (W. L. Gore & Associates, Inc., Elkton, MD) is a wind-impermeable cloth that permits the escape of humidity. It is used in the fabrication of wraps. Gore-tex makes a cooler, more flexible wrap than nylon. For the Red Poncho and Pneumosuit (J. H. Emerson Co., Cambridge, MA) or NuMo Suit (Respironics, Inc., Murrysville, PA), the wrap is formed into arms and pant legs that separately seal each extremity and is closed with a long anterior, air-tight zipper. This design optimizes lower limb mobility and may discourage venous stasis in the lower limbs, but it is inconvenient for toileting.

Chest shells are made of thermomolded plastic. Chest-shell ventilators are the only NPBVs that can be used in the sitting position. Custom shells can be molded to the patient's body to accommodate scoliosis or other deformities. Because the chest-shell ventilator covers less of the chest and abdomen than the other NPBVs, much higher negative pressures must be generated under the shell to ventilate the lungs. Absolute pressures greater than – 60 cmH$_2$O are often too uncomfortable to be tolerated and may not be adequate for ventilatory support. The highest and least effective subshell pressures are often required for patients with scoliosis.

Negative-pressure generators include the 33-CR (J. H. Emerson Co., Cambridge, MA), NEV-100 (Respironics, Inc., Murrysville, PA), and Maxivent (Mallincrodt, Pleasanton, CA). The two latter ventilators can alternately deliver either negative or positive pressure. This feature is especially useful for patients who depend on both NPBVs and noninvasive IPPV methods at different times during the day. The NEV-100 and 33-CR permit use of CNEP. The ventilation modes, alarms, and other options available on these ventilators have been described elsewhere.[6]

High-frequency chest-wall oscillation enhances gas mixing in the lung periphery and during expiration improves gas mixing in the airways. Thus, it can increase the effectiveness of alveolar ventilation and improve gas exchange.[7-9] In normal people, it increases breath-to-breath variability, prolongs expiratory pauses, decreases carbon dioxide, and, in some cases, produces short apneas.[10] High-frequency chest-wall oscillation improved ventilation in bronchoconstricted rabbits, whereas high-frequency ventilation via the trachea did not.[9,11]

The Hayek Oscillator (Breasy Medical Equipment, Inc., Stamford, CT) is an oscillator as well as a NPBV. It can oscillate at up to 17 Hz around a negative pressure (CNEP), positive pressure, or atmospheric pressure baseline as well as work like a standard chest-shell ventilator at normal respiratory rates. It can alternate positive and negative pressure cycles or oscillations at pressures from $+ 70$ to $- 70$ cmH$_2$O. Adjustment of the inspiratory/expiratory (I/E) ratio can create an expiratory bias that may assist in elimination of airway secretions. For example, an I:E ratio of 2:1 can create airway pressures of $+ 6$ to $- 3$ cmH$_2$O, which should favor the migration of airway secretions towards the mouth.

The chest shell of the Hayek Oscillator is a light, moldable, clear plastic, flexible cuirass with soft foam rubber and Velcro closures that comfortably form a tight seal. It is the most comfortable chest shell currently on the market. Although the Hayek Oscillator has been reported to be effective in augmenting alveolar ventilation and improving blood gases in humans in respiratory failure when used at the high frequencies of 1–8 Hz,[12–14] high-frequency chest wall oscillation is uncomfortable in the long-term and does not effectively maintain alveolar ventilation in patients with primarily ventilatory impairment or when inspiratory muscle impairment is severe. When used during sleep in normal people, it resulted in a decrease in spontaneous ventilation, a decrease in total sleep time, and an increase in apneas and hypopneas.[15]

NPBVs are suitable for overnight ventilatory support and have been used for decades to ventilate the lungs of patients with little or no vital capacity despite frequent transient oxyhemoglobin desaturation due to apparent episodes of airway collapse.[16] With aging and decreasing pulmonary compliance or airway stability, NPBVs can become ineffective and may be associated with the development of systemic hypertension. Such patients benefit from switching to the more effective noninvasive IPPV.[17,18] Furthermore, except for the iron lung and Porta-Lung, NPBVs are generally not useful in patients with severe scoliosis or weight extremes. As for custom-molded chest shells, back discomfort can be intolerable when negative pressures must exceed $- 60$ cmH$_2$O in patients with scoliosis.

Although NPBVs continue to be used in a few centers, including ours, as a bridge to noninvasive IPPV during extubation of unweanable patients,[19,20] it is debatable whether long-term use is ever warranted. Only one center has continued to use iron lungs in acute and long-term care. From 1975 to 1991, this center used iron lungs to manage respiratory failure in 2011 of 2116 patients (95%) with chronic obstructive pulmonary disease (COPD).[20] During the same period 604 patients who suffered primarily from ventilatory impairment were managed with iron lungs.[20] The hospitalization mortality rate was 10% for the patients with COPD and 8.9% for the others. The mean length of stay was 10.5 ± 9.5 days. Hypoxic hypercapnic coma was managed by iron lung for 180 patients. Only 13 patients required intubation, and 41 patients (23%) died.

One of the two body ventilators that apply force directly to the body to allow gravity to move the abdominal contents and diaphragm is the rocking bed ventilator (J. H. Emerson Company, Cambridge, MA) (see Fig. 12 of Chapter 3). Although it is still used and can provide tidal volumes of as much as 1000 ml for some patients with no measurable vital capacity, it is, like NPBVs, primarily of historical interest. It is usually less effective than NPBVs,[21] but many patients like it because it relieves constipation and facilitates sexual intercourse.[22]

Noninvasive IPPV. IPPV can be noninvasively delivered via mouthpieces, nasal, and oral-nasal interfaces for nocturnal ventilatory support. Although in acutely ill patients noninvasive ventilation should be introduced in the hospital setting, the great majority of patients begin noninvasive IPPV in the clinic and home setting.

Mouthpiece IPPV. Many patients who have little or no measurable vital capacity and no upper extremity function have used mouthpiece IPPV without alarms for years, including during sleep, without losing the mouthpiece and dying of asphyxia. The best option is a simple 15- or 22-mm angled mouthpiece (Respironics, Inc., Murrysville, PA) held between the teeth. However, they invariably have disturbed sleep architecture and many nocturnal episodes of oxyhemoglobin desaturation. When mouthpiece IPPV is used during sleep, a lipseal retention system with two cloth straps with Velcro closures

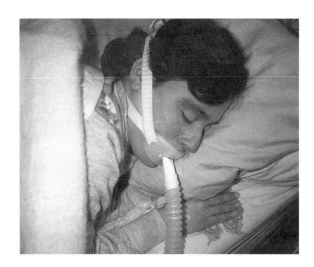

FIGURE 5. Noninvasive IPPV with lipseal retention of mouthpiece used since 1978 by patient with spinal cord injury at birth (June, 1949).

is strongly recommended (Mallincrodt, Pleasanton, CA) (see Fig. 18 of Chapter 3). The retention straps of an Adam circuit (Mallincrodt Inc., Pleasanton, CA) can be substituted for the cloth straps.

The lipseal can provide an essentially closed system of noninvasive ventilatory support. Mouthpiece IPPV with lipseal retention (Fig. 5) is delivered during sleep with little insufflation leakage from the mouth and virtually no risk of losing the mouthpiece. The strap-retained lipseal is becoming increasingly difficult to obtain, but a new strapless lipseal system called the Oracle (Fisher-Paykel, Inc.) should soon be on the market. Another newly described lipseal is made of transparent silicon. It has no intraoral mouthpiece but a similar retention strap system (Masque Buccal, Metamed, France).[23] Orthodontic bite-plates and custom-fabricated acrylic lipseals (see Fig. 19 of Chapter 3) can also increase comfort and efficacy and eliminate the orthodontic deformity that otherwise may occur in some long-term users of continuous IPPV (Fig. 6).

Generally, symptoms from nasal insufflation leakage during lipseal IPPV remain subclinical because the typically used high ventilator insufflation volumes of 1000–2000 ml compensate, at least in part, for nasal leakage. While using nocturnal nasal or lipseal IPPV

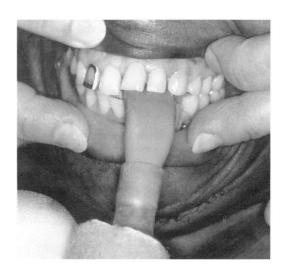

FIGURE 6. Orthodontic deformity caused by 15 years of 24-hour mouthpiece IPPV without a custom bite-plate. (Courtesy of Augusta Alba, M.D.)

in a regimen of 24-hour noninvasive ventilatory support, 3–10% of patients (5 of 161 in one study[24]) with no breathing tolerance have episodes of excessive insufflation leakage and transient oxyhemoglobin desaturation and periods of hypercapnia during sleep—despite the maintenance of normal daytime alveolar ventilation. These episodes can result in arousals with shortness of breath. The patient also may complain of recurrence of morning headaches, fatigue, and perhaps nightmares and anxiety. The nasal ventilation user can be switched to lipseal IPPV, and lipseal IPPV systems can be "closed" by clipping the patient's nostrils or plugging them with cotton and covering them with a Band-aid during sleep. Another practical solution is to set the ventilator's low-pressure alarm at a level that stimulates the patient sufficiently to shorten periods of excessive insufflation leakage during sleep. A low-pressure alarm setting of 10–20 cmH_2O is commonly used for this purpose, and the patient develops conditioned reflexes to prevent prolonged oxyhemoglobin desaturation and hypoventilation associated with excessive leak.

Nasal IPPV Nasal IPPV is preferred to lipseal IPPV by more than two-thirds of patients who use IPPV only for sleep.[25] Nasal IPPV with PEEP can be provided by portable pressure- or volume-cycled ventilators. Numerous nasal interfaces (CPAP masks) are commercially available (Table 1). Each interface design applies pressure differently to the paranasal area. One cannot predict which model will be most effective and preferred by a particular patient (Figs. 7 and 8). Nasal bridge pressure and insufflation leakage into the eyes are common complaints with several of these generic models. Such difficulties resulted in the fabrication of interfaces that mold themselves to facial tissues and custom-molded interface designs (Fig. 9).[25–30] No patient should be offered and expected to use only one nasal interface any more than a patient should be offered only lipseal or oral-nasal interfaces. Alternating IPPV interfaces nightly alternates skin pressure sites, minimizes discomfort, and should be encouraged.

Excessive insufflation leakage via the mouth is prevented by keeping ventilatory drive intact by maintaining normal daytime carbon dioxide and avoiding supplemental oxygen and sedatives (see Chapter 5). However, in the presence of daytime hypercapnia and excessive nocturnal oxyhemoglobin desaturation and bothersome arousals, a chin-strap or

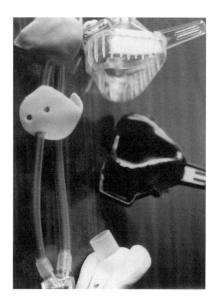

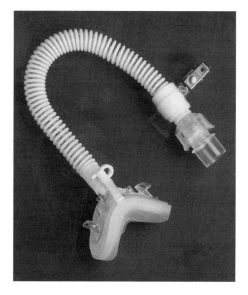

FIGURE 7. Various nasal interfaces.   **FIGURE 8.** Respironics Monarch Mini-Mask.

TABLE 1. Interfaces

Manufacturer	Interface Model	Headgear Mode	Interface Sizes	Headgear Sizes	Interface Material in Contact with Patient	Customizeable Features	Facial Coverage	Comments
AirSep	Ultimate Nasal Mask	Y type or Polynet type	S, M, L	S, M, L	Translucent silicone rubber Optional Gel Ultimate Seal	Malleable nose strap, optional Ultimate Seal (gel interface)	Small nasal mask	
Fisher Paykel	Aclaim	Aclaim		Comes with mask	Silicone rubber		Oronasal	
Fisher Paykel	Oracle	No headgear is needed	One size	NA	Silicone rubber		Oral	
Hans Rudolph	Nasal CPAP Mask	Meshnet headgear or strap-only	S, M, L	S, M, L	Silicone rubber	Nose strap, Comfort Seal, Ultimate Seal, chin strap	Small nasal mask	
Hans Rudolph	Face Mask	Meshnet	Premie, neonate, infant, Ped S, Ped L, Adult S, M, L	4 sizes	Silicone rubber	Comfort Seal, Ultimate Seal	Covers mouth, nose, and chin	Ultimate Seal (hydrogel material) Comfort Seal (soft foam) has wound healing properties Single piece, molded design—no bonded pieces Can wash in dishwasher
Mallincrodt-Puritan-Bennett	Lipseal	2 Velcro straps			Plastic		Covers mouth	
Metamed	Masque buccal	Straps			Silicone		Mouth and lips	

(Continued on following page)

TABLE 1. Interfaces *(Continued)*

Manufacturer	Interface Model	Headgear Mode	Interface Sizes	Headgear Sizes	Interface Material in Contact with Patient	Customizeable Features	Facial Coverage	Comments
ResMed	Full Face Mirage	Full Face Headgear	S, M, L		Silicone rubber	Adjustable arms so nasal cushions can sit closer or further from face	Standard nasal with forehead assembly	Are masks shipped clear or sterile or needing cleaning? Mask may be high level disinfected or sterilized Mask may be purchased with or without nasal partition (making it a mouth breathing mask only); with or without female leur lock, oxygen leak hole (?); can wash in dishwasher
ResMed	Sullivan Mirage Nasal Mask	Mirage Headgear	Standard, large, shallow	Comes with mask	Silicone rubber	Angle of forehead pads can be adjusted	Standard nasal with forehead assembly	Standard, large, shallow (lower nasal bridge, e.g., Japanese customers) or very high nasal bridge (e.g., American Indian and mustaches and patients who take dentures out at night) The instructions say the mask must be disassembled for cleaning. It is difficult to separate the elbow from the mask
						None noted	Covers mouth, nose, and part of cheeks and chin	
ResMed	Ultra Mirage Nasal Mask	Ultra Mirage Headgear	Standard, large, shallow	Comes with mask	Silicone rubber	Removable gel spacer	Standard nasal mask with 1 forehead pad	Includes antiasphyxia valve in case flow generator stops Valve membrane must be changed every 6 months Also has "quick-release" tab to quickly remove mask in case of emergency

Manufacturer	Product	Headgear	Sizes	Fit	Material	Features	Interface type	Comments
Respironics	Contour Deluxe	Any 4-point attachment headgear	S, M, L		Silicone rubber	Spacers, support ring, chin strap, comfort flap	Standard nasal mask	The exhalation port is included in the mask
Respironics	Reusable Contour	Any 4-point attachment headgear	P, S, M/S, M, M/W, L, L/N		Silicone rubber			Must also purchase exhalation port
Respironics	Mini Monarch and Monarch		1 size each	1 size fits all	Silicone rubber	Spacers, support ring, and mask may be boiled to adjust to facial contours	Standard nasal mask	
Respironics	Angled mouth-piece		15 mm; 22 mm		Silicone rubber		Mouthpiece	
Respironics	Profile Lite	Any 4-point attachment headgear	P, S, M/S, M, M/W, L, LN		Soft polyurethane film over pliable gel material	Hose may be worn up or down, comes with stability clip	Small nasal	Stability clip is provided for attaching hose to maskstrap or bed clothing to relieve tension on hose. The exhalation port is included in the mask
Respironics	Simplicity	Simplicity nasal mask headgear	S, M	1 size fits all	Silicone rubber	Forehead pad and comfort flap (optional, included)	Covers mouth and nose and some of the chin	
Respironics	Soft Series	Any 4-point attachment headgear	Ped, S, M, MW, MN, L, LN		Silicone rubber	None noted	Covers entire face	Must also purchase an exhalation port. Mask includes a Fresh Air Entrainment valve in case blower unit fails; the patient can draw in room air. An NG tube sealing pad is an optional accessory to maintain mask seal when NG tube is in place

(Continued on following page)

TABLE 1. Interfaces *(Continued)*

Manufacturer	Interface Model	Headgear Mode	Interface Sizes	Headgear Sizes	Interface Material in Contact with Patient	Customizeable Features	Facial Coverage	Comments
Respironics	Spectrum Reusable Full Face Mask	Convertible Headgear, Softcap, simple strap, reusable headgear	P, S, M, L		Silicone rubber		Oronasal	The system pressure and oxygen therapy must be modified for this mask vs. standard interfaces. Fresh air entrainment valve contains a magnet, so do not use near MRI
Respironics	Total Face Mask	Total Face Mask Headgear	1 size	1 size	Silicone rubber		Oronasal	
SleepNet	Phantom	Phantom Headgear	1 size	1 size (comes with 2 strap lengths)	Soft polyurethane film over pliable gel material	Nose clip, strap length; design allows tubing to attach to either side	Standard nasal plus covers part of cheeks	
SleepNet	IQ	EZ Cap Headgear	1 size	S, M, L	Soft polyurethane film over pliable gel material	Pliable ring molded into flexible shell; tubing can be worn up or down	Standard nasal	
Sunrise Medical	DeVillbiss Serenity	Strap-Style or Cap-Style	S, MS, M, L	1 size	Silicone rubber		Standard nasal	
Tiara	AirPilot Nasal Mask	AirPilot Headgear	1 size	1 size	Silicone rubber	Forehead pad height adjustment	Standard nasal mask plus forehead assembly	
Tiara	CoolCap	Blue Horizon Headgear	1 size	S, M, L, XL	Soft polyurethane film over pliable gel material	Nose clip, and strap length; designs allow tubing to attach to either side	Standard nasal plus covers part of cheeks	
Tiara	Comfort System Mask	CoolCap	1 size	S, M, L, XL	Silicone rubber	Pliable ring molded into flexible shell; tubing can be worn up or down	Standard nasal	
Tiara	IQ	CoolCap	1 size	S, M, L, XL	Soft polyurethane film over pliable gel material	Optional spacer pad	Standard nasal	

			Sizes	Material	Adjustability	Type
Tyco	Adam Ciruit (nasal pillows)	SnugFit	Pillows come in S, M, L, XL; dilator pillows come in S, M, L	Pillows are silicone rubber	Different pillow sizes	Nasal
Tyco	Breeze Sleepgear with Nasal Pillows Assembly	Breeze Sleepgear	Pillows come in S, M, L, XL; dilator pillows come in S, M, L	Pillows are silicone rubber	Comes with S, M, and L nasal pillows; other sizes can be purchased. Dilator pillows are also available in S, M, L. Straps can be adjusted to various configurations (height, length, and angle of the headgear)	Nasal
Tyco	Breeze Sleepgear with Dreamseal Assembly	Breeze Sleepgear	1 size	Silicone gear	Straps can be adjusted to various configurations (height, length, and angle of the headgear)	Standard nasal mask
Tyco	Companion Vinyl Mask	Snugfit	S, M, L	Vinyl	Foam forehead pads and forehead clip (used to hold pad)	Standard nasal mask
Tyco	SoftFit	Snugfit	SN, S, SW, M, MW, L		Foam forehead pads and forehead clip (used to hold pad)	Standard nasal mask
Tyco	SoftFit Ultra	Snugfit	SN, S, SW, M, MW, L		Foam forehead pads and forehead clip (used to hold pad)	Standard nasal mask
Tyco	Mouth Seal	Strap Assembly	1 size	1 size	None noted	Minimal—covers lips only

S = small, M = medium, L = large, P = pediatric, Ped S = pediatric small, Ped L = pediatric large, NA = not applicable, SW = small wide, MW = medium wide, MN = medium narrow, LN = large narrow, XL = extra large, NG = nasogastric, MRI = magnetic resonance imaging.

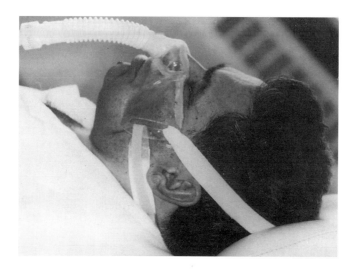

FIGURE 9. Patient with severe chronic alveolar hypoventilation due to kyphoscoliosis who uses a low-profile custom acrylic nasal interface for nocturnal nasal IPPV.

plugged lipseal without mouthpiece can be used to decrease oral leakage for patients not wishing to switch to lipseal IPPV. In the presence of nasal congestion, patients either use decongestants to permit nasal IPPV or switch to mouthpiece and lipseal IPPV or, on rare occasions, use a body ventilator. Most often the patient continues nasal IPPV using decongestants.

Oral-Nasal Interfaces. Oral-nasal interfaces can have strap retention systems like those for mouthpiece or nasal IPPV. Respironics, Inc. (Murrysville, PA) and HealthDyne (Minneapolis, MN) produce comfortable strap-retained oronasal interfaces. Respironics, Inc., manufactures a transparent full-face mask with an inner gasket that creates a hermetic seal around the nose and mouth and was reported in one center to be more comfortable and to provide a better seal than other commonly available nasal interfaces.[31] Custom-prepared strap-retained oral-nasal interfaces are also available.[32,33] These oronasal delivery systems can be comfortable alternatives to lipseal or nasal IPPV (see Fig. 21 of Chapter 3). However, because effective ventilatory support usually can be provided by either nasal or mouthpiece/lipseal IPPV, strap-retained oral-nasal interfaces have been used for long-term ventilatory assistance in few centers. They are used more frequently in the intensive care setting.[34]

Strapless acrylic oral-nasal interfaces (SONIs) with bite-plate retention can require 10 hours or more to construct. However, these interfaces provide more air-tight seal for the delivery of IPPV, and simple tongue thrust is all that is needed to expel them.[35] They also permit better speech than lipseal use. The bite-plate retention is important for patients living alone who are unable to don straps independently (Figs. 10 and 11).[36,37] Adequate and stable dentition is necessary for their use.

Mouthpiece and nasal IPPV typically are used as open systems, and the user relies on central nervous system reflexes to prevent excessive insufflation leakage during sleep (see Chapter 5).[25,36,38] Essentially closed noninvasive IPPV systems include lipseal with nasal pledgets (Fig. 12), strap-retained oral-nasal interfaces (Fig. 13), and SONIs. For an essentially leakless system using a SONI, however, the user must be observed while sleeping and the final touches applied to the acrylic shell and bite-plate to eliminate any insufflation leakage created by loosening of the interface seal as facial soft tissues shift during sleep.[28]

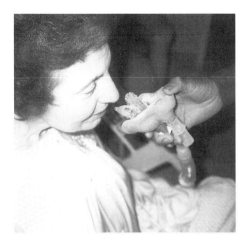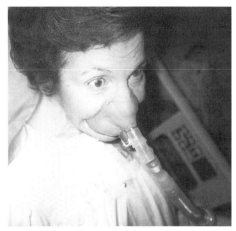

FIGURE 10 *(left).* Patient with poliomyelitis who has used daytime mouthpiece IPPV and noctur-nal IPPV via a strapless oral-nasal interface (seen here) since 1984.

FIGURE 11 *(right).* Oronasal interface that requires no strap retention.

Interface Choice. Because everyone's face and especially nose (Fig. 14) have differ-ent anatomy, one cannot predict which interface will provide the best seal and least insuf-flation leakage or with which interface a particular patient will be most comfortable. A small study comparing a generic nasal "mask" with nasal prongs and full-face interface re-ported significantly higher minute ventilation and greater decreases in $PaCO_2$ with the full-face interface. Nevertheless, patients should be offered a variety of interfaces and, to a large degree, allowed to choose. The same study found no differences in tolerance to ven-tilation, blood gases, or breathing patterns with assist-control or pressure-assist modes. The authors concluded that, regardless of the underlying pathology, the type of interface affects the noninvasive ventilation outcomes more than the ventilatory mode.[39]

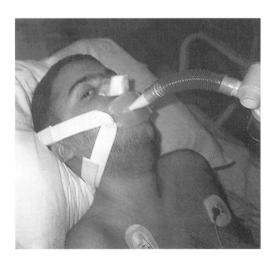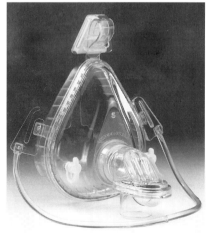

FIGURE 12 *(left).* A 29-year-old patient with Duchenne muscular dystrophy using lipseal IPPV with nasal pledgets.

FIGURE 13 *(right).* Respironics Full-Face Mask.

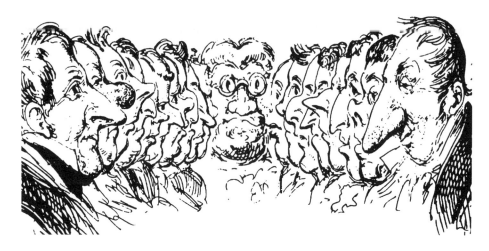

FIGURE 14. Different styles of noses for interface fit. (Drawing by George Cruikshank, 1792–1878.)

Daytime Inspiratory Muscle Aids

Body Ventilators. The chest-shell ventilator is cumbersome, inconvenient, and often not highly effective for the sitting patient. The intermittent abdominal pressure ventilator (IAPV), on the other hand, can be quite effective. It involves the intermittent inflation of an elastic air sac that is contained in a corset or belt worn beneath the patient's outer clothing (Fig. 15) (Exsufflation Belt, Respironics, Inc., Murrysville, PA). The sac is cyclically inflated by a positive-pressure ventilator. The most effective one currently on the market for this purpose is the Achieva (Mallincrodt, Pleasanton, CA). Bladder inflation moves the diaphragm upward. During bladder deflation gravity causes the abdominal contents and diaphragm to return to the resting position, and inspiration occurs passively. A trunk angle of 30° or more from the horizontal is necessary for the device to be effective. Patients who

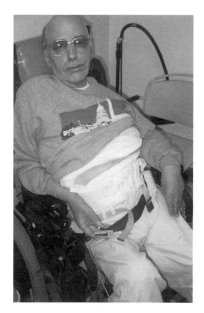

FIGURE 15. A 51-year-old man with muscular dystrophy who has used the intermittent abdominal pressure ventilator (Exsufflation Belt, Lifecare International, Inc., Westminster, CO) during the day and lipseal IPPV during the night since 1979.

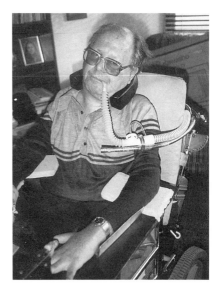

FIGURE 16. Patient with poliomyelitis who used 24-hour mouthpiece IPPV from 1958 until 1995 when he died from leukemia. He kept the small, flexed mouthpiece in place without any other retention despite the fact that he had no upper limb function.

have any inspiratory capacity or are capable of GPB can add volumes of air autonomously taken in to the volume taken in mechanically. The IAPV generally augments tidal volumes by about 300 ml, but volumes as high as 1200 ml have been reported.[40] Patients with less than one hour of breathing tolerance usually prefer to use the IAPV rather than noninvasive IPPV during daytime hours.[40] The IAPV is usually inadequate in the presence of scoliosis or obesity. Recently, an IAPV was created from two blood pressure cuffs.[41]

Mouthpiece IPPV. Mouthpiece IPPV is the most important method of daytime ventilatory support. Some patients keep the mouthpiece between their teeth all day (Fig. 16). Most patients prefer to have the mouthpiece held near the mouth. A metal clamp attached to a wheelchair can be used for this purpose (Fig. 17), or the mouthpiece can be fixed onto motorized wheelchair controls (most often, sip and puff; see Figure 17 of Chapter 3) or chin or tongue (Fig. 18) controls. The ventilator is set for large tidal volumes, often 1000–2000 ml. The patient grabs the mouthpiece with his or her mouth and supplements or substitutes for inadequate autonomous breath volumes. The patient varies the volume of

FIGURE 17. Patient with Duchenne muscular dystrophy using mouthpiece IPPV with the mouthpiece supported by "gooseneck clamp" within reach of the patient's lips.

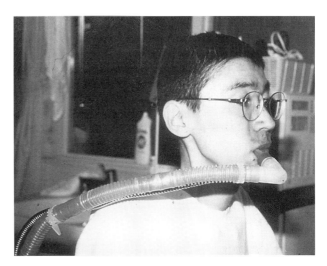

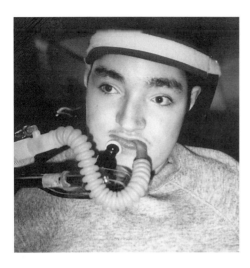

FIGURE 18. Patient with Duchenne muscular dystrophy who has used 24-hour mouthpiece IPPV for 20 years. He now has less than 1 minute of breathing tolerance. The mouthpiece is fixed adjacent to the chin controls for his motorized wheelchair.

air taken from ventilator cycle to ventilator cycle and breath to breath to vary speech volume and cough flows as well as to air-stack for full expansion of the lungs.

To use mouthpiece IPPV effectively and conveniently, adequate neck rotation and oral motor function are necessary to grab the mouthpiece and receive IPPV without insufflation leakage. To prevent leakage, the soft palate must move posterocaudally to seal off the nasopharynx. In addition, the patient must open the glottis and vocal cords, dilate the hypopharynx, and maintain airway patency to receive the air. These normally reflexive movements may require a few minutes to relearn for patients who have been receiving IPPV via a tracheostomy tube, especially one with an inflated cuff, because reflexive abduction of the hypopharynx and glottis is lost during tracheostomy IPPV. Often patients are thought to have tracheal stenosis or other reasons for upper airway obstruction before they learn to reopen the glottis to permit IPPV.

Because the low-pressure alarms of volume-cycled ventilators often cannot be turned off, an angled mouthpiece (Fig. 19) for IPPV or an in-line regenerative humidifier can be used to prevent alarm sounding during routine daytime IPPV when the patient does not receive every delivered volume. These devices create 2–3 cmH$_2$O back pressure, which is usually adequate to prevent low-pressure alarm sounding.

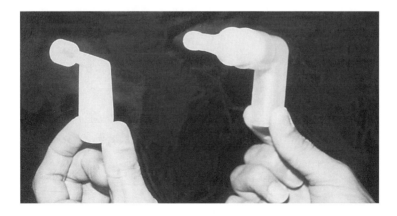

FIGURE 19. Simple mouthpieces for daytime IPPV (Respironics Inc., Murrysville, PA).

Nasal IPPV. Because patients prefer mouthpiece IPPV or an IAPV for daytime use,[25,40] nasal IPPV is most practical only for nocturnal use. Daytime nasal IPPV is indicated for infants and patients who cannot grab or retain a mouthpiece because of oral muscle weakness, inadequate jaw opening, or insufficient neck movement. Twenty-four-hour nasal IPPV, nevertheless, can be a viable and desirable alternative to tracheostomy even for some patients with severe lip and oropharyngeal muscle weakness.[25] Nasal IPPV users learn to close the mouth or seal off the oropharynx with the soft palate and tongue to prevent oral insufflation leakage.

COMPLICATIONS OF NONINVASIVE IPPV AND BAROTRAUMA

In addition to orthodontic deformities and skin pressure from the interface, other potential difficulties include allergy to the plastic lipseal or silicone interfaces (13 vs. 5% for nonsilicone interfaces), dry mouth (65%), eye irritation from air leakage (about 24%), nasal congestion (25%) and dripping (35%), sinusitis (8%), nose bleeding (4 to 19%), gum discomfort (20%) and receding from nasal interface or lipseal pressure, maxillary flattening in children, aerophagia,[29,42] and, as for invasive ventilation, barotrauma. In addition, occasional patients express claustrophobia. Proper interface selection eliminates or minimizes discomfort.

Pressure drop-off through the narrow air passages of the nose is normally between 2 and 3 cmH_2O. Suboptimal humidification dries out and irritates nasal mucus membranes, causes sore throat, and results in vasodilatation and nasal congestion. Increased airflow resistance to 8 cmH_2O can be caused by the loss of humidity due to unidirectional airflow with expiration via the mouth during nasal CPAP or IPPV.[43] This problem cannot be ameliorated by using a cold passover humidifier, but the increase in airway resistance can be reduced by 50% by warming the inspired air to body temperature and humidifying it with a hot-water bath humidifier.[43] Decongestants also can relieve sinus irritation and nasal congestion. Switching to lipseal IPPV can relieve most, if not all, difficulties associated with nasal IPPV. There is also one report of a unilateral orbital herniation after initiation of noninvasive ventilation for obstructive sleep apnea syndrome (OSAS) diagnosed after an intracranial hemorrhage.[44] Relative contraindications to the long-term use of noninvasive inspiratory muscle aids are considered in Table 2.[6]

Abdominal distention tends to occur sporadically in noninvasive IPPV users. Normally the gastroesophageal sphincter can withstand peak airway pressures up to 25 cmH_2O without stomach dilatation. Aerophagia usually occurs only when ventilator-delivered volumes meet with airway obstruction, resulting in peak pressures over 25 cmH_2O. Aerophagia may occur or be exacerbated when patients assume the supine position, especially when the patient reclines in the hour or so after meals.[45] The air usually passes as flatus once the patient arises or is placed into a wheelchair in the morning. Severe aerophagia can present as intestinal pseudo-obstruction with diminished bowel sounds and increased ventilator

TABLE 2. Relative Contraindications for Long-Term Noninvasive IPPV

1. Lack of cooperation or use of heavy sedation or narcotics
2. Need for high levels of supplemental oxygen therapy
3. SpO_2 can not be maintained above 94% (assuming optimal use of assisted coughing techniques when needed)
4. Bulbar muscle function is inadequate for swallowing without aspiration that causes SpO_2 baseline to decrease below 95%
5. Substance abuse or uncontrollable seizures
6. Unassisted or assisted PCFs cannot exceed 2.7 L/sec
7. Conditions that interfere with the use of IPPV interfaces, e.g., facial fractures, inadequate bite for mouthpiece entry, presence of beards that hamper airtight interface seal

dependence. A rectal tube usually can decompress the colon; a gastrostomy tube, when present, can be burped; or a nasogastric tube can be passed to relieve the problem. Although we have never had to discontinue noninvasive IPPV for any patient because of aerophagia first observed after initiation of noninvasive ventilation, in patients with previous aerophagia and severe abdominal distention the distention usually is exacerbated by noninvasive IPPV. For this reason reason, the patient cannot tolerate noninvasive IPPV unless a gastrostomy tube is placed to alleviate the problem. Such patients also may benefit from colostomy or need to undergo tracheostomy.

Barotrauma is lung damage due to overexpansion of lung units. It can occur with invasive or noninvasive ventilation and results from rupture of the boundary between the alveoli and the bronchovascular sheath. Extra-alveolar air entering the lung parenchyma presents as interstitial emphysema and subpleural air cysts. Air also can rupture into the mediastinum, present as subcutaneous emphysema, pneumomediastinum, or pneumoperitoneum, or it can rupture through the fascial planes into the pleural space to result in hemodynamically significant pneumothoraces. The incidence has been cited as 4–15% in intensive-care users of invasive ventilation who suffer primarily from respiratory impairment.[46] One study of 139 patients reported an incidence of 60% in patients with acute respiratory distress syndrome, but barotrauma was not found in patients with congestive heart failure or neurologic disease.[47] Extra-alveolar air also can enter the systemic circulation in patients with a bronchovenous communication and an adequate pressure gradient. Systemic gas embolization is a well-recognized complication in neonatal respiratory distress syndrome.

Pneumothorax in patients receiving IPPV impairs gas exchange and hemodynamics by increasing intrathoracic pressure, decreasing venous return, and increasing afterload to the right side of the heart. The decrease in cardiac output appears to correlate linearly with the volume of pneumothorax.[48] Blood gas alterations may not occur despite the presence of a large pneumothorax, but the airway pressures noted on the ventilator gauge usually increase before blood gas deterioration and acute cardiac decompensation. Computed tomography scans of the chest are as sensitive in diagnosing pneumothoraces as the combination of lateral decubitus, erect, and supine films, and lateral decubitus films can detect pneumothoraces as small as 50 ml. For patients with cardiomyopathies and low left ventricular ejection fractions, sudden evacuation of a pneumothorax can result in hemodynamic collapse.

Numerous investigators have demonstrated that diffuse lung edema, tissue histopathologic changes, and hypoxemia indistinguishable from that which occurs in acute respiratory distress syndrome can develop in normal animals ventilated with moderately high peak airway pressures of 30–50 cmH_2O.[46] Sheep ventilated at 50 cmH_2O pressure developed severely reduced static lung compliance, decreased FRC, hypoxemia, and grossly abnormal lungs within 35 hours.[49] Furthermore, peak inspiratory pressures over 40 cmH_2O are associated with an increased risk of alveolar rupture during mechanical ventilation, and the incidence of barotrauma exceeds 40% in patients exposed to pressures over 70 cmH_2O.[50] However, high airway pressures can be applied to the respiratory system without injury if excessive lung inflation is prevented, as seen in obese patients and patients with decreased abdominal compliance. In such patients, a given change in lung volume is associated with a larger increase in pleural pressures; thus, a greater pressure change at the airway is necessary to inflate the respiratory system. However, because the transmural pressure across the alveolus is no different from that in patients with normal abdominal compliance, the risk of lung injury is not increased.[51] Dreyfuss et al. avoided barotrauma in rats by strapping their chests.[52] The authors also created barotrauma using negative-pressure ventilation that created similar transalveolar pressures. Thus, injury from hyperinflation is due to the extent of the inflation rather than to pressure per se. The risk of barotrauma also is increased by tissue fragility, secretion retention that leads to overexpansion of unobstructed lung units, surfactant depletion, shear forces, and duration of ventilation.[46] Patients ventilated over the long term by increasing dead-space ventilation with high delivered volumes and pressures over 40 cmH$_2$O can develop surfactant depletion, inflammation, and alveolar rupture associated with shear and alveolar distention similar to that seen in adult respiratory distress syndrome.[53,54] However, we have witnessed no barotrauma in patients who suffer primarily from ventilatory impairment (and have essentially normal lung tissues) with multiple daily lung hyperinsufflations to pressures of 60 or 80 cmH$_2$O.

The strategies for diminishing the risk of barotrauma in patients who suffer primarily from respiratory impairment include pressure-cycled ventilation and lowering of pressures by increasing rate, adding PEEP, and permitting hypercapnia. In patients with COPD, however, the lungs may be hypercompliant and require low IPAPs for assisted ventilation; PEEP can counter the effects of air trapping; and hypercapnia may be necessary for ventilator weaning. Any ventilator use may only increase air trapping, and prognosis is generally poor. For patients who suffer primarily from ventilatory impairment, on the other hand, this approach is inappropriate. Permitting hypercapnia increases the risk of morbidity and mortality.[55] Air trapping is not a problem, and PEEP only decreases the extent of respiratory muscle rest (lowering the IPAP–EPAP span). No increased incidence of barotrauma has been reported by using volume- rather than pressure-cycled ventilators (see Table 2 of Chapter 6). We have observed few pneumothoraces in the over 800 ventilator users whom we have managed, many of whom used noninvasive IPPV at airway pressures of 30–45 cmH$_2$O for up to 50 years. Limiting ventilation volumes at the cost of increasing breathing rate and hypercapnia results only in increased pulmonary and chest-wall restriction (see Chapters 5 and 6).

Inspissated secretions are often considered a "life-threatening" complication of noninvasive ventilation.[56,57] However, except for patients with assisted PCF less than 160 L/m who cannot effectively use assisted coughing and have essentially respiratory rather than ventilatory impairment, secretion encumberment is a complication more often of the clinician's failure to teach assisted coughing than of noninvasive ventilation. Because there are 10^{12}–10^{17} bacteria per milliliter of saliva,[58] chronic aspiration of saliva to the extent of lowering baseline SpO$_2$ can overwhelm normally sterile airways and lead to pneumonia,[59] tracheitis, bronchitis,[60] and chronic lung disease.[59] Thus, the only respiratory indication for tracheostomy is assisted PCF less than 160 L/m and SpO$_2$ baseline less than 95% due to chronic airway secretion aspiration. This finding is rare except in for averbal patients with bulbar ALS.

Goal Three: Provide Functional Coughs by Assisting Expiratory Muscles

Why Are Expiratory Muscle Aids Needed?

Bulbar, inspiratory, and expiratory muscles are needed for effective coughing. The expiratory muscles are predominantly the abdominal and intercostal muscles (see Chapter 2). Clearing airway secretions and airway mucus can be a continual problem for patients with airways diseases, certain lung diseases, or generalized muscle weakness and for patients who cannot swallow saliva or food without aspiration. For patients with respiratory muscle dysfunction and functional bulbar musculature, secretion clearance becomes a problem during chest infections, after general anesthesia, and during any other period of bronchial hypersecretion.

Manually Assisted Coughing

The importance of manually assisted coughing to permit effective long-term use of noninvasive ventilation is increasingly recognized by MDA clinic physicians[61] and others.[61,62] PCF is increased by manually assisted coughing. If the vital capacity is under 1.5 L, insufflating the patient to the MIC is especially important to optimize cough flows.[63] Once the patient takes a breath to at least 1.5 L or is insufflated to the MIC, an abdominal thrust is timed to glottic opening as the patient initiates the cough. It was recognized as early as 1966 that assisted PCF could be doubled and readily exceed 6 L/sec in patients receiving maximal insufflations prior to manual thrusts.[64] In 364 evaluations of our patients with NMD who were able to air stack, the mean vital capacity in the sitting position was 996.9 ml, the mean MIC was 1647.6 ml, and, although PCF was 2.3 L/sec (less than 2.7 L/sec or the minimum needed to eliminate airway secretions), mean assisted PCF was 3.9 L/sec.

Although an optimal insufflation followed by an abdominal thrust provides the greatest increase in PCF, PCF also can be significantly increased by providing only a maximal insufflation or an abdominal thrust without a preceding maximal insufflation. Of interest, PCF is increased significantly more by maximal insufflation than by abdominal thrust (see Fig. 1). In data from Ishikawa's center in Hokkaido, 21 patients with DMD had unassisted PCF of 160 ± 88 L/min, PCF with an abdominal thrust of 242 ± 92 L/min, PCF from the MIC of 274 ± 80 L/min, and PCF from the MIC with an abdominal thrust (assisted PCF) of 356 ± 88 L/min (personal communication). Techniques of manually assisted coughing involve different hand and arm placements for expiratory cycle thrusts (Fig. 20). An epigastric thrust with one hand while counterpressure is applied with the other arm and hand across the chest to avoid paradoxical chest expansion further increases assisted PCF for 20% of patients.[63]

Manually assisted coughing requires a cooperative patient, good coordination between the patient and caregiver, and adequate physical effort and often frequent application by the caregiver. It is usually ineffective in the presence of severe scoliosis because of a combination of restricted lung capacity and the inability to effect diaphragm movement by abdominal thrusting because of severe rib cage and diaphragm deformity.

Abdominal compressions should not be used for 1–1.5 hours after a meal, but chest compressions can be used to augment PCF (Fig. 21). Chest-thrusting techniques must be performed with caution in the presence of an osteoporotic rib cage. Unfortunately, because it is not widely taught to health care professionals,[65] manually assisted coughing is underutilized.[66] When PCF is inadequate, especially when inadequacy is due to difficulty with air-stacking, the most effective alternative for generating optimal PCF and clearing airway secretions is the use of mechanical insufflation-exsufflation (MI-E).

The inability to generate over 2.7 L/sec or 160 L/min of assisted PCF despite a vital capacity or MIC greater than 1 L usually indicates fixed upper airway obstruction or severe

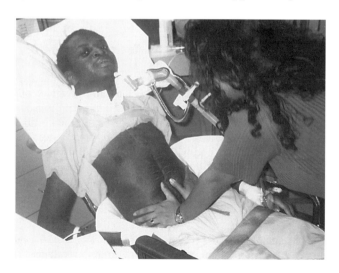

FIGURE 20.   Hand placement for manually assisted coughing.

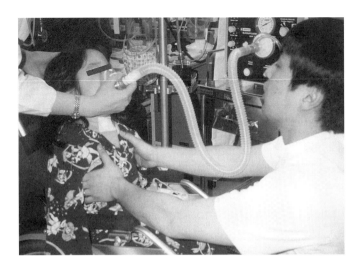

FIGURE 21.   Tussive squeeze applied to the chest during the exsufflation cycle of mechanical insufflation-exsufflation.

bulbar muscle weakness and hypopharyngeal collapse during coughing attempts. Vocal cord adhesions or paralysis may have resulted from a previous translaryngeal intubation or tracheostomy.[67] Because some lesions, especially obstructing granulation tissue, can be corrected surgically, laryngoscopic examination is warranted.

Sir Patrick: Don't misunderstand me, my boy, I'm not belittling your discovery. Most discoveries are made regularly every fifteen years; and it's fully a hundred and fifty since yours was made last. That's something to be proud of. . .

George Bernard Shaw
The Doctor's Dilemma

Mechanical Insufflation-Exsufflation

Introduction of MI-E.   Mechanical insufflator-exsufflators (Cough Assist, J. H. Emerson Co., Cambridge, MA) (see Fig. 21) deliver deep insufflations followed immediately by deep exsufflations. The insufflation and exsufflation pressures and delivery times are independently adjustable. Insufflation to exsufflation pressures of + 40 to – 40 cmH$_2$O are usually the most effective and are preferred by most patients. Onset of insufflation generates a insufflation flow peak (Fig. 22) and a lung insufflation of over 2 liters. A second insufflation flow notch occurs when exsufflation terminates and is due to the reversal of air flow as air re-enters the lung and the lung volume returns to its functional residual capacity. Mechanical exsufflation generates two exsufflation flow notches. One occurs when the insufflation pressure stops and is due to the elastic recoil of the lung. The second flow notch, a bit greater, is caused by the exsufflation pressure itself. Except after a meal, an abdominal thrust is applied in conjunction with the exsufflation (MAC). Mechanical insufflaftion-exsufflation can be provided via an oral-nasal mask, a simple mouthpiece, or a translaryngeal or tracheostomy tube. When MI-E is delivered via tracheostomy, the cuff, if present, should be inflated.

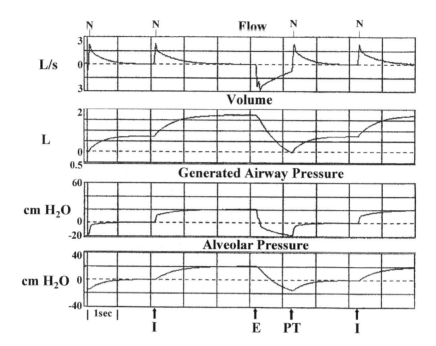

FIGURE 22. Pressure, volume, and flow relationships of mechanical insufflation-exsufflation for insufflation to exsufflation pressures of 20 to –20 cmH₂O, insufflation time of 3 seconds, exsufflation time of 1 second, and pause time of 2 seconds. I denotes onset of insufflation. E denotes onset of exsufflation. PT denotes onset of pause between insufflation and exsufflation.

The Cough Assist can be cycled manually or automatically. Manual cycling facilitates care giver-patient coordination of inspiration and expiration with insufflation and exsufflation, but it requires hands to deliver an abdominal thrust, to hold the mask on the patient, and to cycle the machine. Although the Cough Assist is the only commercially available device that performs MI-E, it is possible to devise less expensive systems. One such system devised in Israel is essentially a double-cylinder valve mechanism simultaneously connecting a vacuum cleaner and a manual resuscitator to a face mask. A simple sliding mechanism operated by the caregiver or patient shifts between the vacuum cleaner and manual resuscitator (personal communication with Eliezer Be'eri, M.D., Jerusalem).

One treatment consists of about five cycles of MI-E or MAC followed by a short period of normal breathing or ventilator use to avoid hyperventilation. Insufflation and exsufflation pressures almost always from + 35 to + 60 cmH₂O to – 35 to – 60 cmH₂O. Most patients use pressures of 35–45 cmH₂O for insufflations and exsufflations. In experimental models, pressures of + 40 to – 40 cmH₂O have been shown to provide maximal forced deflation vital capacity and flows.[68] Insufflation and exsufflation times are adjusted to provide maximal chest expansion and lung emptying, respectively. In general, 2–4 seconds are used. In a recent study in a lung model with normal human compliance, insufflation volumes exceeded 90% of predicted inspiratory capacity when insufflation times were over 5 seconds. In reality, because of lung inertial factors, pressures of 40 cmH₂O can take a full minute to inflate lung tissues fully.[2]

Multiple treatments are given in one sitting until no further secretions are expelled, and any secretion- or mucus-induced oxyhemoglobin desaturation is reversed. Use can be required as frequently as every few minutes around the clock during chest infections when the user is awake. Although no medications are usually required for effective MI-E in neuromuscular ventilator users, liquefaction of sputum using heated aerosol treatments may facilitate exsufflation when secretions are inspissated.

We have routinely used MI-E via translaryngeal and tracheostomy tubes in children with spinal muscular atrophy under 1 year of age. We use pressure settings of +35 to +70 to –35 to –70 through the narrow-gauge pediatric tubes. The severe pressure drop-off caused by the narrow gauge may not always permit the generation of optimal exsufflation flows. However, even at these apparently inadequate pressures secretions can be expulsed and SpO_2 normalized. How to compensate for the pressure drop-offs through narrow tubes needs to be determined.

A recent study measured flow-pressure relationships through endotracheal and tracheostomy tubes of various diameters.[69] Although only positive pressures were used and exsufflation is created by a drop from positive to negative pressure, drop-offs in pressures and flows with tube narrowing are comparable, whether only positive or negative pressures are used. Flows up to 200 L/min, only one third of the maximal flows emanating from MI-E, were measured. Providing 40 cmH_2O of air pressure through a tracheostomy tube with a diameter of 8.5 mm resulted in flows of 170 L/min, whereas the same pressure via a 4.5-mm tube (size of a mini-tracheostomy tube, 0.5 mm smaller than a small adult tube) resulted in a flow of only about 65 L/min. The same 40-cmH_2O pressure via an 8.5-mm endotracheal tube achieved a flow of 200 L/min, whereas a 40-cmH_2O pressure via a 5-mm tube resulted in only 70 L/min and via a 4.5-mm tube in only 55 L/min. Because infant tubes are even narrower, drop offs would be even greater. Whereas in adult airways, 160 L/min measured at the mouth appears to be the critical level for effective coughing,[70] no one has determined the critically effective level for children. However, lower flows may be effective in the airways of small children because cough effectiveness is more a function of the velocity of air rather than its flow.

The use of MI-E via the upper airway can be effective for children as young as 11 months of age. Such patients can become accustomed to MI-E and permit its effective use by not crying or closing their glottis. Between 2.5 and 5 years of age, most children become able to cooperate and cough on cue with MI-E. Exsufflation-timed abdominal thrusts are also used for infants.

Whether via the upper airway or via indwelling airway tubes, routine airway suctioning misses the left mainstem bronchus about 90% of the time. MI-E, on the other hand, provides the same exsufflation flows in both left and right airways without the discomfort or airway trauma of tracheal suctioning and can be effective when suctioning is not (see Case 14 in Chapter 15). Patients almost invariably prefer MI-E to suctioning for comfort and effectiveness and find it less tiring.[71] Deep suctioning, whether via airway tube or the upper airway, can be discontinued for most patients.

Efficacy of Mechanical Insufflation-Exsufflation. The efficacy of MI-E was demonstrated both clinically and in animal models.[72] Flow generation is adequate in both proximal and distal airways to eliminate respiratory tract debris effectively.[73,74] Despite some $dSpO_2$ during MI-E, vital capacity, pulmonary flow rates, and abnormal SpO_2 improve immediately with clearing of airway secretions and mucus by MI-E.[65,75] An increase in vital capacity of 15–42% was noted immediately after treatment in 67 patients with "obstructive dyspnea," and a 55% increase in vital capacity was noted after MI-E in patients with neuromuscular conditions.[76] We have observed improvements of 15–400% (200–800 ml) in vital capacity and normalization of SpO_2 as MI-E eliminates airway mucus for ventilator-assisted patients with NMD and chest infections.[63]

Significant increases in PCF also were demonstrated by use of MI-E in patients with poliomyelitis, bronchiectasis, asthma, and pulmonary emphysema.[77] After instillation of a mucin-thorium dioxide suspension into the lungs of anesthetized dogs, bronchograms revealed virtually complete elimination of the suspension after 6 minutes of MI-E.[72] The technique was shown to be equally effective in expelling bronchoscopically inserted foreign bodies.[72] The use of MI-E through an indwelling tracheostomy tube was demonstrated to be effective in reversing acute atelectasis associated with productive airway secretions;[18] however, PCF was noted to be greater when MI-E was applied via a mask.[79] Barach and Beck demonstrated clinical and radiographic improvement in 92 of 103 patients with upper respiratory infections with the use of MI-E.[76] Included were 72 patients with bronchopulmonary disease and 27 with skeletal or neuromuscular conditions, including poliomyelitis.[78] MI-E was more effective for the latter than for the former.[76]

MI-E has been noted to be effective in the elimination of tenacious sputum before bronchography and of contrast medium after bronchography in patients with bronchial asthma and bronchiectasis. Thus, it has been suggested that MI-E may improve the results of bronchoscopy.[76] Williams and Holaday reported that MI-E could effectively eliminate airway secretions and ventilate patients in the minutes following generalized anesthesia.[80] They applied MI-E both to cooperative and unconscious patients and reported normalization of blood gases in all seven patients, including two with advanced pulmonary emphysema. In addition, improved breath sounds, increased percussion resonance, reduced respiratory rate, clearing of cyanosis, and reversal of right lower lobe collapse were reported for particular patients as a direct result of MI-E. A recent study reported that MI-E was not only effective by comparison with tracheal suctioning and chest physical therapy but also less expansive.[81]

In our practice, MI-E has permitted consistent extubation of patients with NMD after general anesthesia despite their lack of breathing tolerance and subsequent management with noninvasive IPPV. MI-E also has permitted avoidance of intubation or quick extubation of patients with NMD in acute ventilatory failure with no breathing tolerance and profuse airway secretions due to chest infections. In a protocol with manually assisted coughing, oximetry feedback, and home use of noninvasive IPPV, MI-E effectively decreased hospitalizations and respiratory complications and mortality for patients with NMD (see Chapter 9).[75] It may not be effective if the patient cannot cooperate sufficiently to keep the airway open, if a fixed upper or lower airway obstruction is present, or if airways are collapsible on exsufflation so that PCF in adults cannot exceed 160 L/min.[82] This problem is seen most often in patients with advanced bulbar ALS.

Safety of Mechanical Insufflation-Exsufflation. Colebatch observed that applying negative pressure of 40–50 cmH$_2$O is unlikely to have any deleterious effects on pulmonary tissues.[83] He noted that because the negative pressure applied to the airways is analogous to positive pressure on the surface of the lungs during a normal cough, it is improbable that this negative pressure can be more detrimental to the lungs than the normal cough pressure gradient. Furthermore, since FEV$_1$ has been reported only to increase after MI-E, no sustained airway obstruction is caused by the exsufflation cycle of MI-E.[63] Bickerman found no evidence of parenchymal damage, hemorrhage, alveolar tears, or emphysematous blebs in the lungs of animals treated with MI-E.[72] Barach and Beck reported no serious complications in 103 patients treated with over 2000 courses of MI-E, and for no patient did MI-E have to be discontinued.[76] They noted that the initial transient appearance of blood-streaked sputum in a few patients probably originated from the bronchial wall sites after detachment of mucus plugs. Immediately after the initial elimination of blood-streaked sputum, the profuse outpouring of mucopurulent sputum indicated that "obstruction of the atelectatic area had been relieved." In one study, 1 of 19 patients complained of transient nausea associated with the initiation of MI-E. The nausea passed with continued use.[84] Patients with wounds of the abdomen or chest reported less wound pain during MI-E than during spontaneous coughing. No incidence of aspiration of gastric contents has been found either in humans[80] or anesthetized dogs.[72] No reports of damaging side effects have been disclosed in more than 6000 treatments in over 400 patients using MI-E, most of whom suffered primarily from lung disease.[83,85] No publications contradict the reports of effectiveness or describe significant complications of MI-E. Even when used after abdominal surgery and extensive chest-wall surgery, no disruption of recently sutured wounds was noted.[80]

We, too, have observed no serious complications of MI-E in thousands of applications for hundreds of patients, mostly with neuromuscular weakness, many of whom have regularly used MI-E for over 50 years either with the Cof-flators (see Chapter 3) available since 1952 or with the In-exsufflators that came onto the market in 1993. Of interest, before 1993 patients unable to procure Cof-flators often air-stacked, then used vacuum cleaners for exsufflation. We have a number of patients who have depended on continuous noninvasive IPPV at inspiratory positive airway pressures of over 40 cmH$_2$O for longer than 45 years. Thus, the use of equivalent pressures for brief periods of MI-E is very unlikely to cause harm. A recent study using the same pressures on baby monkeys also demonstrated no barotrauma.[68] Borborygmus and abdominal distention are infrequent and can be eliminated by decreasing insufflation (not exsufflation) pressures. As with tracheal suctioning, MI-E can be associated with bradycardias in patients with acute spinal cord injury and spinal shock. Insufflation and exsufflation pressures are increased gradually for such patients. Anticholinergics are used for premedication. The use of high insufflation pressures can cause acute rib cage muscle pulls for patients with low vital capacity who have not routinely received maximal insufflations. Insufflation pressures are also increased gradually for such patients.

Physiology of Mechanical Insufflation-Exsufflation. Physiologic effects of MI-E have been studied in depth.[86] Peripheral venous pressures, as measured in the anterior cubital vein, are slightly raised (i.e., by 5.8 cmH$_2$O) during exsufflation. This is about one-third the increase seen during normal coughing. Blood pressure is increased by an average of 8 mmHg in systole and 4 mmHg in diastole. The pulse can increase or decrease during MI-E, and EKG changes reflect the rotation of the heart at peak inspiratory volumes. The increase in intragastric pressure is 26 mmHg during MI-E and 85 mmHg during normal coughing.[87] With hyperinflation only, falls in cardiac output correlate with increases in tidal volume but not with increases in peak inspiratory pressure, and output can take up to 15 minutes to recover to baseline values.[88]

Dayman[89] found that, in patients with emphysema, the production of high intrathoracic pressures during the glottic-closure phase of unassisted coughing and the subsequent pressure drop result in an even greater pressure difference between the alveoli and lumen of the bronchioles than in normal people. The resulting high alveolar-bronchial pressure gradient can result in closure of bronchioles and obstruction of air exiting the alveoli. Bronchographic appearance of tracheobronchial collapse is much greater during cough than during forced exsufflation.[90] Coughing is, thus, less effective. Part of the benefit of MI-E for patients with COPD was explained by the fact that high expiratory flows occur with lower intrathoracic pressures.[76] It was suggested that patients with COPD or severe intrinsic lung disease should practice passive MI-E[85] (i.e., they should leave the airways passively open and not attempt to cough during exsufflation).

Indications for Mechanical Insufflation-Exsufflation. Because MI-E has been on the market only since February of 1993, there continues to be misinformation and confusion about its indications. Of the three muscle groups required for effective coughing, MI-E can take the place only of the inspiratory and expiratory muscles. Thus, it cannot be used to avert tracheostomy for very long if bulbar function is inadequate to prevent airway collapse, as is often the case in advanced bulbar ALS. On the other hand, patients with completely intact bulbar muscle function, such as most ventilator users with traumatic tetraplegia, can usually air-stack to volumes of 3 L or more, and, unless the patient is quite scoliotic or obese, a properly delivered abdominal thrust can often result in assisted PCF of 6–9 L/sec. These flows should be more than adequate to clear the airways and prevent pneumonia and respiratory failure without the need for MI-E. Thus, patients who need MI-E the most are those whose bulbar muscle function can maintain adequate airway patency but is insufficient to permit optimal air-stacking for assisted PCF over 250–300 L/min. This finding is typical of most patients with nonbulbar ALS/MND. Patients with DMD are the most typical example of those who can consistently avoid hospitalization and respiratory failure by using MI-E during chest colds. Patients with respiratory muscle weakness complicated by scoliosis and inability to capture the asymmetric diaphragm by abdominal thrusting also greatly benefit from MI-E. Its use in pediatrics is reviewed in Chapter 10.

OTHER TECHNIQUES THAT ASSIST RESPIRATORY MUSCLE EFFORT

For patients with paralyzed abdominal musculature (e.g., patients with spinal cord injury) but a well-functioning diaphragm, a thoracoabdominal corset limits the increase in FRC that occurs when the patient assumes the upright position. The resulting mild increase in vital capacity can increase PCF in the upright position. The binder also can help to maintain blood pressure and trunk stability,[64] decrease the subjective effort of breathing, relieve accessory neck and upper intercostal muscle use, decrease respiratory rate, and increase tidal air with a lowering of the total pulmonary ventilation for patients with spinal cord injury and some patients with NMD or pulmonary emphysema.[78]

A 4-inch wide abdominal belt with hand grips or handles has been designed as a postoperative coughing aid.[91] When the patient needs to cough, he or she passes one handle through the other and pulls with both hands. This maneuver instantaneously applies pressure to the abdomen and facilitates a pain-free cough.

An abdominal binder with functional electrical stimulation electrodes (Quik Coff Belt Company, Sunnyvale, CA) has become available to enhance the coughs of patients with spinal cord injury. It has been shown to increase maximal expiratory pressure at the mouth from 30 cmH_2O for spontaneous coughing to 60 cmH_2O. This finding compares favorably with the 80 cmH_2O obtained during manually assisted coughing. Although its use cannot generate the flows of manually assisted coughing, the patient does not require personal assistance, and stimulation can be provided at regular intervals. Further studies are needed to determine the possible clinical utility of this apparatus.[92]

Functional magnetic stimulation has the advantage of stimulating the expiratory muscle of patients with spinal cord injury without the discomfort of electrical stimulation. In a recent study, maximal expiratory pressure at total lung capacity was increased by 29% in trained patients.[93] The effect of this improvement on PCF was not measured.

GLOSSOPHARYNGEAL BREATHING

Both inspiratory and, indirectly, expiratory muscle function can be assisted by GPB.[94] For patients with weak inspiratory muscles and no vital capacity or breathing tolerance, GPB can provide normal alveolar ventilation and perfect safety when they are not using a ventilator or in the event of sudden ventilator failure during the day or night.[94,95] The technique involves the use of the glottis to add to an inspiratory effort by projecting (gulping) boluses of air into the lungs. The glottis closes with each gulp. One breath usually consists of 6–9 gulps of 40–200 ml each (Fig. 23). During the training period the efficiency of GPB can be monitored by spirometrically measuring the milliliters of air per gulp, gulps per breath, and breaths per minute. A training manual[96] (Fig. 24) and numerous videos are available,[97] the best of which was produced in 1999.[98]

Although severe oropharyngeal muscle weakness can limit the usefulness of GPB, Baydur et al.[99] reported success in two ventilator users with DMD. We have managed nine ventilator users with DMD who had no breathing tolerance other than by GPB. Approximately 60% of ventilator users with no autonomous ability to breathe and good bulbar muscle function[95,100] can use GPB for breathing from minutes up to all day. Although potentially extremely useful, GPB is rarely taught because few health care professionals are familiar with the technique. GPB is also rarely useful in the presence of an indwelling tracheostomy tube. It cannot be used when the tube is uncapped, as it is during tracheostomy IPPV; even when the tube is capped, the gulped air tends to leak around the

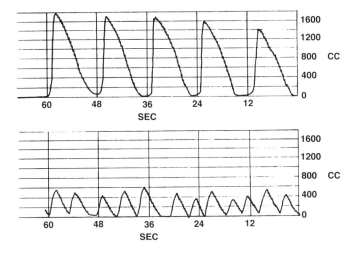

FIGURE 23. *Top*, Patient with a vital capacity of 0 ml. With glossopharyngeal breathing (GPB), his maximal minute ventilation was 8.39 L/min; inspirations averaged 1.67 L, with 20 gulps (84 ml/gulp) for each breath. *Bottom*, The same patient with regular GPB minute ventilation of 4.76 L/min, 12.5 breaths, average of 8 gulps per breath (47.5 ml/gulp) performed over a 1-minute period. (Courtesy of the March of Dimes.)

outer walls of the tube and out the stoma as airway volumes and pressures increase during the GPB air-stacking process. The safety and versatility afforded by GPB are key reasons to eliminate tracheostomy in favor of noninvasive aids (Table 3).

ELECTROPHRENIC RESPIRATION

Although electrophrenic respiration (EPR) is not a noninvasive aid, it can serve as a complement to noninvasive methods in certain patients. Since 1972, over 1000 phrenic nerve pacers have been implanted into patients with central hypoventilation and high-level spinal cord injury, occasionally with highly favorable results.[101]

EPR involves the transmission of a radio-wave signal by an antenna placed on the skin to an implanted receiver. The signal is converted to electrical impulses that are carried to electrodes in contact with the phrenic nerves. The impulses can be delivered in a manner that simulates the natural recruitment of phrenic nerve fibers to stimulate the diaphragm.

The in-hospital training period is at least 4–6 weeks, often much longer, and total initial costs often exceed $300,000. Problems include operative risks, infection, and trauma to the easily damaged phrenic nerves. Unilateral pacing causes paradoxical diaphragmatic movement and microatelectasis. Tidal volumes cannot be routinely modified nor precisely controlled, and voice quality is poorer than for patients using noninvasive methods of support or GPB. Patients using EPR are also subject to potential complications from the tracheostomy. A tracheostomy is maintained in at least 90% of patients using EPR[101] because of the upper airway collapse that often occurs during sleep and possible sudden operational failure[102] and because physicians prescribing EPR are not familiar with noninvasive respiratory aids (else they would not prescribe EPR in the first place).[102] EPR can also be hazardous because of the lack of internal alarms and the inability to use GPB effectively with the tracheostomy tube in place. Neuromuscular fatigue also can lead to irreparable phrenic nerve damage and myopathic changes of the diaphragm.[102,103]

Although EPR has few indications; is invasive, expensive, suboptimally effective, or ineffective for over 60% of patients[104]; and usually entails complications associated with an indwelling tracheostomy, it is indicated for patients with complete C1 to C2 spinal cord

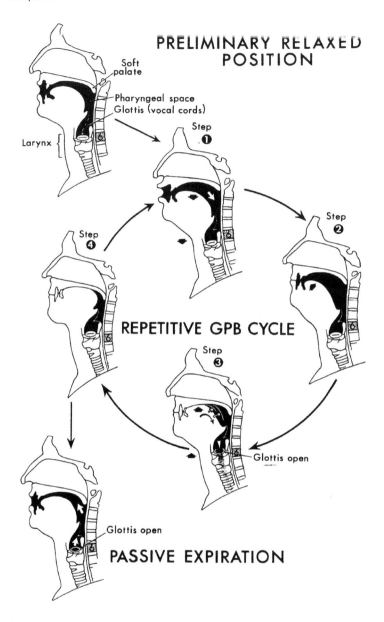

PRELIMINARY RELAXED POSITION

Soft palate

Pharyngeal space
Glottis (vocal cords)

Larynx

Step ❶

Step ❷

Step ❸

Step ❹

REPETITIVE GPB CYCLE

Glottis open

Glottis open

PASSIVE EXPIRATION

FIGURE 24. Demonstration of glossopharyngeal breathing from a classic training manual.[96]

injury who have no measurable vital capacity and inadequate neck rotation or labial strength to use mouthpiece IPPV. Such patients can use EPR for daytime aid and nasal IPPV overnight. This approach permits decannulation and GPB. EPR also can be useful during tracheostomy site closure for transition to noninvasive nasal IPPV. Considering the difficulties with EPR, the fact that virtually all patients with pacemakers and the ability to grab a mouthpiece prefer noninvasive aids and discontinue their pacemakers, and the fact that small children are obligate nose breathers and can use nasal IPPV successfully, there are no other indications for EPR.

TABLE 3. Uses of Glossopharyngeal Breathing

- For back-up in the event of ventilator failure
- For increased breathing tolerance
- Ventilatory support during transfer between different methods of noninvasive ventilatory support
- For a deeper breath to improve cough effectiveness
- To increase speech volume or shout
- To normalize the volume and rhythm of speech
- To improve or maintain pulmonary compliance
- To prevent microatelectasis

THE BATTLE

by Jamys Moriarty

Today I celebrate a victory, the joyous existence of life.
For only four weeks ago, my body was burdened in strife.
It happened unexpectedly, and much to my chagrin;
  I was bitten by the Flu bug, and the battle did begin.
      My lymphocytes assembled to bolster a strong defense;
  On the battlefield within lungs, the combat grew intense.
An army of antibiotics dispersed with a trumpeting call.
  Unrelenting were the invaders, affixed to my bronchial wall.
My chest muscle mechanics tried to expectorate those bugs;
  Still, germs swarmed my airways, building dams of mucus plugs!
Then I recalled reading in Quest, of Physiatrist John Bach;
  His creative understanding make him a most inventive Doc!
He's pioneered ventilation with a noninvasive technique,
  And reestablished a coughing machine: The In-Exsufflator unique!
Now the battle still stormed, and my lungs began to tire.
  I had to take some action, as it was difficult to respire.
A trip to the hospital, was a journey I wanted to resist,
  Hence I dialed up Emerson, to ask if they'd assist.
It was to my advantage—a most fortunate quirk;
  That the person I spoke with was New England Rep. Kirk.
As a Respiratory Therapist, he knew I was in vital need;
  So he brought down the In-Exsufflator to me top speed!
The machine was a Wonder, I could cough and expel!
  My lungs breathed deeply as the virus bid fare-well!
Today I celebrate good health and pause for reflection,
Many thanks to all who helped me Evict that infection!
Conclusion
No Need to fear.
Should a virus adhere.
My lungs will stay clear.
With the In-Exsufflator near.

Written August 9, 1995

. . . dicen que hacerse poeta es enfermedad incurable y contagiosa. (. . . they say that becoming a poet is an incurable and contagious disease.)

La Sobrina de Quijote

ACKNOWLEDGMENT

The author thanks the American College of Chest Physicians for permission to republish passages from his article: Update and perspectives on noninvasive respiratory muscle aids. Part 1: The inspiratory muscle aids. Chest 105:1230–1240, 1994.

REFERENCES

1. Woollam CHM: The development of apparatus for intermittent negative pressure respiration. I: 1832–1918. Anaesthesia 31:537–547, 1976.
2. Conference on Respiratory Problems in Poliomyelitis, March 12–14, 1952, Ann Arbor, National Foundation for Infantile Paralysis-March of Dimes, White Plains, NY, 1952.
3. Bach JR: Amyotrophic lateral sclerosis: Predictors for prolongation of life by noninvasive respiratory aids. Arch Phys Med Rehabil 76:828–832, 1995.
4. Miller WF: Rehabilitation of patients with chronic obstructive lung disease. Med Clin North Am 51:349–361, 1967.
5. Marrery M: Chest development as a component of normal motor development: Implications for pediatric physical therapists. Pediatr Phys Ther 3:3–8, 1991.
6. Bach JR: Update and perspectives on noninvasive respiratory muscle aids. Part 1: The inspiratory muscle aids. Chest 105:1230–1240, 1994.
7. Eisenmenger R: Suction and pressure over the belly: Its action and application [in German]. Wien Med Wochenschr 31:807–812, 1939.
8. Harf A, Zidulka A, Chang HK: Nitrogen washout during tidal breathing with superimposed high-frequency chest-wall oscillation. Am Rev Respir Dis 132:350–353, 1985.
9. Isabey D, Piquet J: The ventilatory effect of external oscillation. Acta Anaesthesiol Scand 33(S90):87–92, 1989.
10. Khoo M, Gelmont D, Howell S, et al: Effects of high-frequency chest-wall oscillation on respiratory control in humans. Am Rev Respir Dis 139:1223–1230, 1989.
11. Piquet J, Isabey D, Chang HK, Harf A: High-frequency transthoracic ventilation improves gas exchange during experimental bronchoconstriction in rabbits. Am Rev Respir Dis 1986;133:605–608, 1986.
12. Delaubier A: Traitement de l'insuffisance respiratoire chronique dans les dystrophies musculaires. In Memoires de certificat d'etudes superieures de reeducation et readaptation fonctionnelles. Paris, Universite R Descarte, 1984, pp 1–124.
13. al-Saady NM, Fernando SS, Petros AJ, et al: External high-frequency oscillation in normal subjects and in patients with acute respiratory failure. Anaesthesia 50:1031–1035, 1995.
14. Calverley PMA, Chang HK, Vartian V, Zidulka A: High-frequency chest wall oscillation: Assistance to ventilation in spontaneously breathing subjects. Chest 89:218–223, 1986.
15. Dolmage TE, Eisenberg HA, Davis LL, Goldstein RS: Chest wall oscillation at 1 Hz reduces spontaneous ventilation in healthy subjects during sleep. Chest 110:128–135, 1996.
16. Bach JR, Penek J: Obstructive sleep apnea complicating negative pressure ventilatory support in patients with chronic paralytic/restrictive ventilatory dysfunction. Chest 99:1386–1393, 1991.
17. Bach JR: Inappropriate weaning and late onset ventilatory failure of individuals with traumatic quadriplegia. Paraplegia 31:430–438, 1993.
18. Bach JR, Alba AS, Bohatiuk G, et al: Mouth intermittent positive pressure ventilation in the management of post-polio respiratory insufficiency. Chest 91:859-864, 1987.
19. Frederick C: Noninvasive mechanical ventilation with the iron lung. Crit Care Nurs Clin North Am 6:831–840, 1994.
20. Corrado A, Gorini M, De Paola E, et al: Alternative techniques for managing acute respiratory failure. Semin Neurol 15:18–24, 1995.
21. Goldstein RS, Molotiu N, Skrastins R, et al: Assisting ventilation in respiratory failure by negative pressure ventilation and by rocking bed. Chest 92:470–474, 1987.
22. Bach JR, Bardach JL: Neuromuscular diseases. In Sipski ML, Alexander CJ (eds): Sexual Function in People with Disability and Chronic Illness: A Health Practitioner's Guide. Gaithersburg, MD, Aspen, 1997, pp 147–160.
23. Lherm T: Ventilation postopratoire non invasive par masque buccal. Ann Fr Anesth Ranim 17:344-347, 1998.
24. Bach JR, Alba AS, Saporito LR: Intermittent positive pressure ventilation via the mouth as an alternative to tracheostomy for 257 ventilator users. Chest 103:174–182, 1993.
25. Bach JR, Alba AS: Management of chronic alveolar hypoventilation by nasal ventilation. Chest 97:52–57, 1990.
26. Bach JF, Alba A, Mosher R, Delaubier A: Intermittent positive pressure ventilation via nasal access in the management of respiratory insufficiency. Chest 92:168–170, 1987.
27. Leger P, Jennequin J, Gerard M, Robert D: Home positive pressure ventilation via nasal mask for patients with neuromuscular weakness or restrictive lung or chest-wall disease. Respir Care 34:73–79, 1989.
28. McDermott I, Bach JR, Parker C, Sortor S: Custom-fabricated interfaces for intermittent positive pressure ventilation. Int J Prosthodont 2:224–233, 1989.

29. Leger SS, Leger P: The art of interface: Tools for administering noninvasive ventilation. Med Klin 94:35–39, 1999.
30. Sekino H, Ohi M, Chin K, et al: Long-term artificial ventilation by nasal intermittent positive pressure ventilation: 6 cases of domiciliary assisted ventilation. Nihon Kyobu Shikkan Gakkai Zasshi 31:1377–1384, 1993.
31. Criner GJ, Travaline JM, Brennan KJ, Kreimer DT: Efficacy of a new full face mask for noninvasive positive pressure ventilation. Chest 106:1109–1115, 1994.
32. Schonhofer B, Kohler D: Intermittent self-ventilation: Therapy of chronic respiratory pump fatigue. Fortschr Med 113:46–48, 1995.
33. Netzer N, Sorichter S, Bosch W, ete al: The clinical use of an individually fitted nasal mask ("Freiburg Respiratory Mask") within the scope of a case report of controlled BiPAP ventilation. Pneumologie 51(Suppl 3):798–801, 1997.
34. Meduri GU, Abou-Shala N, Fox RC, et al: Noninvasive face mask mechanical ventilation in patients with acute hypercapnic respiratory failure. Chest 100:445–454, 1991.
35. Viroslav J, Sortor S, Rosenblatt R: Alternatives to tracheostomy ventilation in high level SCI [abstract]. J Am Parapleg Soc 14:87, 1991.
36. Bach JR, Robert D, Leger P, Langevin B: Sleep fragmentation in kyphoscoliotic individuals with alveolar hypoventilation treated by nasal IPPV. Chest 107:1552–1558, 1995.
37. Choi JW, Saunders TR, Tebrock O, Hansen NA: Comparison of different mechanical ventilators for patients with poliomyelitis. Mil Med 160:293–296, 1995.
38. Bach JR, Alba AS: Sleep and nocturnal mouthpiece IPPV efficiency in post-poliomyelitis ventilator users. Chest 106:1705–1710, 1994.
39. Navalesi P, Fanfulla F, Frigerio P, et al: Physiologic evaluation of noninvasive mechanical ventilation delivered with three types of masks in patients with chronic hypercapnic respiratory failure. Crit Care Med 28:1785–1790, 2000.
40. Bach JR, Alba AS: Total ventilatory support by the intermittent abdominal pressure ventilator. Chest 99:630–636, 1991.
41. Dougherty G, Davis GM, Gaul M, Diana P: Pneumobelt assisted home ventilation in Duchenne's muscular dystrophy. Fourth International Conference on Home Mechanical Ventilation: Book of Abstracts. Lyon, France, Enterprise Rhone Alpes International, 1993.
42. Pepin JL, Leger P, Veale D, et al: Side effects of nasal continuous positive airway pressure in sleep apnea syndrome: Study of 193 patients in two French sleep centers. Chest 107:375–381, 1995.
43. Richards GN, Cistulli PA, Gunnar Ungar R, et al: Mouth leak with nasal continuous positive airway pressure increases nasal airway resistance. Am J Respir Crit Care Med 154:182–186, 1996.
44. Lazowick D, Meyer TJ, Pressman M, Peterson D: Orbital herniation associated with noninvasive positive pressure ventilation. Chest 113:841–843, 1998.
45. Yamada S, Nishimiya J, Kurokawa K, et al: Bilevel nasal positive airway pressure and ballooning of the stomach. Chest 119:1965–1966, 2001.
46. Marcy TW: Barotrauma: Detection, recognition, and management. Chest 104:578–584, 1993.
47. Gammon RB, Shin MS, Buchalter SE: Pulmonary barotrauma in mechanical ventilation. Chest 102:568–572, 1992.
48. Bitto T, Mannion JD, Stephenson LW, et al: Pneumothorax during positive-pressure mechanical ventilation. J Thorac Cardiovasc Surg 89:585–591, 1985.
49. Kolobow T, Moretti MP, Fumagalli R, et al: Severe impairment in lung function induced by high peak airway pressures during mechanical ventilation: An experimental study. Am Rev Respir Dis 135:312–315, 1987.
50. Haake R, Schlichtig R, Ulstad DR, Henschen RR: Barotrauma: Pathophysiology, risk factors, and prevention. Chest 91:608–613, 1987.
51. Manning HL: Peak airway pressure: why the fuss? Chest 105:242–247, 1994.
52. Dreyfuss D, Soler P, Basset G, Saumon G: High inflation pressure pulmonary edema: Respective effects of high airway pressure, high tidal volume, and positive end-expiratory pressure. Am Rev Respir Dis 137:1159–1164, 1988.
53. Kolobow T, Moretti MP, Fumagalli R, et al: Severe impairment in lung function induced by high peak airway pressure during mechanial ventilation: An experimental study. Am Rev Respir Dis 135:312–315, 1987.
54. Dreyfuss D, Basset G, Soler P, Saumon G: Intermittent positive-pressure hyperventilation with high inflation pressures produces pulmonary microvascular injury in rats. Am Rev Respir Dis 132:880–884, 1985.
55. Bach JR, Rajaraman R, Ballanger F, et al: Neuromuscular ventilatory insufficiency: The effect of home mechanical ventilator use vs. oxygen therapy on pneumonia and hospitalization rates. Am J Phys Med Rehabil 77:8–19, 1998.
56. Wood KE, Flaten AL, Backes WJ: Inspissated secretions: A life-threatening complication of prolonged noninvasive ventilation. Respir Care 45:491–493, 2000.
57. Hill NS: Complications of noninvasive ventilation. Respir Care 45:480–481, 2000.

58. Laraya-Cuasay L, Mikkilimeni S: Respiratory conditions and care. In Rosenthal SR, Sheppard JJ, Lotze M (eds): Dysphagia and the Child with Developmental Disabilities. San Diego, Singular Publishing, 1995, pp 227–252.

59. Arvedson J, Rogers B, Buck G, et al: Silent aspiration prominent in children with dysphagia. Int J Pediatr Otorhinolaryngol 28:173–181, 1994.

60. Loughlin GM: Respiratory consequences of dysfunctional swallowing and aspiration. Dysphagia 3:126–130, 1989.

61. Bach JR, Chaudhry SS: Management approaches in muscular dystrophy association clinics. Am J Phys Med Rehabil 79:193–196, 2000.

62. Ishikawa Y, Ishikawa Y, Minami R: The effect of nasal IPPV on patients with respiratory failure during sleep due to Duchenne muscular dystrophy. Clin Neurol 33:856–861, 1993.

63. Bach JR: Mechanical insufflation-exsufflation: Comparison of peak expiratory flows with manually assisted and unassisted coughing techniques. Chest 104:1553–1562, 1993.

64. Kirby NA, Barnerias MJ, Siebens AA: An evaluation of assisted cough in quadriparetic patients. Arch Phys Med Rehabil 47:705–710, 1966.

65. Bach JR, Smith WH, Michaels J, et al: Airway secretion clearance by mechanical exsufflation for post-poliomyelitis ventilator assisted individuals. Arch Phys Med Rehabil 74:170–177, 1993.

66. Sortor S, McKenzie M: Toward Independence: Assisted Cough [video]. Dallas, BioScience Communications of Dallas, Inc, 1986.

67. Richard I, Giraud M, Perrouin-Verbe B, et al: Laryngo-tracheal stenosis after intubation or tracheostomy in neurological patients. Arch Phys Med Rehabil 77:493–497, 1996.

68. Newth CJL, Asmler B, Anderson GP, Morley J: The effects of varying inflation and deflation pressures on the maximal expiratory deflation flow-volume relationship in anesthetized Rhesus monkeys. Am Rev Respir Dis 144:807–813, 1991.

69. Operator's and Technical Reference Manual: 840 Ventilator System. Carlsbad, CA, Nellcor Puritan Bennett, 1998, pp 10–11.

70. Bach JR, Saporito LR: Criteria for extubation and tracheostomy tube removal for patients with ventilatory failure: A different approach to weaning. Chest 110:1566–1571, 1996.

71. Garstang SV, Kirshblum SC, Wood KE: Patient preference for in-exsufflation for secretion management with spinal cord injury. J Spinal Cord Med 23:80–85, 2000.

72. Bickerman HA: Exsufflation with negative pressure: elimination of radiopaque material and foreign bodies from bronchi of anesthetized dogs. Arch Intern Med 193:698–704, 1954.

73. Leiner GC, Abramowitz S, Small MJ, et al: Expiratory peak flow rate. Standard values for normal subjects. Am Rev Respir Dis 88:644, 1963.

74. Siebens AA, Kirby NA, Poulos DA: Cough following transection of spinal cord at C-6. Arch Phys Med Rehabil 45:1–8, 1964.

75. Bach JR, Ishikawa Y, Kim H: Prevention of pulmonary morbidity for patients with Duchenne muscular dystrophy. Chest 112:1024–1028, 1997.

76. Barach AL, Beck GJ: Exsufflation with negative pressure: Physiologic and clinical studies in poliomyelitis, bronchial asthma, pulmonary emphysema and bronchiectasis. Arch Intern Med 93:825–841, 1954.

77. Barach AL, Beck GJ, Smith RH: Mechanical production of expiratory flow rates surpassing the capacity of human coughing. Am J Med Sci 226:241–248, 1953.

78. Beck GJ, Barach AL: Value of mechanical aids in the management of a patient with poliomyelitis. Ann Int Med;40:1081–1094, 1954.

79. Beck GJ, Graham GC, Barach AL: Effect of physical methods on the mechanics of breathing in poliomyelitis. Ann Intern Med 43:549–566, 1955.

80. Williams EK, Holaday DA: The use of exsufflation with negative pressure in postoperative patients. Am J Surg 90:637–640, 1955.

81. Sammon K, Menon S, Massery M, Cahalin I: A pilot investigation comparing the effects of the mechanical in-exsufflator to suctioning and chest physical therapy in persons with difficulty mobilizing pulmonary secretions [abstract]. Cardiopulm Phys Ther 9:22–23, 1998.

82. Kobavashi I, Perry A, Rhymer J, et al: Relationships between the electrical activity of genioglossus muscle and the upper airway patency: A study in laryngectomised subjects. Respir Crit Care Med 149:A148, 1994.

83. Colebatch HJH: Artificial coughing for patients with respiratory paralysis. Austr J Med 10:201–212, 1961.

84. Cherniack RM, Hildes JA, Alcock AJW: The clinical use of the exsufflator attachment for tank respirators in poliomyelitis. Ann Intern Med 40:540–548, 1954.

85. Barach AL: The application of pressure, including exsufflation, in pulmonary emphysema. Am J Surg 89:372–382, 1955.

86. Beck GJ, Scarrone LA: Physiological effects of exsufflation with negative pressure. Dis Chest 29:1–16, 1956.

87. Freitag L, Long WM, Kim CS, Wanner A: Removal of excessive bronchial secretions by asymmetric high-frequency oscillations. J Appl Physiol 67:614–619, 1989.

88. Singer M, Vermaat J, Hall G, et al: Hemodynamic effects of manual hyperinflation in critically ill mechanically ventilated patients. Chest 106:1182–1187, 1994.

89. Dayman HG: Mechanics of airflow in health and emphysema. J Clin Invest 30:1175–1190, 1951.
90. DiRienzo S. Functional bronchial stenosis. Surgery 1950;27:853 861.
91. Rennie H, Wilson JAC: A coughing-belt. Lancet i:138–139, 1983.
92. Linder SH: Functional electrical stimulation to enhance cough in quadriplegia. Chest 103:166–169, 1993.
93. Lin VW, Nsiao IN, Zhu E, Perkash I: Functional magnetic stimulation for conditioning of expiratory muscles in patients with spinal cord injury. Arch Phys Med Rehabil 82:162–166, 2001.
94. Bach JR, Alba AS, Bodofsky E, et al: Glossopharyngeal breathing and non-invasive aids in the management of post-polio respiratory insufficiency. Birth Defects 23:99–113, 1987.
95. Bach JR: New approaches in the rehabilitation of the traumatic high level quadriplegic. Am J Phys Med Rehabil 70:13–20, 1991.
96. Dail C, Rodgers M, Guess V, Adkins HV: Glossopharyngeal Breathing. Downey, CA, Rancho Los Amigos Department of Physical Therapy, 1979.
97. Dail CW, Affeldt JE: Glossopharyngeal Breathing [video]. Los Angeles, Department of Visual Education, College of Medical Evangelists, 1954.
98. Webber B, Higgens J: Glossopharyngeal Breathing—What, When and How? [video]. Holbrook, England, Aslan Studios Ltd., 1999.
99. Baydur A, Gilgoff I, Prentice W, eet al: Decline in respiratory function and experience with long-term assisted ventilation in advanced Duchenne's muscular dystrophy. Chest 97:884-889, 1990.
100. Bach JR, Alba AS: Noninvasive options for ventilatory support of the traumatic high level quadriplegic. Chest 98:613–619, 1990.
101. Glenn WWL, Brouillette RT, Dentz B, et al: Fundamental considerations in pacing of the diaphragm for chronic ventilatory insufficiency: A multicenter study. PACE 11:2121–2127, 1988.
102. Oakes DD, Wilmot CB, Halverson D, Hamilton RD: Neurogenic respiratory failure: A 5-year experience using implantable phrenic nerve stimulators. Ann Thorac Surg 30:118–122, 1980.
103. McMichan JC, Piepgras DG, Gracey DR, et al: Electrophrenic respiration. Mayo Clin Proc 54:662–668, 1979.
104. Bach JR, O'Connor K: Electrophrenic ventilation: a different perspective. J Am Parapleg Soc 14:9–17, 1991.

8 —— Respiratory Muscle Aids: Patient Evaluation and the Oximetry-Respiratory Aid Protocol

JOHN R. BACH, M.D.

Lorsque les chiens aboient, nous comprenons que nous allons au galop.
(When the dogs bark, you know you are on the move.)

Gustav Mahler, *Briefe*

STATE OF AFFAIRS FOR THE NEUROMUSCULAR PATIENT WITH VENTILATORY INSUFFICIENCY

Only about 31% of ventilator users in acute hospitals have neuromuscular ventilatory failure, whereas 60% of ventilator users have cardiopulmonary disorders. But because neuromuscular ventilator users have a better prognosis and tend to use ventilators much longer, they constitute over 50% of home mechanical ventilator users in the United States.[1] The population of home mechanical ventilator users, in fact, has more than doubled since 1987,[1] and the percentage of neurologists who treat patients with NMD and are biased against ventilator use has decreased from 38% to 22%.[2] The number of home ventilator users is also greatly increasing in England, Scandinavia, and probably elsewhere.[3]

Since 1987, the steady increase in the use of noninvasive ventilation has been mostly in the form of nocturnal-only, low-span positive inspiratory pressure plus positive end-expiratory pressure (PIP + PEEP) via nasal access.[2] A 1997 survey of MDA clinic directors found that nocturnal PIP + PEEP was used in 88% of clinics and body ventilators in 14%; yet the vital provision of mouthpiece intermittent positive-pressure ventilation (IPPV) was reported in only 20% of clinics.[2] Furthermore, much of the reported use of mouthpiece IPPV may have resulted from confusion with intermittent positive-pressure breathing (IPPB). In only 15% of clinics were both pressure- and volume-cycled ventilators used for noninvasive IPPV. Furthermore, the vital use of manually assisted coughing was reported in only 18% and mechanical insufflation-exsufflation (MI-E) in only 5% of clinics. Thus, failure to provide effective nocturnal ventilatory support, mouthpiece IPPV, and assisted coughing continues to make respiratory failure inevitable for the great majority of people

165

with NMD. Most such patients remain uninformed about noninvasive options when they consent to or refuse endotracheal intubation or tracheotomy.

The decision to accept or reject tracheotomy has been commonly called the "crisis decision"[4–7]—whether to live on a respirator for the rest of one's life or to die of suffocation. However, no crisis decision needs to be made, and patients do not "refuse respiratory support" when noninvasive aids are first used for lung expansion (range of motion) (see Chapter 7). Patients naturally increase the use of insufflation therapy via a mouthpiece and thereby use mouthpiece IPPV with increasing frequency as they feel the need with advancing weakness.[8] The only neuromuscular diseases (NMDs) for which the crisis decision about tracheotomy still needs to be made are bulbar amyotrophic lateral sclerosis (ALS) and, infrequently, spinal muscular atrophy (SMA) type 1.

EVALUATION OF RESPIRATORY MUSCLE DYSFUNCTION

The patient evaluation includes a survey for symptoms of chronic alveolar hypoventilation (Table 1), physical examination, manual muscle testing, and four painless and simple pulmonary tests. Although severe diaphragm weakness and loss of the ability to breathe can occur without extremity weakness, Nathanson et al. reported that proximal upper limb weakness is a significant predictor of respiratory muscle dysfunction for patients with Charcot-Marie-Tooth disease.[9] We have found this to be the case for patients with other NMDs as well.

The patient is observed for paradoxical breathing. Typically, patients with spinal cord injury and childhood-onset myopathies or SMA have very weak intercostal muscles and breathe predominantly with the diaphragm. Chest-wall volumes decrease during inspiration,[10] and vital capacity in the sitting position is less than or equal to vital capacity in the supine position. On the other hand, patients with paralyzed diaphragms who breathe to a large degree with accessory breathing or abdominal muscles and patients whose diaphragms are too weak in the supine position to move the abdominal contents to ventilate the lungs can have a much lower vital capacity and less breathing tolerance in the supine position. They also may occasionally have chest expansion with abdominal retractions during inspiration. Patients with certain myopathies typically fall into this category (see Chapter 2).

Lung auscultation, spirometry, oximetry, peak cough flow (PCF), and end-tidal carbon dioxide measurements are made. A spirometer is used to measure vital capacity in sitting, recumbent, and sidelying positions and with a thoracolumbar brace in place and removed, if applicable. A well-constructed thoracolumbar brace can increase vital capacity for scoliotic patients, whereas a poorly prepared or poorly fitting brace can decrease vital capacity and impair breathing. The spirometer is also used to measure the maximal insufflation capacity (MIC) for patients who have a vital capacity at least 30% less than predicted normal levels

TABLE 1. Symptoms of Chronic Alveolar Hypoventilation and Sleep-disordered Breathing*

Fatigue	Irritability
Dyspnea (particularly when capable of ambulation)	Anxiety
Morning or continuous headaches	Nocturnal urinary frequency
Multiple nocturnal awakenings with dyspnea/tachycardia	Polycythemia
Difficult arousals	Impaired intellectual function
Hypersomnolence	Depression
Difficulty with concentration	Decreased libido
Frequent nightmares	Weight loss or gain
Nightmares about breathing difficulties (e.g., suffocation, drowning)	Muscle aches
	Memory impairment
Congestive heart failure	Poor control of airway secretions
Lower extremity edema	

* In order of appearance.[52]

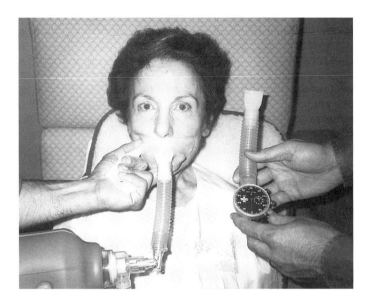

FIGURE 1. Patient air-stacking via lipseal for spirometric measurement of maximal insufflation capacity.

and are trained in air-stacking (see Chapter 7). Usually a manual resuscitator is used for the patient to air-stack via a mouthpiece for MIC measurements. If the lips are too weak or the soft palate cannot seal off the nasopharynx and the patient cannot air-stack optimally via a mouthpiece, the patient air-stacks via a lipseal (Fig. 1) or uses a nasal interface (Fig. 2). An oronasal interface also can be used for patients with weak buccal muscles, but MIC measurement may need to be done without removing the interface from volumes exhaled at the expiratory valve on the interface tubing.

FIGURE 2. Patient air-stacking via nasal interface for spirometric measurement of maximal insufflation capacity.

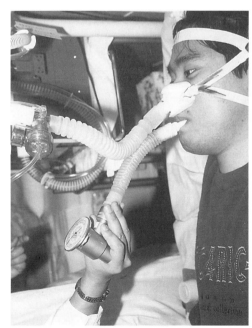

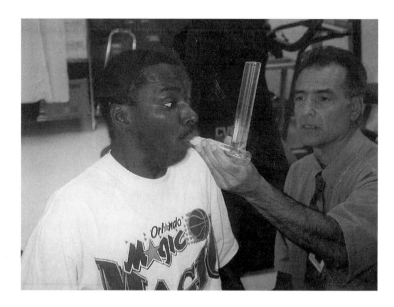

FIGURE 3. Patient coughing via simple mouthpiece into peak flow meter.

Unassisted PCF is measured by having the patient cough as hard as possible through a peak flow meter (Fig. 3). The PCF is then measured with the patient coughing from a maximally air-stacked volume (MIC). The patient coughs via an oronasal interface if there is a tendency for insufflated air to leak out of the nose (Fig. 4). Finally, fully assisted PCF is measured from the MIC with an abdominal thrust timed to glottic opening.[11] The most important PCF measurement is usually the latter because the patient must often use the manually assisted cough to clear airway secretions and avoid respiratory failure. Patients unable to close the glottis can generate the latter but not the former.

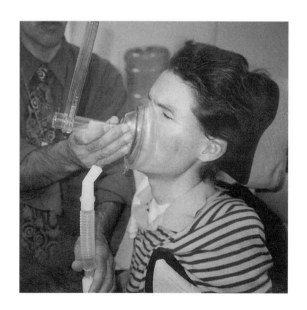

FIGURE 4. Patients with a soft palate incompetent to prevent nasal insufflation leakage (or weak lips) can cough into a peak flow meter via oronasal interface after air-stacking to approach maximal insufflation capacity. Concurrent abdominal thrust timed to cough permits the measurement of "assisted peak cough flows."

End-tidal carbon dioxide has been shown to correlate with lung underventilation, cardiac output, and lung perfusion pressures. End-tidal carbon dioxide correlates closely with $PaCO_2$ (r = 0.94–0.98) except in patients with severe concomitant lung or vascular disease and congestive hear failure or impaired lung diffusion or perfusion, in which case it is low.[12,13] End-tidal carbon dioxide approximates $PaCO_2$ when significant physiologic dead space is not present.[14] A recent decrease in end-tidal carbon dioxide without introduction of ventilator use often signals asymptomatic congestive heart failure and an early shock state.

Measurements of end-tidal carbon dioxide and transcutaneous carbon dioxide measurements are extremely close in efficacy among older children and adults.[15,16] With currently available sensors, the transcutaneous carbon dioxide has been shown to correlate extremely well with $PaCO_2$ over a range of 26–71 mmHg.[15] Although both can be accurate in assessing stable $PaCO_2$ during mechanical ventilation, both also can underestimate increases in hypercapnia briefly after cessation of ventilatory support.[17] End-tidal carbon dioxide measurements are more accurate during full expiratory maneuvers than during tidal expiration[18] (Fig. 5). We record the maximal observed end-tidal carbon dioxide and have all patients exhale completely from their vital capacity several times to see if this maneuver will increase or decrease end-tidal carbon dioxide readings as a result of hyperventilation.

Studies comparing end-tidal carbon dioxide and $PaCO_2$ in patients extubated immediately after general anesthesia have reported somewhat contradictory results.[19,20] Whereas one study found end-tidal carbon dioxide unreliable,[19] the other found identical means and standard deviations of 38.9 ± 5.7 mmHg for both values in 65 measurements. In another study of extubated postoperative adult patients, the end-tidal carbon dioxide was lower than $PaCO_2$ by 2.8 ± 2.6 mmHg.[21] Patients, however, have had wide discrepancies between end-tidal carbon dioxide and $PaCO_2$ values.[20] Large discrepancies also were reported for infants and toddlers using invasive mechanical ventilation. These small patients had differences in end-tidal carbon dioxide and $PaCO_2$ of 6.8 ± 5.1 mmHg, whereas the differences between transcutaneous carbon dioxide and $PaCO_2$ were 2.3 ± 1.3 mmHg. The absolute difference between transcutaneous carbon dioxide and $PaCO_2$ was 4 mmHg or less in 96 of 100 values, whereas the difference between end-tidal carbon dioxide and $PaCO_2$ was 4 mmHg or less in only 38 of 100 values.[22]

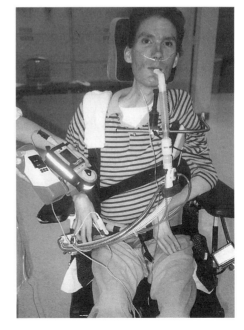

FIGURE 5. Measurement of end-tidal carbon dioxide with sensor at the nose and oxyhemoglobin saturation with pick-up electrode on the thumb for 24-hour noninvasive ventilation user.

Routine arterial blood gas analyses are not justified for such patients. Pain from the arterial stick causes hyperventilation and can cause falsely low carbon dioxide tensions in 30% of cases.[23] A single glimpse at PaO_2 and SpO_2 is much less useful as a guide for assisted ventilation and airway secretion elimination than continuous SpO_2 monitoring. The chronicity of hypoventilation can be assessed from venous bicarbonate levels.

SpO_2 may be normal despite end-tidal carbon dioxide levels in the low 60s. However, once hypercapnia causes the SpO_2 to decrease below 95%, patients tend to develop symptoms of alveolar hypoventilation (see Chapter 2). If the SpO_2 baseline is found to be below 95%, the patient is asked to increase breathing effort. If this effort normalizes SpO_2, the low baseline SpO_2 is usually due in large part to underventilation. When increasing or normalizing alveolar ventilation does not normalize SpO_2, severe ventilation-perfusion mismatching is present (see Chapter 2).

If the vital capacity is at least 30% more in the sitting than in the supine position, if symptoms of sleep-disordered breathing or chronic alveolar hypoventilation are present, if dyspnea is present in the supine position, or if daytime end-tidal carbon dioxide is greater than 45 mmHg, significant nocturnal hypoventilation is a strong possibility, and nocturnal SpO_2 monitoring is performed. An Ohmeda oximeter (Louisville, KY) collates data by the hour and for the entire night and provides hourly means, percentages of time that SpO_2 is less than 90%, 85%, 80%, and 70%, and hourly lows. Such quantifiable data can be used to demonstrate objectively the need for nocturnal noninvasive IPPV and ameliorations with treatment. If the patient is symptomatic but has an essentially normal vital capacity as well as normal SpO_2 and end-tidal carbon dioxide during the day and night, polysomnography is used to evaluate for sleep-disordered breathing. In addition to data about SpO_2, oximetry also provides information about heart rate and, therefore, the success of certain cardiac medications such as beta blockers. The pulse waveform also correlates significantly with systolic pressures and can be a sensitive indicator of hypovolemia.[24]

INTRODUCTION OF RESPIRATORY MUSCLE AIDS AND MONITORING FOR ADOLESCENTS AND ADULTS

As noted in Chapter 7, noninvasive IPPV is ideally introduced as daily air-stacking. The introduction of air-stacking, maximal insufflations, noninvasive IPPV, and assisted coughing is best done in the outpatient setting. Others, too, have found hospitalization unnecessary for introduction of noninvasive IPPV.[25]

Mouthpiece and nasal ventilation are introduced with the patient in any comfortable position. A variety of nasal and lipseal interfaces and headgear can be tried and individually adapted (see Chapter 7). Because all interface air leakage need not be eliminated and comfort and avoidance of excessive skin pressure are important, the straps should not be tightly applied. If no ventilator is conveniently available, the interfaces and headgear can be conveniently tested by using a manual resuscitator. One or more interfaces are selected on the basis of fit, comfort, seal around the nostrils, and hours of daily use.

For hospitalized patients using volume-cycled ventilators with expiratory volume alarms, the alarms are set at a minimum of 10 ml. Even this setting, however, does not prevent alarms from sounding during interface trials and noninvasive IPPV. Hospitalized patients usually must be switched to portable ventilators without expiratory volume alarms before trying noninvasive ventilation.

Selection of the ventilator is relatively easy for the outpatient setting. All patients whose MICs exceed vital capacity need to air-stack to maximal insufflations. Thus, they require volume-cycled ventilators to achieve this goal independently. A portable volume-cycled ventilator eventually is needed for daytime IPPV as the disease progresses. It is tempting to set delivered volumes according to some formula. However, because noninvasive ventilation is an open system and patients can take as much of the delivered air as they want, we generally initiate IPPV at the relatively high volumes of 600–1000 ml before raising them to more effective levels (see Chapter 7). Frequent sighs or air-stacking is also promoted.

Some patients may continue to use high-span PIP + PEEP overnight and reserve volume-cycled ventilators for daytime use only. When PIP + PEEP is used, the initial spans of inspiratory and expiratory positive airway pressure (IPAP and EPAP) are 10–15 and 2 cmH_2O, respectively. IPAP is increased to 15–20 cmH_2O or more as needed to maintain normal end-tidal carbon dioxide. EPAP is left at the minimum unless the patient has auto-PEEP or is being treated for documented obstructive sleep apnea. For patients without volume-cycled ventilators who use only nocturnal high-span PIP + PEEP, air-stacking can be provided by manual resuscitators or regular maximal insufflations by Cough-Assist (J. H. Emerson Co., Cambridge, MA).

The first signs of successful use of noninvasive ventilation are decreases in respiratory rate and accessory respiratory muscle use; increased chest expansion; breathing synchrony with pressure-cycled ventilators or ventilator gauge pressures of 18–25 cmH_2O with exhalation via the exhalation valve of volume-cycled ventilators; normalization of end-tidal carbon dioxide and SpO_2; and relief of dyspnea. In addition, however, because the goal is to rest respiratory muscles, lung insufflation volumes compatible with ventilatory support are used, whether the ventilator is pressure- or volume-cycled.

Supplemental oxygen is avoided for patients with primarily ventilatory impairment but may be beneficial for patients with lung disease whose SpO_2 cannot be normalized by improving alveolar ventilation and airway secretion clearance. Humidification must be considered (see Chapter 13). Air leaks, interface retention, and strap tension are monitored periodically. Sedation is avoided or at least minimized. Noninvasive IPPV efficacy is monitored by end-tidal carbon dioxide, oximetry, observing the ventilator pressure gauge for adequate airway pressures, and monitoring expiratory volumes by attaching a spirometer to the expiratory valve when volume-cycle ventilation is used. Blood gas monitoring is unnecessary except to correlate end-tidal carbon dioxide with $PaCO_2$ for patients who suffer primarily from respiratory impairment and require supplemental oxygen or who have severe cardiovascular impairment.

For a patient with chronic daytime as well as nocturnal hypercapnia and oxyhemoglobin desaturation who has not been using ventilatory support, introduction to and use of mouthpiece or nasal IPPV can be facilitated by oximetry feedback. Oximetry feedback serves as a guide to indicate how much noninvasive IPPV is required per day. Patients are instructed to normalize SpO_2 or end-tidal carbon dioxide by autonomously increasing lung ventilation— an activity that they quickly find fatiguing. They are then taught to take mouthpiece-assisted breaths as necessary to normalize and maintain normal SpO_2. Initially, an oximetry alarm can be set at 94% to remind the patient to take assisted breaths (Fig. 6). The patient sees that by taking slightly deeper or assisted breaths the SpO_2 will go above 94% within seconds. After a few weeks of maintaining normal SpO_2 by assisting ventilation around the clock, reversal of compensatory metabolic alkalosis, normalization of ventilatory drive, and respiratory muscle rest often result in the ability to maintain normal SpO_2 and ventilation most, if not all, of the day without daytime assisted breathing. Over the passage of years, however, noninvasive IPPV use becomes continuous as autonomous breathing ability is lost with advancing weakness and age. The restoration of central ventilatory drive and normalization of daytime blood gases also guarantee the effectiveness of noninvasive IPPV during sleep (see Chapter 5).

Once the maximal assisted PCF decreases below 270 L/min or 4.5 L/sec, risk of pneumonia is high during episodes of airway encumberment (see Chapter 2), and the patient is trained in manually and mechanically assisted coughing.

An oximeter is prescribed for home use, and the patient is provided with rapid access to MI-E and a portable volume ventilator to use during chest infections if they are not already available.[26] If the patient is told simply to call the physician when a cold develops, he or she often waits too long. The SpO_2 baseline often will have decreased below 80%, the vital capacity may have decreased by 50–80% from baseline, and pneumonia may already be

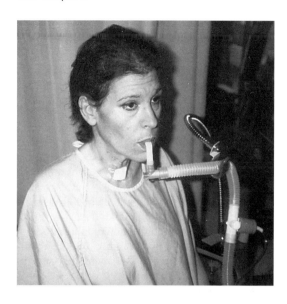

FIGURE 6. After decannulation a 24-hour ventilator-dependent patient with hypercapnia and muscular dystrophy used oximetry as feedback to normalize alveolar ventilation with mouthpiece IPPV.

present. In this case there is often no recourse to hospitalization and translaryngeal intubation. For this reason, after the manual resuscitator, an oximeter is the next device to be prescribed, and the patient and care providers are taught the outpatient oximetry feedback protocol (see below) before respiratory failure can develop.

If the patient is symptomatic or if he or she does not appear to be symptomatic despite hypercapnia (see Table 1) but has a vital capacity below 50% and a mean SpO_2 below 95% for 1 or more hours of sleep or multiple episodes of oxyhemoglobin desaturation of 4% or more per hour during sleep, a trial of nocturnal noninvasive IPPV is arranged. Once they try nocturnal noninvasive IPPV, such patients often feel relief of fatigue and other symptoms that they did not recognize. The nocturnal oximetry is repeated with the patient using noninvasive IPPV. Typically, nocturnal SpO_2 means an increase from lower levels to 94–95% with treatment. For such patients, withdrawing nasal IPPV often results in decreases in mean nocturnal SpO_2, increases in daytime symptoms, and worsening of blood gases[27,28] until nocturnal nasal IPPV is re-instituted. If there is no improvement in symptoms or mean nocturnal SpO_2 using nasal IPPV, little or no benefit is derived from its nocturnal use.

Clinicians often fail to appreciate how and why noninvasive ventilation can be effective during sleep in the absence of respiratory muscle function. To understand this, recognizing the importance of keeping the central ventilatory drive intact (see Chapter 5) is essential. Such clinicians often are tempted to monitor the efficacy of noninvasive IPPV by regular blood gas analyses, nocturnal end-tidal carbon dioxide or transcutaneous carbon dioxide monitoring, chest radiographs, traditional pulmonary function analyses, measurements of expiratory volume, and polysomnographs. However, because the efficacy of noninvasive IPPV depends on the intactness of central nervous system asphyxia avoidance reflexes, there is no need for any of these measures in patients who do not receive supplemental oxygen.

The consideration of insufflation pressures or pressure-volume curves of the lungs and thorax can be useful. Increases in pressure can signal pulmonary edema, pneumonia, bronchospasm, intubation of a mainstem bronchus, atelectasis, airway mucus accumulation, or space-occupying lesions such as pneumothoraces. Pressure decreases, generally below 18 cmH_2O, signal inadequate ventilator-delivered volumes, interface leakage, or temporary insufflation leakage to avoid hyperventilation. Electromyography of respiratory muscles during sleep has also been used for optimizing inspiratory muscle rest by adjusting nocturnal noninvasive IPPV settings.[29,30]

OXIMETRY FEEDBACK–RESPIRATORY MUSCLE AID PROTOCOL

Headaches, fatigue, a little bit lazy . . .
Too much CO_2 can make me feel crazy.

Richard L. Clingman, Sr., Webmaster for DoctorBach.com

Because supplemental oxygen is avoided for patients with NMD, the patient and care providers are instructed that, once artifact is ruled out,[31] SpO_2 below 95% is due to one of three causes: hypercapnia (hypoventilation), airway encumberment (secretions), or, if these are not managed properly, intrinsic lung disease, usually pneumonia. The oximetry feedback-respiratory muscle aid protocol consists of using an oximeter for feedback to maintain SpO_2 greater than 94% by maintaining effective alveolar ventilation and airway secretion elimination.

The protocol is most important during respiratory tract infections and extubation of patients with little or no breathing tolerance. Because respiratory muscles are weakened and bronchial secretions are profuse during chest infections and after general anesthesia,[32] patients often need to use noninvasive IPPV continuously, both to maintain alveolar ventilation and to increase PCF by air-stacking. If, when noninvasive IPPV is used at adequate delivered volumes, the SpO_2 is not above 94%, the desaturation is due not to hypoventilation but to airway mucus accumulation. Indeed, sudden episodes of oxyhemoglobin desaturation in ventilator users during chest infections are almost always due to mucus accumulation. Manually assisted coughing with air stacking as needed and MAC are then used until the mucus is expelled and SpO_2 returns to normal or baseline levels.

If the baseline SpO_2 decreases below 95% despite ventilatory support and aggressive assisted coughing, the outpatient is asked to present for a formal evaluation. A clear radiograph in the presence of a baseline SpO_2 of 92–94% usually denotes microscopic atelectasis. Radiographic evidence of pneumonia accompanied by oxyhemoglobin desaturation and ventilator dependence warrants admission and possibly intubation. Despite hyperpyrexia and elevated white blood cell counts, baseline SpO_2 to 92% can typically return to normal and hospitalization can be avoided when patients use respiratory muscle aids with oximetry feedback.[26] As the SpO_2 baseline returns to normal, most patients gradually wean to nocturnal-only noninvasive IPPV or, at times, to no daily use of respiratory muscle aids until the next chest infection.

Even in the event of hospitalization, however, the patient's primary care providers are asked to continue to use MAC with oximetry feedback to eliminate airway secretions and avoid intubation. This approach is recommended because we have found it impossible to expect nursing and respiratory therapy staff to clear airway secretions as often as needed either to avoid intubation or after extubation. It is most practical and efficacious to let the family and care providers administer the respiratory muscle aids, even when the patient is in intensive care. Overnight, provided that sedatives, narcotics, and excessive oxygen therapy are avoided, heavy mucus accumulation will arouse the patient and he or she will request MAC. The family or primary care providers quickly learn that, since they are doing most of the work, patients usually receive the best and safest care at home.

INTUBATION AND EXTUBATION

Noninvasive IPPV can be used to avoid intubation in patients who suffer primarily from respiratory impairment in about 70% of cases (see Chapter 11). Properly managed patients should rarely require intubation for ventilatory or respiratory failure. However, we are often called to manage such patients who are intubated because they have not been introduced to noninvasive respiratory aids or the oximetry feedback protocol. Some who use only nocturnal nasal IPPV develop respiratory failure because of lack of knowledge of daytime assisted ventilation methods and assisted coughing or because of inadequate home care to help them with assisted coughing. In addition, some patients have mixed ventilatory and respiratory impairment.

Intubation is a clinical decision. Patients presenting in respiratory distress with pneumonia and low baseline SpO_2 often require intubation. They are managed conventionally in respect to antibiotic therapy, hydration, and nutrition. Chest physical therapy and the use of an Intrapulmonary Percussive Ventilator (Percussionaire Corp., Sandpoint, ID) can be useful. These methods may mobilize deep secretions, but they cannot expel them because they do not compensate for an ineffective cough.

Once the patient is intubated, minute ventilation is increased as needed to maintain $PaCO_2$ between 30 and 40 cmH$_2$O. So long as $PaCO_2$ is below 40 mmHg and the SpO_2 remains below 95% despite aggressive MAC, supplemental oxygen can be provided to titrate the SpO_2 to approach but not exceed 95%. Too often in emergency department and hospital settings, oxygen delivery is increased instead of using assisted coughing to eliminate airway mucus-associated episodes of oxyhemoglobin desaturation or adequate assisted ventilation to eliminate hypercapnia.

MAC is used via the tube to eliminate mucus whenever the SpO_2 decreases below 95% or baseline, whenever the patient requests it, or on a regular frequent schedule until SpO_2 baseline has returned to normal. Pressures from + 40 to – 40 cmH$_2$O are typically used. For patients with profuse airway secretion, MAC may be needed every few minutes around the clock. Because intensive care nursing and respiratory staff usually cannot provide this service as often as needed, even here it is often best to employ the patient's primary care providers.

Unlike with conventional management in which supplemental oxygen is delivered and ventilator weaning is attempted at the expense of hypercapnia—an approach tantamount to "weaning the patient to death"—ventilator weaning must never be attempted at the expense of hypercapnia for patients who suffer primarily from ventilatory impairment. Before extubation of weanable patients, we use the assist-control mode with minimal pressure support (to compensate for airway resistance due to the presence of the airway tube) to maximize breath volumes while minimizing breathing rate.

The patient is extubated when the following criteria are satisfied: no supplemental oxygen requirement to maintain SpO_2 greater than 94%, chest radiograph abnormalities cleared or clearing, respiratory depressants discontinued, airway secretions less than on admission, and nasal congestion cleared. The nasogastric tube is first removed to facilitate postextubation nasal IPPV. Patients who used air stacking, PIP + PEEP, or noninvasive IPPV before intubation are extubated directly to noninvasive IPPV. Thus, once the patient is afebrile with a normal white blood cell count and the SpO_2 is normal on room air the patient is extubated to up to full-time noninvasive support on room air, whether or not he or she is able to breathe. The patient is weaned, as feasible, by taking fewer and fewer assisted breaths, usually via a mouthpiece, as ventilatory function is recovered. Thus, the need to fulfill "weaning criteria" is irrelevant because the patient self-weans, if possible, after extubation or decannulation.[33,34] MAC is then provided via the upper airway, and the oximetry feedback protocol is followed. MI-E is usually provided via an oral-nasal interface but some patients with excellent bulbar muscle function use a simple mouthpiece.

After extubation it is best to have the patient's care providers provide MAC with oximetry feedback. Just as is done at home, the care provider performs MAC every few minutes while the patient is awake, as necessary, to keep the SpO_2 baseline above 94%.

This protocol facilitates successful extubation, and the care providers become expert at how to prevent respiratory decompensation and hospitalization in the future.

Extubation succeeds when postextubation PCF can reach 160 L/min.[8] In a study of 67 consecutive extubations, the inability to achieve unassisted or assisted PCF of 160 L/min invariably resulted in reintubation within 48 hours, whereas vital capacity and the ability to breathe were almost irrelevant because of the use of noninvasive IPPV after extubation. One patient with no measurable vital capacity was successfully extubated to continuous noninvasive IPPV. His assisted PCF was adequate. On the other hand, a patient with a vital capacity of 2000 ml, although breathing comfortably after extubation with normal SpO_2, had maximal assisted PCF of 120 L/min and required reintubation for secretion encumberment 24 hours later. It was discovered that he had tracheal stenosis.

Acutely ill patients may require supportive therapies. Once adequate hydration is established and patients are comfortable with noninvasive IPPV, they may be encouraged to eat puréed food or drink fluids through a straw. Swallowing is facilitated by first delivering a few quick, deep, assisted breaths. Episodic desaturations for the first 1–2 hours after a meal are managed by MI-E without abdominal thrusts. Gastrostomy feedings are suspended if abdominal thrusts are required to supplement MI-E.

We have extubated numerous patients with no significant breathing tolerance. Many had used noninvasive IPPV continuously for years when requiring surgery and general anesthesia. Postoperatively they were extubated to their usual method of noninvasive IPPV. Others used only nocturnal noninvasive IPPV and daily air stacking when an intercurrent chest infection or surgical anesthesia caused the development of pneumonia and respiratory failure[26,35] (see Case 13 in Chapter 15). Other patients who had never been taught air-stacking or noninvasive aids were referred to us already intubated and incapable of ventilator weaning (see Case 17 in Chapter 15). Untrained patients are the most difficult to extubate to noninvasive IPPV. Body ventilators can be used to support lung ventilation during and immediately after extubation so that the patient can be trained in noninvasive IPPV. Once the technique is mastered, the body ventilators can be discontinued in favor of continued use of noninvasive IPPV.[36,37] The greatest number of patients with a specific diagnosis whom we have extubated despite absence of breathing tolerance and inability to cooperate were diagnosed with infantile SMA[38] (see Chapter 10). As can be seen from reported data, extubation of ventilator-dependent patients following the principles cited above and in Chapter 10 is almost always successful, even under these most difficult circumstances.[38]

An instructive example is provided by a patient with DMD who, despite symptomatic hypercapnia, refused consistent use of nocturnal noninvasive IPPV because of "fear that [he] would become addicted to it." The patient had an oximeter and Cough Assist at home but did not use them when he developed an upper respiratory tract infection and was admitted to a local hospital in December of 1996. In March of 1997, he was hospitalized again and intubated for a respiratory tract infection and respiratory failure. When he failed extubation, he was transferred to our service. When asked why he had not used MI-E, he said that he "forgot how to use it." We used our respiratory aid extubation protocol, but he failed extubation twice with postextubation assisted PCF below 160 L/min. Fortunately, the third extubation attempt (fifth overall) succeeded, and he has been using 20 or more hours per day of noninvasive IPPV for over 5 years. Because of the episodes of respiratory failure and the close brush with tracheotomy, he has become a strong advocate for using the oximetry protocol and noninvasive IPPV.

Another center described the use of noninvasive IPPV delivered from volume-cycled ventilators after extubation in 43 patients with chronic ventilatory failure once hypercapnia (pCO_2 greater than 48 mmHg) developed after 24 hours of spontaneous breathing in ambient air. It was believed that postextubation nocturnal noninvasive IPPV "stabilized the weaning process" for at least 40% of the extubated patients, whereas the other 60% did not require ongoing ventilatory assistance.[39]

In addition to the benefits of using noninvasive IPPV for postextubation weaning,[40] there have been reports of avoidance of intubation by use of noninvasive IPPV[41] and extubation of unweanable patients with mixed ventilation and oxygenation impairment to noninvasive IPPV.[42] Forty-six conscious trauma patients with acute respiratory failure were managed with noninvasive IPPV and supplemental oxygen. Thirty-three were eventually weaned. However, nine with hypercapnic and four with hypoxemic respiratory failure required intubation. Of the 13 who failed noninvasive IPPV, nine died after switching to invasive ventilation after 10 ± 3 days, whereas death was reported in no patient using noninvasive IPPV. Mean IPAP/EPAP were 12/4.5 cmH$_2$O. Twenty-two patients had decreases in PaCO$_2$ from 53 ± 8 to 42 ± 8 mmHg and normalization of pH.[41] In another study, 25 intubated patients without breathing tolerance were extubated to noninvasive IPPV.[42]

DECANNULATION AND CONVERSION TO NONINVASIVE RESPIRATORY AIDS

With the trach removed
I much better can breathe
The only cuff that remains
I wear on my sleeve

Richard L. Clingman, Sr., Webmaster for DoctorBach.com

Any patient with an indwelling tracheostomy tube who is capable of understandable speech when the tube cuff is deflated is evaluated for decannulation. Patients without severe speech and swallowing impairment are usually good candidates. Because noninvasive ventilatory support is successful even for patients with no ability to breathe, decannulation indications depend primarily on bulbar function and, in particular, on the ability to clear airway secretions noninvasively.

The ability to effect glottic closure and then to maintain airway patency during the cough is critical for successful decannulation. Cross-sectional anatomy of the airway can be assessed by CT scan. Flow-volume loops also provide information about airway patency but do not assess for glottic closure and, therefore, do not correlate with the ability to cough (PCF). Airway patency can be quantitated for patients with tracheostomies by measuring upper airway airflow resistance. This technique uses either a body plethysmograph or an oral pneumotach to measure airflow while pressure is measured in the stoma through a sealed tracheostomy tube. Resistance to flow in cmH$_2$O/L/sec is equal to the change in pressure (cmH$_2$O) across the resistor per unit volume of air over time (L/sec). The patient breathes with the mouth wide open to eliminate nasal or oral resistance. The pressure gradient is determined from the trachea to the atmosphere. Airflow is measured, pressure-flow curves are generated, and resistance is calculated 50 times per second. Normal resistance is under 1 cmH$_2$O/L/sec.[43] It is unclear what values correspond to ineffective cough flows.

The most important criterion for safe decannulation is the ability to achieve assisted PCF of about 160 L/min (see Case 4 in Chapter 15). Somewhat lower flows are acceptable with the tube in place because air-stacking is usually impossible and there is airflow obstruction from the tube as well as air leakage around the tube and out of the tracheostomy site during measurements of PCF. The problem of tube obstruction can be alleviated by placing a fenestrated tube to increase airflow between the upper airway and the lungs. Any cuff must be deflated and the tube capped as the patient receives IPPV via mouthpiece or nasal interface and attempts to air-stack. If the tube fits snugly into the tracheostomy tract and is capped, air-stacking occasionally can be done to some degree, and the assisted PCF better reflects post-tracheostomy site closure levels. If the fit is not snug, a manual cough assist must be done without providing a deep insufflation.

If PCF is much lower than 160 L/min with the tube in place, it is removed, at least temporarily, and the site is covered by hand or with a tracheostomy button (Olympic Medical, Inc., Seattle). The button clears the airway entirely. This technique decreases obstruction to upper airway airflows, allowing more accurate measurement of assisted PCF, and facilitates the use of noninvasive IPPV as well as autonomous breathing. On button placement or ostomy site covering, patients with no breathing tolerance are immediately placed on noninvasive IPPV (Fig. 7). If, despite air stacking and coordinated abdominal thrusts, levels still fail to approach 160 L/min, vocal cord paralysis, hypopharyngeal collapse, tracheal stenosis, or other reasons for fixed airway obstruction are considered, and the patient is referred for fiberoptic evaluation of the upper airway. If the tracheostomy tube is replaced after the PCF measurement and the patient has a considerable amount of airway secretions, a fenestrated cuffed tracheostomy tube may be warranted. Although cuffs are deflated for IPPV, inflation increases the effectiveness of MI-E.

Patients who are accustomed to tracheostomy IPPV and have never used noninvasive IPPV lose the reflex glottic opening that normally occurs at the initiation of inspiration. Thus, the patient may have to relearn how to open the vocal cords and glottis to receive IPPV noninvasively. This process can take a few minutes or longer during trials of noninvasive IPPV. It may necessitate frequent, brief reconnecting to tracheostomy IPPV or a body ventilator until the patient "breathes" with the delivered air and prevents excessive insufflation leakage out of the mouth or nose. Occasionally, as soon as air enters from a mouthpiece or nasal interface, the patient reflexly opens the mouth to allow the air leak. This reflex can occur whether the tube is left in the airway or the airway is clear and the site is capped. Thus, it may take practice to be ventilated noninvasively (Fig. 8).

Airway obstruction from an indwelling tracheostomy tube, even a cuffless one with a fenestration, often can make it difficult for patients to be adequately ventilated via the

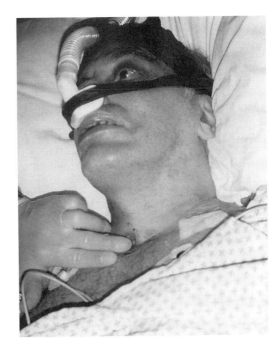

FIGURE 7. Tracheostomy tube is removed and the site occluded for assessment of maximal insufflation capacity, assisted peak cough flows, and training in noninvasive IPPV.

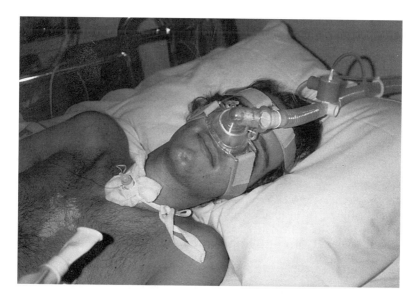

FIGURE 8.   Patient with high-level spinal cord injury and no breathing tolerance practicing nasal IPPV and mouthpiece IPPV with tracheostomy tube capped before decannulation.

upper airway. High, uncomfortable oropharyngeal pressures can be generated in this manner. If such pressures are not excessive, it may be helpful to let the patient use noninvasive IPPV for about 24 hours before removing the tube or button and letting the site close. Often when the tracheostomy tube has been removed for the more accurate measurement of PCF and noninvasive IPPV no longer induces high oropharyngeal pressures, the patient quickly becomes accustomed to it and the tracheostomy tube is simply not replaced. We no longer use body ventilators as a bridge to ventilate the patient's lungs while facilitating training in noninvasive IPPV and tracheostomy site closure.[36,44] Because we have rarely had to replace a tracheostomy tube, we now usually decannulate patients who meet the criterion, convert them directly to noninvasive IPPV, and let the tracheostomy sites close immediately on decannulation. Thus, whereas the ability to achieve adequate PCF is critical, the ability to sustain alveolar ventilation autonomously is unnecessary because ventilatory support can be provided noninvasively.[8] In addition to noninvasive IPPV, IAPVs can be used (see Chapter 7).

While the clinician is gaining confidence in using noninvasive IPPV for patients with little or no breathing tolerance, use of noninvasive ventilation with a tracheostomy button is advisable for a few days. In this way the tracheostomy tube can be replaced in the event of tracheal edema or some other development that makes recannulation desirable.

Soft silicon material with a 2-inch diameter in the form of a plugged donut (Respironics, Inc., Murrysville, PA) (Fig. 9) or a cane tip (Fig. 10) cut short is placed over an occlusive tracheostomy site dressing (Tegaderm, 3M Company, St. Paul, MN) (Fig. 11). The cane tip decreases any tendency for silicon slippage and prevents airway secretions from wetting and loosening the overlying gauze and elastic dressing. Four-by-four inch sterile gauze is placed over the silicon donut and may can be covered and fixed in place with adhesive tape. Insufflation leakage through the site can be further countered by placing an elastic figure-of-eight strap. The strap crosses anteriorly under the neck, under the axillae, over the shoulders, and across the back and inserts into an elastic band in front of the neck[45] (Fig. 12). This approach minimizes skin maceration from secretions that leak through the tracheostomy site and minimizes the amount of adhesive tape applied to the skin, thereby

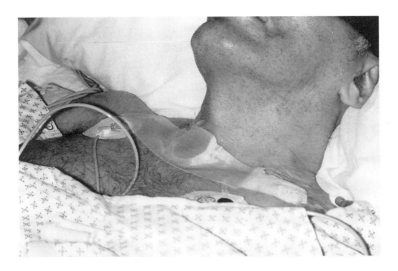

FIGURE 9.   Soft silicon occlusive pressure dressing (Respironics, Inc., Murrysville, PA) to permit continued noninvasive IPPV after decannulation and before ostomy closure

optimizing comfort and facilitating visualization of the ostomy as it closes. The tracheostomy site usually closes in 24–72 hours, but if it is not closed after 2 weeks, it is usually sutured. Once the tracheostomy site is closed, assisted PCF can be maximized and measured accurately, the patient can be taught GPB, and MI-E use via the upper airway can be assessed more accurately.

In 1990 we summarized the steps for the respiratory management and decannulation of patients with high-level spinal cord injury admitted to an acute rehabilitation facility as follows:

1. The patients were medically stabilized, and the use of supplemental oxygen therapy was discontinued or minimized. Aggressive manual and, for some patients, mechanical assisted coughing via the tube were used as alternatives to tracheal suctioning.

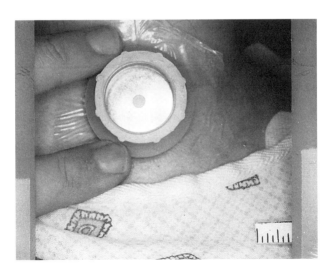

FIGURE 10.   Cane tip cut short and placed over an occlusive tracheostomy site dressing (Tegaderm, 3M Company, St. Paul, MN).

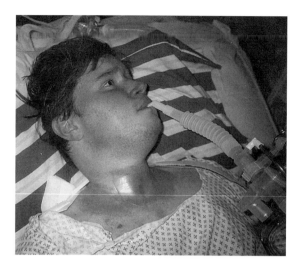

FIGURE 11. Occlusive tracheostomy site dressing (Tegaderm, 3M Company, St. Paul, MN) under cane tip or silicon plug.

2. All of the patients were placed on portable volume or, if the patient preferred, pressure-cycled ventilators. The cuffs were completely deflated for increasing periods hourly, until cuff deflation could be tolerated throughout the day. Partial-to-complete cuff deflation was used overnight. To ensure adequate alveolar ventilation, the delivered insufflation volumes were increased to maintain the same airway pressures as with the cuff inflated. When necessary, the diameter of the tracheostomy tube was changed to permit sufficient leakage for speech while maintaining adequate fit to permit effective assisted ventilation with delivered ventilator volumes generally of 1–2 liters. The set volumes on assist-control mode (rate: 10–12) were titrated to maintain pCO_2 levels between 35 and 40 mmHg. Tracheal integrity, tracheostomy tube width, and volitional glottic and vocal cord movements determined the amount of delivered air that entered the lungs and the amount that "leaked" through the vocal cords with each delivered volume. The insufflation leakage was used for inspiratory cycle speech. SpO_2 was maintained above 94% during daytime hours with a mean of 94% or greater during sleep.

Speech depended on crescendo/decrescendo pattern with the rhythm dependent on the cycling ventilator. A low speech volume indicated inadequate insufflation volume, a

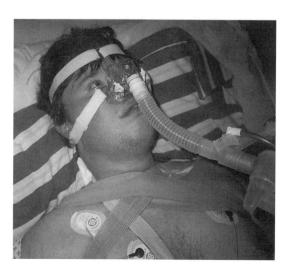

FIGURE 12. Postdecannulation pressure covering of occlusive ostomy dressing for patient with Duchenne muscular dystrophy and no autonomous breathing tolerance (see Fig. 8).

tracheostomy tube that was too wide, or subglottic obstruction, usually by granulation tissue. For such patients, optimal insufflation volumes for normal ventilation and more effective speech were obtained by cuff removal, by placing a tracheostomy tube with a narrower diameter, or by surgical ablation of the granulation tissue, when indicated. The expiratory valve was occasionally capped, permitting continuous speech without the expense of a Passy-Muir valve.

3. Patients were advanced to the use of 24-hour tracheostomy IPPV with a deflated cuff. The prolonged use of partial cuff deflation was discouraged because the nursing staff tended to gradually increase the amount of air in the cuff with time. Some patients were introduced to noninvasive ventilatory support by using an iron lung or chest-shell ventilator with the tracheostomy tube open. Care was taken to maintain the tracheostomy tube above the iron lung collar.

4. All patients were trained in the use of mouthpiece IPPV for daytime ventilatory support with the tracheostomy tube capped. Each patient learned to close off the nasopharynx with the soft palate to prevent nasal leakage. Temporarily pinching the nostrils helped the patient to understand why this technique was necessary. Patients who had their cuffs inflated for long periods initially maintained the vocal cords in full adduction during attempts at mouthpiece IPPV. Each patient was unaware that he was obstructing flow. This phenomenon was not infrequently mistaken for tracheal stenosis. Each patient successfully relearned the reflexive vocal cord abduction that permitted effective mouthpiece IPPV. Nasal IPPV is also used successfully before decannulation. For nasal IPPV users with no breathing tolerance, end-tidal carbon dioxide can be evaluated by sampling end-tidal air under the interface and as close to the nostrils as possible (Fig. 13).

Once daytime mouthpiece IPPV was mastered, body ventilators were occasionally used for nocturnal support with the ostomy covered. Body ventilator use facilitated tracheostomy site closure by relieving the stoma of the positive expulsive pressures that occur during IPPV; in addition, early use of a body ventilator for patients with no breathing tolerance facilitated training in mouthpiece and nasal IPPV by alleviating fear of dyspnea during early trials.

Mouthpiece IPPV normalized speech rhythm, provided normal daytime ventilation, and permitted air-stacking for volitional sighing, shouting, and assisted coughing when the tube fit tightly in the tracheostomy tract. The change to a fenestrated tracheostomy tube and its capping and cuff deflation often improved the efficacy of mouthpiece IPPV as well

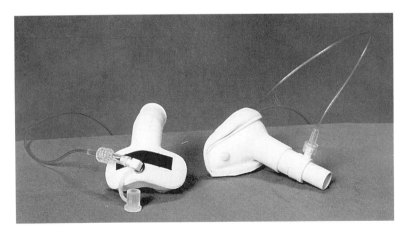

FIGURE 13.   End-tidal sampler passed via nasal prongs interface for measurements of end-tidal carbon dioxide during nasal ventilation.

as the effectiveness of body ventilator use. It also improved speech volume during use of mouthpiece IPPV or autonomous breathing, whenever possible. The fenestration of the commercially available tubes, however, was at times malpositioned against the posterior tracheal wall. Invagination of the tracheal mucosa into the fenestration rendered it ineffective, caused bleeding, and had the potential to exacerbating granulation formation. Proper positioning of the fenestration was accomplished by ordering a custom-made fenestrated tube or changing to a smaller tube.

5. Patients were advanced to the use of cuffless tracheostomy tubes. The great majority of patients did not require a change in tracheostomy diameter to maintain optimal ventilation and speech volume; however, ventilator volumes often needed to be as much as doubled to compensate for increased leakage. Patients were given trials of ventilatory support by the IAPV. Several trials were often necessary to determine the optimal belt size and position and the optimal buckle or Velcro strap pressures. The patient also had to learn to coordinate breathing with the IAPV.

6. Ventilator weaning was facilitated by mouthpiece IPPV. The mouthpiece was fixed adjacent to the mouth and was accessible to the patient by neck rotation. Patients took fewer and fewer assisted breaths as they weaned. This technique relieved the anxiety that most ventilator users feel when disconnected from tracheostomy IPPV. Mouthpiece IPPV also was used overnight with a lipseal. Secure dressings were used to minimize stomal leakage around the capped tracheostomy tube.

7. When the efficacy of noninvasive IPPV was observed, the tracheostomy tube was at times replaced by a tracheostomy button for 1 or 2 days before the tracheostomy site was allowed to close definitively.

8. In general, patients tried a variety of methods of noninvasive IPPV and were allowed to use the techniques that they preferred. Few patients using overnight mouthpiece/lipseal IPPV required nasal cotton pledgets to prevent excessive nasal leakage.

With mask or with pillows
I breathe through my nose
And the hole in my throat
Is ready to close

Richard L. Clingman, Sr., Webmaster for DoctorBach.com

OUTCOMES OF DECANNULATION

Five centers have reported tracheostomy tube removal for conversion to noninvasive respiratory muscle aids. One center reported transition from tracheostomy to noninvasive IPPV and site closure for one nocturnal ventilator user with poliomyelitis.[46] A second center reported the decannulation of 9 nocturnal-only assisted ventilation users and surgical stomal closure to nocturnal-only noninvasive ventilation.[47]

We reported the management of 80 consecutively admitted patients with spinal cord injury, including 74 who arrived using 24-hour tracheostomy IPPV with a tracheostomy tube cuff inflated up to 24 hours/ day and 4 who arrived intubated.[36,37] Of the 74 tracheostomy IPPV users, all 73 with intact oropharyngeal muscles were successfully converted to fenestrated tubes and used mouthpiece IPPV with the tubes plugged for increasing periods of daytime ventilatory support. Seventy of the 74 patients were also successfully converted to up to 24-hour tracheostomy IPPV with completely deflated cuffs with tubes of optimal diameter. All of these patients had effective speech during the ventilator inspiratory cycle. Three patients slept with partially inflated cuffs without placement of wider-gauged tubes. Three of the four patients who maintained at least partial cuff inflation did so because of severe tracheomalacia due to prolonged cuff use. The fourth patient had significant head trauma with bulbar muscle involvement that precluded cuff deflation or progression to noninvasive IPPV.

Of the 70 patients who had advanced to 24-hour tracheostomy IPPV with completely deflated cuffs, 28 were discharged using some combination of tracheostomy IPPV and IAPV, and 27 were weaned. Thirteen of the remaining 15 patients were decannulated and converted to noninvasive IPPV. Two of the 15 had severe tracheal stenosis and could not be decannulated. A small-gauge tube had to be left in place, but was it not used for assisted ventilation. Twelve of the 15 patients had life-threatening complications related to the tracheostomies or simply wished to have the tubes removed. In four of these patients, tracheostomy sites were closed despite a supine vital capacity of 50, 430, 740, and 560 ml and no significant breathing tolerance. In an additional three patients, respiratory failure was managed only by noninvasive IPPV; they were never tracheostomized. Thus, a total of 18 patients were supported by noninvasive IPPV without tracheostomy.

Another six patients, including three initially tracheostomized patients whose sites were allowed to close but who developed late-onset failure, were managed from onset of chronic ventilatory insufficiency without tracheostomy. Three were supported by mouthpiece IPPV, which they required for up to 24 hours/day, and three by wrap ventilators for nocturnal aid. One of these patients had been converted directly from IPPV via nasotracheal intubation to mouthpiece IPPV.

In all, 31 patients have regained independent respiration for a mean of 2.4 + 2.2 years (1 month to 8 years, median of 1.7 years) after onset of injury. At least five of the weaned patients required and routinely used mouthpiece IPPV during intercurrent chest infections to aid in ventilation and facilitate coughing. Two of these patients used mouthpiece IPPV 24 hours/day (including overnight) with a lip seal during chest infections for 28 and 39 years, respectively. The second patient died from metastatic cancer in 1997. Twenty of the 25 noninvasive IPPV users were discharged to private residences. Five patients were discharged to chronic care facilities.

The seven patients for whom noninvasive IPPV was the definitive method of continuous ventilatory support had a mean age at onset of injury of 25.1 ± 12.1 years. They have used 24-hour noninvasive IPPV for 22.6 ± 6.3 years. Two of these patients have died. One patient died from septicemia associated with massive decubiti after 8 years of noninvasive IPPV, including 7 years of continuous mouthpiece IPPV. The other patient died from seizure-induced apnea while using mouthpiece IPPV after 5 years of noninvasive ventilation. The 25 patients who continued 24-hour tracheostomy IPPV had a mean age of 30.2 ± 20 years at onset of injury. They used 24-hour tracheostomy IPPV for a mean of 7.1 ± 5.1 years. Five of these patients are currently lost to follow-up. Ten of the remaining 20 patients died after 3.8 ± 2.8 years of ventilatory support. Four deaths were associated with pneumonia, two with cancer, two with accidental tracheostomy disconnection, and one each with aspiration from tracheal hemorrhage, ventilator malfunction, and unknown cause.

Five patients mastered GPB sufficiently after tracheostomy site closure to use it for breathing tolerance during the day and as a back-up in the event of ventilator failure overnight. The longest duration of total dependence on noninvasive ventilation in a patient with spinal cord injury was that of a 17-year-old boy who fell from a horse in a school gymnasium on March 10, 1967, and sustained a fracture dislocation of C1–C2 and complete C2 tetraplegia. He was immediately and permanently dependent on supported ventilation with no breathing tolerance. On September 27, 1967, phrenic pacemakers were placed bilaterally but were ineffective. He remained in a local intensive care unit for 10 months with multiple pulmonary infections. He was transferred for rehabilitation in February of 1968 with a Rausch tracheostomy tube of 16-mm diameter and cuff inflated with 12 ml. He had severe trachiectasis with a cuff-to-trachea diameter ratio of 3:1. He continued to have frequent purulent mucus plugging, which led to an episode of respiratory arrest that resulted in partial blindness. He also had two other episodes of near arrest. Because of these difficulties he was highly motivated for tracheostomy closure.

The patient began daytime mouthpiece IPPV on April 17, 1968. He also began to use an iron lung for nocturnal aid on July 3, 1968. The iron lung provided a delivered volume of 660 ml, minute volume of 11.8 L, and normal blood gases. The Rausch tube was replaced by a metal cuffless tube with the orifice plugged by a custom-made prosthesis during use of the mouthpiece IPPV and iron lung. Even with the tube plugged, tracheal site leakage prevented more than 5 minutes of breathing tolerance by combined GPB and use of accessory muscles. In April of 1969, the tracheostomy site was allowed to close after another two episodes of pneumonia. Breathing tolerance increased to greater than 3 hours with GPB, and the patient had a GPB maximal single breath capacity of 1700 ml. Vital capacity increased to 420 ml with accessory muscle use in the sitting position. He had trials of the chest-shell ventilator and IAPV, neither of which worked as well for him as mouthpiece IPPV and the iron lung. He was discharged to a chronic care facility, where he was converted from the iron lung to a wrap ventilator overnight. He continued to use mouthpiece IPPV during the daytime and the Pulmowrap (Respironics, Inc., Murrysville, PA) ventilator overnight until July 1999 when he decided to withdraw from ventilatory support and died using morphine and supplemental oxygen. This patient used the IAPV during dental procedures. He had had only two episodes of pneumonia resulting from chest colds over the last 30 years of his life.

A fourth center practicing decannulation of patients with high-level SCI and other patients with neuromuscular weakness is the Dallas Rehabilitation Institute.[48] By 1991, 13 patients who were apparently unweanable from tracheostomy IPPV (mean age: 29.8 + 18.4 years) and four other patients in respiratory failure had mastered mouthpiece IPPV, and all but two were placed on body ventilators for overnight ventilatory support. These two patients were converted directly from tracheostomy IPPV to 24-hour mouthpiece IPPV. Mouthpiece IPPV was mastered on the first day by about one-half of patients. The average vital capacity at the time of tracheostomy closure and/or conversion to solely non-invasive methods of ventilatory support was about 600 ml with a range of 0- 1100 ml. Most patients had less than 3 hours of breathing tolerance; seven had no breathing tolerance; and two had no measurable vital capacity when the tracheostomy sites were allowed to close.

Six patients with spinal cord injury, less than 600 ml of vital capacity, and no significant breathing tolerance learned GPB. Five of the six had a mean GPB maximal single breath capacity of 2205 ml despite an average vital capacity of 402 ml and used GPB successfully for breathing tolerance.

Since 1990 the Dallas center has successfully decannulated 30–40 other patients with high-level spinal cord injury and no significant breathing tolerance. We have decannulated 11 patients with non-Duchenne muscular dystrophy, 15 with high-level spinal cord injury, 3 with nonbulbar ALS, 4 with poliomyelitis, 3 with DMD, 2 with multiple sclerosis, and 2 with SMA despite little or no breathing tolerance. Only two of these patients, both with bulbar ALS, underwent tracheostomy a second time.

In yet another center, 37 patients were decannulated after invasive IPPV for a mean of 57 days. Twenty-nine patients required ongoing home noninvasive IPPV, five underwent repeat tracheostomy, and three were weaned from noninvasive IPPV.[42]

Guidelines for the long-term ventilator management of patients with acute spinal cord injury are presented as a function of level of injury in Table 2. The great majority of patients with spinal cord injury who develop ventilatory failure do so during the first week after injury. Failing ventilatory function in the acute setting at times also can be managed without intubation by using noninvasive IPPV, MAC, and oximetry as feedback.[49]

TABLE 2. Management of Patients with Spinal Cord Injury

Level*	Vital Capacity (L)	Bulbar/Neck Muscles†	Daytime	Nocturnal
Above C1	0	Inadequate/inadequate	TPV	TPV
Above C2	< 0.2	Adequate/inadequate	EPR	EPR/NPV
Below C2	> 0.2	Adequate/adequate	NPV/IAPV	NPV

TPV = tracheostomy intermittent positive pressure ventilation, EPR = electrophrenic pacing, NPV = nasal intermittent positive pressure ventilation, IAPV = intermittent abdomenal pressure ventilator.
* Any patients with assisted PCF less than 160 L/min retain indwelling tracheostomy tubes regardless of ability to breathe unaided.
† Adequate neck function indicates sufficient oral and neck muscular control to rotate, flex, and extend the neck to grab and use a mouthpiece for IPPV; adequate bulbar function is indicated by the ability to generate assisted PCF > 160 L/min and to prevent aspiration of saliva to the degree that the SaO_2 baseline decreases below 95%.

POSTSURGICAL COMPLICATIONS

With age, many patients with poliomyelitis and many others with neuromuscular weakness but no history of respiratory complications experience respiratory difficulties after an unrelated surgical intervention with general anesthesia. Typically they fail to wean from the ventilator in a timely manner, are left intubated, develop pneumonia, and are told that they need tracheostomy tubes. Even otherwise benign procedures, such as colonoscopies performed under conscious sedation with oximetry monitoring and possibly supplemental oxygen administration rather than carbon dioxide monitoring and assisted ventilation, have typically resulted in tracheostomies or deaths from ventilatory failure. For example, the 25% of patients with DMD and low plateau (lifetime maximum) vital capacity[50] invariably develop scoliosis that requires spinal stabilization. Postoperatively they often fail to wean from the ventilator and undergo tracheotomy. However, this procedure is avoidable by training such patients in the use of respiratory muscle aids before surgery so that, even with failure to wean from the ventilator postoperatively, they can be extubated to full non-invasive ventilatory support and assisted coughing with oximetry feedback (see Chapter 8). The avoidance of opioid and muscle relaxant anesthetics also may be beneficial.[51]

All over the place nothing was to be heard except the barking of dogs, which deafened the ears of Don Quixote and troubled the heart of Sancho. "The fact that the dogs are barking, Sancho, means that we are moving forward."

Miguel de Cervantes, *Don Quijote de la Mancha*

REFERENCES

1. Goldberg AI, Frownfelter D: The ventilator-assisted individuals study. Chest 98:428–433, 1990.
2. Chaudhry SS, Bach JR: Management approaches in muscular dystrophy association clinics. Am J Phys Med Rehabil 79:193–196, 2000.
3. Jardine E, O'Toole M, Paton JY, Wallis C: Current status of long term ventilation of children in the United Kingdom: Questionnaire survey. Br Med J 318:295–298, 1999.
4. Hall CD, Howard JF Jr, Donohue JF: The ventilator support of patients with neuromuscular disorders. In Kutscher AH (ed): Muscular Dystrophy and Other Neuromuscular Diseases: Psychosocial Issues. New York, Haworth Press, 1991, pp 185–191.
5. Miller JR: Family response to Duchenne muscular dystrophy. In Kutscher AH (ed): Muscular Dystrophy and Other Neuromuscular Diseases: Psychosocial Issues. New York, Haworth Press, 1991, pp 31–41.
6. Gilgoff IS: End stage Duchenne patients: Choosing between respirator and natural death. In Charash LI (ed): Psychosocial Aspects of Muscular Dystrophy and Allied Diseases. Springfield, IL, Charles C Thomas, 1983, pp 301–307.

7. Gilgoff I, Prentice W, Baydur P: Patient and family participation in the management of respiratory failure in Duchenne's muscular dystrophy. Chest 95:319–324, 1989.
8. Bach JR, Saporito LR: Criteria for extubation and tracheostomy tube removal for patients with ventilatory failure: A different approach to weaning. Chest 110:1566–1571, 1996.
9. Nathanson BN, Yu DG, Chan CK: Respiratory muscle weakness in Charcot-Marie-Tooth disease. Arch Intern Med 149:1389–1391, 1989.
10. Lissoni A, Aliverti A, Molteni F, Bach JR: Spinal muscular atrophy: Kinematic breathing analysis. Am J Phys Med Rehabil 75:332–339, 1996.
11. Kang SW, Bach JR: Maximum insufflation capacity. Chest 118:61–65, 2000.
12. Lindahl SG, Yates AP, Hatch DJ: Relationship between invasive and noninvasive measurements of gas exchange in anesthetized infants and children. Anesthesiology 66:168–175, 1987.
13. Morley TF, Giaimo J, Maroszan E, et al: Use of capnography for assessment of the adequacy of alveolar ventilation during weaning from mechanical ventilation. Am Rev Respir Dis 148:339–344, 1993.
14. Wiedemann HP, McCarthy K: Noninvasive monitoring of oxygen and carbon dioxide. Clin Chest Med 10:239–254, 1989.
15. Janssens JP, Howarth-Frey C, Chevrolet JC, et al: Transcutaneous PCO_2 to monitor noninvasive mechanical ventilation in adults: Assessment of a new transcutaneous PCO_2 device. Chest 113:768–773, 1998.
16. Flanagan JF, Garrett JS, McDuffee A, Tobias JD: Noninvasive monitoring of end-tidal carbon dioxide tension via nasal cannulas in spontaneously breathing children with profound hypocarbia. Crit Care Med 23:1140–1142, 1995.
17. Healey CJ, Fedullo AJ, Swinburne AJ, Wahl GW: Comparison of noninvasive measurements of carbon dioxide tension during withdrawal from mechanical ventilation. Crit Care Med 15:764–768, 1987.
18. Plewa MC, Sikora S, Engoren M, et al: Evaluation of capnography in nonintubated emergency department patients with respiratory distress. Acad Emerg Med 2:901–908, 1995.
19. Kavanagh BP, Sandler AN, Turner KE, etal: Use of end-tidal pCO2 and transcutaneous PCO2 as noninvasive measurement of arterial PCO_2 in extubated patients recovering from general anesthesia. J Clin Monit 8:226–230, 1992.
20. Lenz G, Heipertz W, Epple E: Capnometry for postoperative monitoring of nonintubated, spontaneously breathing patients. J Clin Monit 7:245–248, 1991.
21. Bongard F, Wu Y, Lee TS, Klein S: Capnographic monitoring of extubated postoperative patients. J Invest Surg 7:259–264, 1994.
22. Tobias JD, Meyer DJ: Noninvasive monitoring of carbon dioxide during respiratory failure in toddlers and infants: end-tidal versus transcutaneous carbon dioxide. Anesth Anag 85:55–58, 1997.
23. Cinel D, Markwell K, Lee R, Szidon P: Variability of the respiratory gas exchange ratio during arterial puncture. Am Rev Respir Dis 143:217–218, 1991.
24. Partridge BL: Use of pulse oximetry as a noninvasive indicator of intravascular volume status. J Clin Monit 3:263–268, 1987.
25. Watson L, Colbert F, Topley L, Kinnear W: Initiation of non-invasive ventilation as an out-patient. Eighth Journées Internationales de Ventilation à Domicile, abstract 46, March 7, 2001, Hôpital de la Croix-Rousse, Lyon, France.
26. Bach JR, Ishikawa Y, Kim H: Prevention of pulmonary morbidity for patients with Duchenne muscular dystrophy. Chest 112:1024–1028, 1997.
27. Hill NS, Eveloff SE, Carlisle CC, Goff SG: Efficacy of nocturnal nasal ventilation in patients with restrictive thoracic disease. Am Rev Respir Dis 145:365–371, 1992.
28. Jimenez JFM, Sanchez de Cos Escuin J, Vicente CD, et al: Nasal intermittent positive pressure ventilation: analysis of its withdrawal. Chest 107:382–388, 1995.
29. Goldstein RS, DeRosie JA, Avendano MA, Dolmage TE: Influence of noninvasive positive pressure ventilation on inspiratory muscles. Chest 99:408–415, 1991.
30. Belman MJ, Soo Hoo GW, Kuei JH, Shadmehr R: Efficacy of positive vs. negative pressure ventilation in unloading the respiratory muscles. Chest 98:850–856, 1990.
31. Welch JR, DeCesare R, Hess D: Pulse oximetry: instrumentation and clinical applications. Respir Care 35:584–594, 1990.
32. Mier-Jedrzejowicz A, Brophy C, Green M: Respiratory muscle weakness during upper respiratory tract infections. Am Rev Respir Dis 138:5–7, 1988.
33. Laier-Groeneveld G, Criee CP: Epidemiology and diagnosis of intermittent self-ventilation [in German]. Med Klin 92(Suppl 1):2–8, 1997.
34. Rubini F, Zanotti E, Nava S: Ventilatory techniques during weaning. Monaldi Arch Chest Dis 49:527–529, 1994.
35. Tzeng AC, Bach JR: Prevention of pulmonary morbidity for patients with neuromuscular disease. Chest 118:1390–1396, 2000.
36. Bach JR, Alba AS: Noninvasive options for ventilatory support of the traumatic high level quadriplegic. Chest 98:613–619, 1990.
37. Bach JR: New approaches in the rehabilitation of the traumatic high level quadriplegic. Am J Phys Med Rehabil 70:13–20, 1991.

38. Niranjan V, Bach JR: Spinal muscular atrophy type 1: A noninvasive respiratory management approach. Chest 117:1100–1105, 2000.
39. Schonhofer B, Sonneborn M, Haidl P, et al: Intermittent self-ventilation after respirator weaning [in German]. Med Klin 91(Suppl 2):27–30, 1996.
40. Girault C, Daudenthun I, Chevron V, et al: Noninvasive ventilation as a systemic extubation and weaning technique in acute-on-chronic respiratory failure. Am J Respir Crit Care Med 160:86–92, 1999.
41. Beltrame F, Lucangelo U, Gregori D, Gregoretti C: Noninvasive positive pressure ventilation in trauma patients with acute respiratory failure. Monaldi Arch Chest Dis 54:109–114, 1999.
42. Korber W, Laier-Groeneveld G, Criee CP: Endotracheal complications after long-term ventilation: noninvasive ventilation in chronic thoracic diseases as an alternative to tracheostomy. Med Klin 94:45–50, 1999.
43. Forte V, Cole P, Crysdale WS: Objective assessment of upper airway resistance in the tracheotomized patient. J Otolaryngol 15:359–361, 1986.
44. Bach JR. Alternative methods of ventilatory support for the patient with ventilatory failure due to spinal cord injury. J Am Parapleg Soc 14:158–174, 1991.
45. Bach JR, Saporito LS: Indications and criteria for decannulation and transition from invasive to noninvasive long-term ventilatory support. Respir Care 39:515–531, 1994.
46. Goodenberger DM, Couser JI Jr, May JJ: Successful discontinuation of ventilation via tracheostomy by substitution of nasal positive pressure ventilation. Chest 102:1277–1279, 1992.
47. Hickey SA, Ford GR, Evans JNG, et al: Tracheostomy closure in restrictive respiratory insufficiency. J Laryngol Otol 104:883–886, 1990.
48. Viroslav J, Rosenblatt R, Morris-Tomazevic S: Respiratory management, survival, and quality of life for high-level traumatic tetraplegics. 3:313–322, 1996.
49. Bach JR, Hunt D, Horton JA III: Traumatic tetraplegia: Noninvasive management in the acute setting. Am J Phys Med [in press].
50. Rideau Y, Glorion B, Delaubier A, et al: Treatment of scoliosis in Duchenne muscular dystrophy. Muscle Nerve 7:281–286, 1984.
51. Patrick JA, Meyer-Witting M, Reynolds F, Spencer GT: Peri-operative care in restrictive respiratory disease. Anaesthesia 45:390 395, 1990.
52. Bach JR, Alba AS: Management of chronic alveolar hypoventilation by nasal ventilation. Chest 97:52–57, 1990.

9 —— Respiratory Muscle Aids: Diagnosis-related Outcomes

JOHN R. BACH, M.D.

> *Un artiste créateur est comme un archer qui tire ses flèches dans le noir, sans jamais savoir si elles toucheront le but.*
> *(An artist is like an archer who shoots his arrows in the dark without ever knowing whether or not they will hit the target.)*
>
> Gustav Mahler

Chapter 7 described respiratory muscle aids and the clinical goals of attaining full chest expansion, maintaining alveolar ventilation, and maximizing peak cough flow (PCF). Many of the diagnoses listed in Table 1 of Chapter 1, however, have pathophysiologic features (see Chapter 2) that warrant particular strategies to achieve these goals. Chapter 8 presented an oximetry feedback-respiratory muscle aid protocol. This chapter discusses outcomes related to its use for various common conditions.

NONINVASIVE RESPIRATORY MUSCLE AID OUTCOMES

From 1977 to 1999 the author managed 643 long-term users of noninvasive intermittent positive-pressure ventilation (IPPV) with the diagnoses listed in Table 1. Pulmonary function, extent of ventilator need, duration of use, and prolongation of survival for many of these ventilator users have been published elsewhere.[1-7] Although most patients used mouthpiece IPPV as the primary method, as early as 1990 we reported 43 noninvasive IPPV users, of whom 33 had been using nocturnal nasal IPPV in a regimen of full-time noninvasive IPPV for over 20 months.[4]

Numerous other patients with many of the same diagnoses listed in Table 1 of Chapter 1, including 94 patients reported in a recent publication, avoided hospitalizations during chest infections by having access to the oximetry feedback-respiratory muscle aid protocol. In other words, they became full-time ventilator-dependent without being hospitalized and were able to reverse oxyhemoglobin desaturation associated with airway mucus plugs by using mechanically assisted coughing (MAC) with oximetry feedback during chest colds. Sixteen of the patients avoided 1.02 ± 0.99 hospitalizations per patient per year over a period of 2.1 ± 91.84 years before requiring ongoing ventilator use. Forty-nine part-time ventilator users avoided 0.99 ± 1.12 hospitalizations per patient per year over 3.88 ± 3.45 years; and 18 full-time noninvasive ventilation users avoided 0.80 ± 0.85 hospitalizations per patient per year over 6.54 ± 5.00 years. All comparisons of preprotocol and protocol rates were statistically significant at p <0.004.[1,8] After resolution of chest

TABLE 1. Diagnoses of Long-Term Noninvasive IPPV Users at the Author's Center

Polio	186
Diagnosis not confirmed	93
Duchenne muscular dystrophy	78
Spinal cord injury	59
Non-Duchenne myopathies	61
Amyotrophic lateral sclerosis	41
Spinal muscular atrophy	64
Chronic obstructive pulmonary disease	10
Scoliosis	11
Obesity hypoventilation	9
Multiple sclerosis	5
Myasthenia gravis	5
Phrenic neuropathy	4
Polymyositis	3
Other respiratory disease[†]	3
Myelopathy other than traumatic	2
Charcot-Marie-Tooth disease	2
Miscellaneous[‡]	7
Total	643

* Including Emery-Dreifuss, limb-girdle, and myotonic muscular dystrophies and generalized myopathies including acid maltase deficiency.
† Including pulmonary fibrosis, Milroy's disease, tuberculosis.
‡ Including Friedreich's ataxia, neuropathy associated with cancer, osteogenesis imperfecta, Guillain-Barré syndrome, central alveolar hypoventilation, brainstem astrocytoma, post-curarization paralysis.

infections, patients generally weaned from full-time ventilator use to preinfection regimens until the next respiratory tract infection developed.[1]

Although nine other groups have reported isolated cases of avoidance of respiratory complications and eventual use of up to 24-hour long-term noninvasive ventilatory support,[9] these reports have resulted mostly from patients who refused tracheostomy, continued nasal IPPV into daytime hours, and have not yet had chest infections. The use of crucial noninvasive expiratory muscle aids has not been noted.[10] For example, Baydur et al. reported 46 years of experience using noninvasive ventilation in 79 patients with neuromusculoskeletal disorders.[11] They noted that hospital admissions increased 8-fold once patients began using negative-pressure body ventilators (NPBVs) but decreased by 36% for those using noninvasive IPPV. Because of failure to use expiratory aids and noninvasive IPPV appropriately during daytime hours, 30 patients, including 10 of 15 with Duchenne muscular dystrophy (DMD), underwent tracheotomy. Most certainly none of these patients would have required tracheostomy if managed with the oximetry respiratory aid protocol.[12]

Duchenne Muscular Dystrophy

Because patients with DMD breathe mostly with their diaphragms, vital capacity is usually the same in the sitting and supine positions. As vital capacity decreases below 2000 ml, maximal insufflation lung mobilizations are initiated 3 times/day, using a manual resuscitator. Soon after this point, unassisted PCF tends to decrease below 270 L/sec, and untrained and unequipped patients are at an increasingly greater risk of developing pneumonia and respiratory failure during intercurrent chest infections. Therefore, they are taught MAC and the oximetry protocol. Because respiratory tract infections are frequent in this young population, an oximeter and Cough-Assist are prescribed for home use. Many patients with DMD have airway secretion encumberment, often from chronic aspiration of upper airway secretions or from congestive heart failure, necessitating use of MAC multiple times every day.

Because such patients also may have scoliosis that decreases the efficacy of abdominal thrusts and because their bulbar musculature is dysfunctional, although never entirely impaired, maximal insufflation capacity (MIC) eventually decreases below 1000 ml, but assisted PCF rarely decreases below 160 L/min.

The older the patient, the greater the risk of hypoventilation at higher vital capacities. As the vital capacity decreases below 800 ml, patients with DMD often begin to rock back and forth in their wheelchair to compress the abdomen during exhalation and thus increase tidal volumes. At this point they also tend to develop hypercapnia during sleep and eventually begin to use accessory breathing muscles. They usually remain grossly asymptomatic, however, until vital capacity decreases below 450 ml and hypercapnia extends into daytime hours and causes oxyhemoglobin desaturation below 95%. This first occurs during sleep and eventually when the patient is awake. Around this time nocturnal nasal IPPV with a portable volume-cycled ventilator usually is indicated.

Patients usually require daytime mouthpiece IPPV with the ventilator on the back of the wheelchair and the mouthpiece adjacent to the mouth once vital capacity is less than 350 ml. About 15% of patients eventually lose the ability to use mouthpiece IPPV because of oromotor weakness. Such patients typically prefer to use nasal IPPV around the clock rather than undergo tracheotomy. Often they also can use intermittent abdominal pressure ventilators (IAPVs). Thus, the typical patient eventually requires a volume-cycled ventilator, a Cough-Assist, oximeter, and manual resuscitator and requires noninvasive IPPV on a full-time basis during intercurrent chest infections, for air stacking, and eventually for ventilatory support.

Some patients, even with vital capacity as high as 1500 ml, feel better and less fatigued with nocturnal nasal IPPV or even with low-span positive inspiratory pressure and positive end-expiratory pressure (PIP + PEEP) early in the course of disease. They also may have improvements in nocturnal SpO_2. However, although mild nocturnal hypoventilation may appear and evidence of sleep-disordered breathing usually can be seen in polysomnography studies long before vital capacity has decreased to 700 ml, nightly ventilator use should not be recommended unless the patient has improvements in symptoms. The reason is simple: such patients are likely to use noninvasive IPPV for 20 years or more. Burdening them too early and in the absence of symptoms is probably unwarranted.

When patients are properly equipped and trained and when optimal personal care assistance is available in the home, respiratory complications of DMD can be completely avoided.[1] In our study of patients referred after 1983, 86 patients (mean age: 26.0 ± 7.0 years) had become wheelchair-dependent at 9.7 ± 2.2 years of age. The mean age at first visit was 19.2 + 6.2 years. Fifty-one (59.3%) were still alive at 25.2 ± 5.9 years of age, and 35 (40.7%) died at 27.3 ± 8.2 years of age. The causes of death were respiratory in 17 patients, cardiac in 12, other in two, and unknown in four. Although these early patients used up to full-time noninvasive IPPV, no patient who died of respiratory-related causes had access to oximetry or cough aids. Of the 12 patients who died from congestive heart failure, the nine who used mechanical ventilation died later than the nonventilator users at 26.8 ± 5.5 years of age. Of the 17 patients who died from respiratory complications, 14 died from acute respiratory tract illness and three from ventilatory insufficiency when they were disconnected from the ventilator or slept without using it. These three patients had a vital capacity of 411 ± 391 ml immediately before dying and had been using IPPV for 16.3 ± 6.65 years when they died at 40 ± 10.15 years of age. Thus, in almost all cases, death occurred within days after onset of a chest infection or from congestive heart failure in patients with extremely low cardiac ejection fractions. None of the seven deaths for which autopsies were performed were due to pulmonary emboli or noncardiopulmonary causes.

Of the 34 patients with access to the oximetry protocol, 31 are still alive at 25.7 ± 4.5 years of age. They have been using the protocol for 5.3 ± 4.2 years (range: 1–16 years) and have been using noninvasive IPPV for 5.4 ± 4.0 years, including 1.6 ± 1.6 years of nocturnal-only noninvasive IPPV. None of these patients have died from respiratory causes. The three who died (at 25 ± 2 years of age) had left ventricular ejection fractions below 15%.

The longest period for which our patients with DMD have been using 24-hour noninvasive IPPV has been for 26, 20, and 15 years to ages 43, 34, and 38 years, respectively. We also decannulated three full-time tracheostomy IPPV users and switched them to noninvasive IPPV. Five patients have required full-time noninvasive IPPV for 5 years or more without being hospitalized.[1] None of our patients with DMD have undergone tracheotomy since 1983.

Because they retain adequate assisted PCF at all ages, virtually no properly managed patients with DMD require tracheostomy tubes. If a tube is already placed, it need not always be removed because such patients are usually not good candidates for effective GPB. However, 12 of our patients with a mean vital capacity of 265 + 104 ml and no breathing tolerance using respiratory muscles were able to use GPB to volumes of 1273 ± 499 ml. This technique permitted them a mean of 5.3 ± 4.8 hours of breathing tolerance. Therefore, tubes should be removed if the patient so desires, if there have been complications of tracheostomy, or if tube removal can facilitate social functioning (e.g., deinstitutionalization). Usually decannulation and transition to noninvasive IPPV from 24-hour tracheostomy IPPV result in discontinuance of daytime ventilator use and facilitate returning home (see Case 16 in Chapter 15).

Because respiratory mortality can now be avoided, the limiting factor for survival in our center and others in Japan has become cardiomyopathy. Death from cardiomyopathy can occur as early as 12 years of age but can also be delayed. The Yakumo Byoin National Sanatorium in Hokkaido, Japan, under the direction of Yuka Ishikawa, M.D., and Tatara's center at the Tokushima National Sanatorium Hospital in Tokushima, Japan, have reported survival data for full-time mouthpiece/nasal IPPV users with DMD. Tatara recently reported a 5-year cumulative survival rate of 75% for 34 pediatric patients, including 25 with DMD, who were noninvasive IPPV users. Tokushima is also the home of the rock group Dream Music Directory, pictured on the cover of this book. At Ishikawa's center, 44 patients with DMD have used noninvasive ventilation since 20.3 ± 3.4 years of age. They have 1- and 3-year survival rates of 97.7% and a 10-year survival rate of 93.3%. Before 1991 at the same center, tracheostomy IPPV was begun as the only method of ventilatory support for 26 patients with DMD at age 20.0 ± 4.0 years. The 1-year survival rate was 73.1%; the 3-year survival rate, 53.8%; the 5-year survival, 50%; and the 10-year survival rate, 42.3%. We are aware of no other centers with more than a few patients with DMD who use 24-hour noninvasive IPPV.

Non-Duchenne Myopathies

Patients with non-Duchenne muscular dystrophies and other myopathies are managed similarly to patients with DMD, except that their conditions are usually milder. As a result, they develop ventilatory insufficiency at older ages and at higher vital capacities. In addition, some of these patients, especially those with adult-onset muscular dystrophies and acid-maltase deficiency, develop severe diaphragm weakness and lose breathing tolerance in the supine but not in the sitting position. Often vital capacity in the supine position is less than half the vital capacity in the sitting position. Such patients can require nocturnal ventilatory support for many years before needing daytime aid. Many can walk despite symptomatic daytime hypercapnia. As a result, they do not use assisted ventilation sufficiently during daytime hours to normalize diurnal carbon dioxide levels and thereby optimize nocturnal use (see Chapter 5). Except for an occasional patient with facioscapulohumeral muscular dystrophy (FSH), bulbar muscles usually retain adequate function for effective speech, swallowing, GPB, and assisted coughing. Therefore, few patients require tracheostomy tubes, and those with tubes are usually excellent candidates for decannulation and transition to noninvasive IPPV and GPB (see Chapter 8).

As for patients with DMD, insufflations to the MIC are begun 3 times/day once vital capacity decreases from normal. Younger patients who develop more frequent chest infections require oximeters and Cough-Assists in the home. All patients are trained in assisted coughing and the oximetry feedback protocol once assisted PCF is less than 270 L/min. Older patients who have no history of pneumonia and infrequently develop chest infections may require oximeters in the home but rapid access to mechanical insufflation-exsufflation (MI-E) only during chest infections. Depending on the extent of the myopathic process in the myocardium, many of these patients can use full-time noninvasive IPPV for 30 years or more before cardiomyopathy limits survival.

We reported that respiratory complications and hospitalizations were avoided for 25 ventilator users with non-Duchenne myopathies by use of the oximetry protocol.[8] Because such patients have less bulbar muscle dysfunction and often less cardiomyopathy than patients with DMD, it is not surprising that 17 of our patients with non-DMD myopathy and a mean vital capacity of 363 ml have lived up to 30 years using full-time noninvasive ventilation.[13]

Myotonic Dystrophy

Although myotonic dystrophy is essentially a non-DMD myopathy, it deserves special comment. The chemosensitivity of the respiratory centers, as measured by $P_{0.1}$, is well preserved in patients with myotonic dystrophy as it is in the other muscular dystrophies, but even in the absence of restricted lung volumes, output to breathing is modulated by impaired respiratory mechanics. The result of impaired respiratory mechanics is chronic symptomatic alveolar hypoventilation despite the fact that vital capacity and MIC are generally well preserved until late in the disease course.[14] Even in the absence of obstructive sleep apneas[15] or chronic diurnal hypercapnia, however, these patients can exhibit hypersomnia (see Chapter 2).

In addition, hypersomnia and apneas and hypopneas, when present, can be exacerbated by chronic alveolar hypoventilation due to weak and myotonic inspiratory muscles. Despite severe hypercapnia and nocturnal ventilatory insufficiency, such patients often fail to use assisted ventilation sufficiently either during the day or overnight—probably because they are usually able to walk and because general apathy and perhaps cognitive impairment are often part of the primary pathology. One study reported poor compliance with ventilator use by 62% of 38 patients in comparison with patients with other NMDs.[16] Thus, many patients never cooperate sufficiently to benefit optimally from noninvasive IPPV. Most patients are hospitalized repeatedly before succumbing to cor pulmonale and congestive heart failure. Because of persistent hypercapnia and hypersomnolence, these patients are perhaps the most frustrating to try to treat by noninvasive ventilation. Nevertheless, those who cooperate sufficiently to use at least nocturnal noninvasive IPPV have improved arterial blood gases and improved survival with greater alertness, less sleep disturbance, and fewer morning headaches—if not always less hypersomnolence.[17]

Patients with myotonic dystrophy also have poor prognoses with tracheostomy tubes for the same reasons that they often fail to use noninvasive IPPV adequately. Although no long-term studies address the use of mechanical ventilation by patients with myotonic dystrophy, we have managed a handful of patients with up to full-time dependence on tracheostomy IPPV and eight others with noninvasive IPPV, which prolonged survival by up to 8 years.

Multiple Sclerosis and Myasthenia Gravis

Patients with multiple sclerosis and myasthenia gravis can develop ventilatory failure and may require full-time noninvasive IPPV and the oximetry protocol over the long term as well as during acute exacerbations. Both acutely and over the long term, inordinate diaphragm weakness may manifest itself by inability to breathe in the recumbent position.

Patients benefit from ongoing nocturnal use of noninvasive IPPV so that they can sleep in the supine position. Depending on the extent of bulbar muscle dysfunction, the protocol can sometimes avert the need for intubation. Indeed, the first patient ever to depend on full-time nasal IPPV with no breathing tolerance was diagnosed with multiple sclerosis.[18]

The contribution of chronic upper airway obstruction to hypoventilation may be underestimated. Putman and Wise found that in 12 of 61 patients with myasthenia gravis, pulmonary function testing revealed a pattern of upper airway obstruction.[19] Patients with multiple sclerosis also have a high incidence of symptomatic obstructive sleep apneas, stridor, and hypopharyngeal collapse when coughing or using MI-E. These conditions may contribute to or exacerbate nocturnal hypoventilation and inadequate PCF. Some patients with little or no volitional assisted PCF have excellent reflexive PCF and can clear airway secretions to some degree in this manner. Perhaps because of airway instability, we find that the use of high-span PIP + PEEP is better tolerated and more effective for treating nocturnal breathing disorders, at least when the vital capacity is greater than 2 liters, than the use of portable volume ventilators without PEEP. Patients with less than normal vital capacity also require regular daily maximal insufflations if they are unable to air-stack.

No statistics are available about the number of these patients who have benefited from noninvasive alternatives to avoid intubation and tracheostomy tubes. We have demonstrated the avoidance of respiratory failure and hospitalizations for three such patients with use of the oximetry protocol.[8] We also have seen one patient with myasthenia gravis who was intubated for pneumonia and respiratory failure on four occasions from 1987 to 1992. On the last occasion, she had failed extubation three times with increasingly severe hypercapnia and had remained on full-time IPPV for 4 months when we were consulted. We first weaned her from supplemental oxygen by aggressive MI-E via the translaryngeal tube and then extubated her to full-time noninvasive IPPV (see Table 1 in Chapter 10). Because she had highly functional upper extremities, she became quite adept at self-applying MI-E and has not had any respiratory difficulties despite subsequent chest infections and the need to use MI-E daily. She requires MI-E every morning on rising to clear aspirated airway secretions. An attempt to discontinue nocturnal nasal IPPV in 1995 resulted in a return of symptoms; she continues to use it today.

We have successfully decannulated three patients with multiple sclerosis and one patient with myasthenia gravis. All required IPPV at decannulation and for at least 3 years afterward because of no breathing tolerance. On the other hand, two averbal patients with multiple sclerosis, admitted for respiratory failure, and one patient with multiple sclerosis and severe bulbar dysfunction and chronic aspiration of saliva underwent tracheostomy because of chronic oxyhemoglobin desaturation, distress from secretions, and unmeasurable PCF. One died 3 weeks after tracheotomy; the other two have survived with tubes for 6 months and 4 years, respectively. Although only a minority of patients with multiple sclerosis benefit from ongoing noninvasive IPPV, and only when the condition is quite advanced, many patients with weak expiratory and dysfunctional bulbar muscles need to use the oximetry protocol during intercurrent chest infections.

Poliomyelitis

Of the over 180 postpoliomyelitis ventilator users we have managed, all but 3 required ventilatory support during the acute course of poliomyelitis in the 1930s, 1940s, and 1950s. Most were weaned from ventilator use, but after a period of 15 years or more, they once again required ventilator support—this time for the rest of their lives. Most patients initially require only nocturnal ventilator use; some use it only during daytime hours. Eventually, however, many patients require full-time use, depending on the distribution of respiratory muscle weakness (see Chapter 2).[13] Sixty-one of our patients have required at least nocturnal noninvasive ventilator use since onset of acute poliomyelitis, and 24 have required full-time ventilator assistance for 26.5 + 13.7 years.

Early in the course of disease, most patients used NPBVs. With time, however, NPBV no longer provided optimal ventilation[20] and was associated with obstructive sleep apneas, systemic hypertension,[21] and symptoms of chronic alveolar hypoventilation. Rises in blood pressure after episodes of apneas are not due primarily to oxyhemoglobin desaturation but to apnea duration and may be caused by increased sympathetic activity secondary to arousal.[22] We switched 40 nocturnal users of NPBV to noninvasive IPPV. They experienced a significant improvement in nocturnal SpO$_2$ and alveolar ventilation and relief of symptoms. Five were cured of hypertension. We switched another 34 full-time ventilator users with no breathing tolerance from tracheostomy to noninvasive IPPV with decannulation and ostomy closure. These patients had significantly fewer respiratory complications and hospitalizations with noninvasive IPPV than when they used tracheostomy IPPV.[23] We have seen only one postpoliomyelitis ventilator user who required an indwelling tracheostomy tube. In this patient, severe abdominal distention necessitated colostomy even before ventilator use was required. Thus, because of the adequacy of the bulbar musculature for assisted PCF over 160 L/min, virtually all self-directed postpolio ventilator users with tracheostomy tubes are excellent candidates for decannulation and transition to noninvasive IPPV. They are also excellent candidates for learning GPB for breathing tolerance, provided that invasive management has not caused severe, irreversible airway damage that precludes tube removal by decreasing maximal assisted PCF below 160 L/min.[13,20]

Because postpolio patients tend to be older, they have few chest infections and rarely need Cough-Assists (J. H. Emerson Co., Cambridge, MA) in the home except during chest infections. However, regular, daily maximal insufflations and manually assisted coughing can be important and oximeters and rapid access to Cough-Assists may be needed when assisted PCF is less than 270 L/min. Thus far, over 400 postpolio survivors have benefited from full-time use of noninvasive ventilation for over 7000 patient-years of prolonged survival without resort to tracheostomy.[13,23]

Spinal Cord Injury

Although occasionally avoidable with the use of respiratory muscle aids (see Case 17 in Chapter 15), most ventilator patients with spinal cord injury who require ventilatory support undergo tracheotomy during their acute hospitalization. Like postpolio survivors, unless intubation and tracheostomy resulted in permanent damage to the upper airway, they should be decannulated as part of their rehabilitation. They are excellent candidates for IAPV and noninvasive IPPV as well as for learning GPB to improve breathing tolerance once the tracheostomy sites are closed. Forty-five traumatic tetraplegics were converted from tracheostomy to full-time long-term noninvasive IPPV without complications.[24,25] Over 50 such patients have benefited from prolonged survival and significantly decreased rates of hospitalization and pneumonia using noninvasive rather than tracheostomy IPPV.[23] A discussion of the outcomes of decannulation attempts for patients with spinal cord injury can be found in Chapter 8.

Patients with spinal cord injury can develop late-onset ventilatory failure[26] and require the use of noninvasive IPPV, maximal insufflations, oximeters, and MAC in much the same manner as postpolio patients. The use of noninvasive IPPV and expiratory aids rather than intubation and tracheotomy can especially decrease morbidity and mortality in these patients because of their usually excellent bulbar muscle function.[23] Younger patients with spinal cord injury, who have assisted PCF of less than 270 L/min and who tend to have chest infections more frequently, should have oximeters and Cough-Assists in their homes.

Amyotrophic Lateral Sclerosis/Motor Neuron Disease

Onset of generalized motor neuron disease is almost always after 19 years of age. As a result, patients are generally able to cooperate with the use of noninvasive respiratory muscle aids. There are essentially three types of presentation: bulbar, nonbulbar, and both. Patients with bulbar onset can lose verbal communication and the ability to swallow and develop respiratory failure from aspiration of food or upper airway secretions while vital capacity is still above 1500 ml. In addition, they often demonstrate severe airway collapsibility during inspiration, expiration, or both. Collapsibility during expiration has been shown to be associated with the obstructive apneas of sleep-disordered breathing.[27] Five centimeters of negative pressure applied to the airway during expiration resulted in expiratory flow limitations and oxyhemoglobin desaturation in patients with sleep-disordered breathing but not in normal controls.[27] In patients with amyotrophic lateral sclerosis (ALS), collapsibility can be so severe that it renders assisted PCF unmeasurable and MI-E useless. For patients with severe bulbar disease, the difference between MIC and vital capacity becomes zero and assisted PCF becomes unmeasurable. In addition to airway collapsibility, loss of glottic closure[28] also precludes assisted coughing. Some patients with little or no volitional cough have reflexive cough flows and can clear airway secretions to some degree. For such patients, although reflexive coughing and MAC are at times helpful,[29] eventually only repeated intubation or tracheotomy can maintain survival. As for others, tracheotomy is necessary when assisted PCF is less than 160 L/min and SpO_2 baseline is less than 95%. Usually assisted PCF should be accompanied by laryngeal diversion.

Patients with strictly nonbulbar presentation, on the other hand, retain effective speech and swallowing despite the fact that vital capacity can decrease to under 100 ml and all breathing tolerance can be lost. MIC can remain greater than 3000 ml and assisted PCF much greater than 160 L/min for many years. These patients often can use GPB for breathing tolerance. Tracheostomy tubes are often mistakeningly placed during episodes of acute respiratory failure due to from chest infections because patients are not trained in noninvasive IPPV and assisted coughing.

In one study, 57 ventilator users with ALS had been familiarized with the use of mouthpiece and nasal IPPV, IAPV, and MAC. Twenty-six of the 57 became dependent on 24-hour noninvasive ventilatory support with no breathing tolerance for 23.7 ± 20.3 months. This occurred at 20.2 ± 23.4 months before tracheostomy in 13 patients, 24.1 ± 15.6 months in seven patients who died without being intubated, and 32.2 ± 20.0 months for six patients still using noninvasive support.[3] Thus, noninvasive respiratory muscle aids can delay or eliminate the need for tracheostomy in patients with ALS who retain some bulbar muscle function.

We extubated or decannulated six patients with ALS who had been intubated or had unnecessarily undergone tracheostomy for full-time ventilatory support. All six continued to require full-time ventilatory support after extubation/decannulation. Two continued to use full-time noninvasive IPPV for 4 and 7 years after decannulation. The first patient underwent repeat tracheotomy because of bulbar muscle dysfunction. The second patient continues to use full-time noninvasive IPPV. Another decannulated patient was convinced by local physicians to undergo elective repeat tracheotomy within 2 months of decannulation. Another decannulated noninvasive IPPV user died 6 months after decannulation and use of full-time noninvasive IPPV when bulbar deterioration resulted in severe aspiration. He preferred death to repeat tracheotomy.

The other deceased patient was decannulated despite having absolutely no residual bulbar muscle function and receiving all nutrition via a gastrostomy tube. She subsequently developed respiratory failure and was intubated at a local hospital. Because of full-time ventilator dependence, severe airway mucus encumberment, and refusal of repeat tracheotomy, she was transferred to our service for a trial of extubation to noninvasive IPPV. After aggressive MI-E via the tube had successfully cleared her airways and SpO_2 on room air was normalized, she was extubated to full-time IPPV. However, bulbar muscle dysfunction was too severe for effective nasal or lipseal IPPV; she could not eliminate insufflation leakage during lipseal or nasal IPPV. Therefore, full-time noninvasive IPPV had to be provided via an oral-nasal interface. Unexpectedly, one month after hospital discharge, she gradually weaned to nocturnal-only oral-nasal IPPV until she died suddenly 9 months later, probably of airway mucus-associated asphyxia. Thus, even in the absence of measurable assisted PCF, patients can be extubated to noninvasive IPPV. With such severe bulbar muscle dysfunction, however, long-term prognosis with noninvasive ventilation remains guarded.

Most patients with motor neuron disease develop some combination of bulbar and skeletal muscle weakness. As long as the MIC can exceed the vital capacity and assisted PCF remains greater than 160 L/min, they can benefit from maximal insufflations 3 times/day[3] and the oximetry protocol. At times these patients lose measurable PCF and require gastrostomy tubes, but if they do not aspirate upper airway secretions so much as to decrease SpO_2 baseline below 95%, they do not require invasive management until they experience airway encumberment during chest infections. At least 5 other MDA clinics in the U.S.[12] as well as centers in other countries[30] are successfully using this noninvasive approach for patients with ALS.

For patients with no measurable PCF who drool or aspirate airway secretions, injections of botulinum toxin A into the salivary glands or irradiation of the salivary glands may be considered.[31] This approach may be particularly valuable when chronic aspiration causes a long-term decrease in SpO_2 baseline below 95%, indicating a very high risk of pneumonia and respiratory failure. If reduction in salivary production can decrease aspiration to the point of normalizing baseline SpO_2, the risk of pneumonia is greatly diminished.

Once the patient is intubated, caution must be taken before considering extubation. Tracheostomy is usually warranted when preintubation assisted PCF is unmeasurable. Attempts at ventilator weaning are almost always fruitless and should not be permitted to prolong hospitalization as a substitute for tracheotomy.

In general, patients with ALS and tracheostomy tubes are evaluated for decannulation by measuring assisted PCF, as in patients with other NMDs or spinal cord injury. However, the rate of deterioration should be ascertained by monitoring vital capacity, MIC, assisted PCF, and manual muscle testing every other month for at least 4–6 months. This protocol, along with the patient's history, helps to determine whether bulbar muscle function is sufficiently stable to permit long-term benefit from decannulation. As for other patients with NMD, the MIC of most patients with ALS increases with practice for months to a year or two despite decreasing vital capacity and rapidly progressive disease.[28] For patients with NMD and rapidly decreasing MIC or MIC that equals vital capacity, decannulation should be avoided.

Spinal Muscular Atrophy

Although muscle strength is unchanged during adolescence, physiologic deterioration begins at age 19, and weakness due to adult-onset SMA progresses at an increasingly greater rate in middle age. Nevertheless, patients with SMA rarely lose the ability to speak, assisted PCF remains adequate, and initially ventilator use may be required only during intercurrent chest infections; ongoing nocturnal use may not be needed until many years after onset of muscle weakness. With advancing age, however, full-time noninvasive IPPV is often required, but tracheotomy is rarely needed because of retention of adequate bulbar muscle function. The infantile forms of SMA are discussed in Chapter 10.

Obesity–Hypoventilation

Morbidly obese patients who are intubated for ventilatory support (e.g., during general anesthesia) can be extubated to noninvasive ventilation (see Chapter 8). Acute or chronic ventilatory failure also can be managed without resort to intubation by using mouthpiece IPPV during daytime hours and nasal or lipseal IPPV overnight. Because oxygen supplementation is avoided and cough flows are generally effective, SpO_2 less than 95% is usually due to hypoventilation. Such patients are excellent candidates for oximetry feedback to normalize SpO_2 by increasing alveolar ventilation with mouthpiece IPPV. They can almost always normalize SpO_2 in this manner. However, patients who can walk often do not use noninvasive IPPV sufficiently during daytime hours, have worsening nocturnal assisted ventilation (see Chapter 5), and eventually present with cor pulmonale. Patients with severely morbid obesity who cannot walk tend to use noninvasive IPPV for longer periods during the day and thus can more successfully avoid acute respiratory failure. However, when airway pressures over 35 cmH_2O are required for ventilatory assistance, nasal IPPV is often inadequate and lipseals must be used for effective nocturnal assistance.

DIFFICULTIES IN INITIATING THE USE OF NONINVASIVE AIDS

Paradigm paralysis is the failure to learn new and superior approaches because they differ radically from the generally used methods in which one has invested time and energy.[32] It is the terminal disease of misplaced certainty.[33]

Patients and caregivers prefer noninvasive approaches.[34] Noninvasive methods lower the cost of home mechanical ventilation[35]; can eliminate the need for hospitalization, intubation, tracheostomy, and bronchoscopy[23]; and may shorten hospitalizations. They decrease the need for invasive ventilation[36] and are associated with fewer complications[37] and episodes of pneumonia[38] than invasive ventilation in both the long-term and acute care settings. Despite these advantages as well as long-term safety and efficacy, noninvasive methods are not widely used. They are generally not yet a part of medical or other health professional school curricula, and current invasive approaches are centered on the general tendency to resort to the highest available and most costly technology. Physician and hospital reimbursement is procedure-based and directed toward inpatient management rather than preventive care. One can be remunerated for hospitalizing patients for intubation, tracheostomy, and bronchoscopies, but outpatient management that prevents hospitalization by using noninvasive aids is not recognized and often not fully reimbursed by third-party payors, even though it costs a small fraction of the invasive alternative. Patients require equipment and training, which necessitate letters of justification and explanation. Furthermore, the initial use of noninvasive aids requires a significant time commitment for evaluating the use of various IPPV interfaces to optimize comfort and effectiveness. Some interfaces provide better ventilatory assistance than others.[39] For example, the lipseal and oral-nasal interfaces are more efficacious than nasal interfaces in particular patients.

Even more important than using inspiratory muscle aids is the evaluation of PCF and methods for increasing it. Although expiratory muscle aids must be used for noninvasive ventilation to be effective over the long term, in none of the studies in which the use of nocturnal nasal IPPV or PIP + PEEP ultimately terminated in acute respiratory failure and tracheotomy or death was their use reported.[10,40–43]

Patients with neuromuscular disease are rarely taught to prevent acute respiratory failure before it occurs and leads to intubation—in part because only about 3% of NMD clinics in the U.S. teach expiratory muscle aids and even fewer use the oximetry protocol.[12] Certainly, our experience with NMD has been consistent with the following statement by one of the many physicians knowledgeable about respiratory muscle aids 45 years ago:

As experience with exsufflation with negative pressure increased, bronchoscopy was performed less frequently for the removal of bronchial secretions. At times bronchoscopic aspiration did relieve acute obstructive anoxia; but it is clear from the case reports that bronchoscopy contributed little to the overall control of bronchial secretions.... Had not artificial coughing been available, death might well have followed bronchoscopy in [several cases]. The only possible value of bronchoscopy is to relieve obstruction due to secretions in the trachea and main bronchi. This is usually only of transient benefit, and as the relief can be more easily achieved with exsufflation with negative pressure, bronchoscopic aspiration should rarely, if ever, be performed in patients undergoing artificial respiration.[44]

Thus, the medical community in general has little knowledge of mouthpiece IPPV, IAPVs, and expiratory aids. However, even nasal ventilation, about which many articles have been published, is used suboptimally or incorrectly. This problem is best typified by a recent article, entitled "Randomized trial of preventive nasal ventilation in Duchenne muscular dystrophy,"[43] in an otherwise reputable journal. Seventy patients with DMD, 15–16 years of age, were randomized to nocturnal nasal IPPV or a control group that did not use nasal IPPV. The patients were reported to have a vital capacity of 20–50% of predicted normal but neither hypercapnia nor hypoxia (PaO_2 exceeded 60 mmHg). The 70 patients came from 17 centers. There was no standardization in ventilator use, nasal interface selection, caregiver or patient training, or follow-up. The authors stated that 15 of the 35 nasal IPPV users admitted that they did not use nasal ventilation for the minimal 6 hours per night, and the authors concluded from the history that only 20 were "effectively ventilated." The authors made no effort to substantiate ventilator use by using ventilators that indicate hours of utilization. Indeed, historical claims tend to overestimate ventilator utilization, especially claims by asymptomatic users. This problem is particularly common when patients are told to use ventilators by clinicians who have little or no experience in noninvasive ventilation, prescribe inappropriate ventilator settings, and make little effort to try various styles of interfaces. In our experience, no one interface style, not even the custom-molded interface,[45] is tolerated by a majority of patients. In addition, ventilator adjustments were made during daytime hours, not during sleep when insufflation leakage occurs. Thus, delivered volumes of 15 ml/kg can be grossly inadequate for nocturnal nasal IPPV.[43] The stated goal of lowering the $PaCO_2$ by 10% or to decrease it by "at least 10% of recorded daytime value(s)" is inappropriate when one considers that daytime values were already normal. This goal also shows that the authors did not recognize the importance of monitoring nocturnal gases, normalizing carbon dioxide, and improving nocturnal SpO_2, when abnormal. Furthermore, there is no reason to believe that the patients used nasal ventilation correctly because no effort was made to determine whether the interfaces were sufficiently snug to provide effective IPPV during sleep. Rather than performing painful daytime arterial blood gas sampling for patients with normal pretreatment gases and other inappropriate pulmonary function testing, the authors might have documented efficacy by showing improvements in nocturnal oximetry or transcutaneous or end-tidal carbon dioxide.[4,46]

The tragedy of such a report lies in the perpetuation of misconceptions that dissuade clinicians from appropriate use of noninvasive IPPV.[43] The authors reported that the mortality rate of "nasal IPPV users" may have been increased and even recommended earlier resort to tracheotomy. Although the predominant cause of death was mucus plugging during chest infections, patients were not offered mouthpiece IPPV, air-stacking, or cough assistance. During such episodes, nasal congestion can preclude effective use of nasal ventilation, and patients benefit by being switched to lipseal IPPV. Thus, it is no surprise that the patients died, subjects and controls. For those with "left ventricular hypokinesis," cardiac ejection fractions under 20% are predictive of early mortality,[47] but this factor, too, was not taken into account.

Thus, this study perpetuated the following misconceptions about noninvasive ventilation: (1) nasal ventilation is the only noninvasive method to be considered (IPPV via mouthpieces, lipseals, or oral-nasal interfaces and body ventilators are ignored); (2) when nocturnal use of nasal ventilation is no longer adequate, one must resort to tracheotomy; (3) simple prescription of nasal ventilation can be enough without the participation of a specifically trained respiratory therapist to evaluate IPPV trials with various interfaces and to train patients in assisted coughing and oximetry feedback; and (4) the primary difficulty in preventing mortality in patients with DMD lies in assisting nocturnal ventilation rather than in assisted coughing and treatment of cardiomyopathy.

Finally, it must be recognized that portable volume-limited ventilators are useful not only for IPPV via tracheostomy tubes but also for mouthpiece and nasal IPPV and IAPV use. Likewise, BiPAP-ST machines are useful not only for providing nasal ventilation but also for tracheostomy and mouthpiece ventilation. Paradigms are difficult to break.

. . . y no hay que hacer caso de estas cosas de encantamientos, ni hay que tener cólera ni enojo por ellas, porque, como son invisibles y fantásticas, no hallaremos de quien vengarnos. (. . . there is no reason to pay attention to these matters of spells nor to feel anger or annoyance at them, because, as they are invisible and fanciful, we cannot know on whom to take revenge.)

Miguel de Cervantes, *Don Quijote de La Mancha*

REFERENCES

1. Bach JR, Ishikawa Y, Kim H: Prevention of pulmonary morbidity for patients with Duchenne muscular dystrophy. Chest 112:1024–1028, 1997.
2. Bach JR. Management of neuromuscular ventilatory failure by 24-hour noninvasive intermittent positive pressure ventilation. Eur Respir Rev 3:284–291, 1993.
3. Bach JR: Amyotrophic lateral sclerosis: Predictors for prolongation of life by noninvasive respiratory aids. Arch Phys Med Rehabil 76:828–832, 1995.
4. Bach JR, Alba AS: Management of chronic alveolar hypoventilation by nasal ventilation. Chest 97:52–57, 1990.
5. Bach JR, Wang TG: Noninvasive long-term ventilatory support for individuals with spinal muscular atrophy and functional bulbar musculature. Arch Phys Med Rehabil 76:213–217, 1995.
6. Niranjan V, Bach JR: Spinal muscular atrophy type 1: A noninvasive respiratory management approach. Chest 117:1100–1005, 2000.
7. Bach JR: Amyotrophic lateral sclerosis: Communication status and survival with ventilatory support. Am J Phys Med Rehabil 72:343–349, 1993.
8. Tzeng AC, Bach JR: Prevention of pulmonary morbidity for patients with neuromuscular disease. Chest 118:1390–1396, 2000.
9. Cantas-Yamsuan M, Sanchez I, Kesselman M, Chernick V: Morbidity and mortality patterns of ventilator-dependent children in a home care program. Clin Pediatr 32:706–713, 1993.
10. Leger P, Bedicam JM, Cornette A, et al: Nasal intermittent positive pressure ventilation: Long-term follow-up in patients with severe chronic respiratory insufficiency. Chest 105:100–105, 1994.
11. Baydur A, Layne E, Aral H, et al: Long term non-invasive ventilation in the community for patients with musculoskeletal disorders: 46 year experience and review. Thorax 55:4–11, 2000.
12. Chaudhry SS, Bach JR: Management approaches in muscular dystrophy association clinics. Am J Phys Med Rehabil 79:193–196, 2000.
13. Bach JR, Alba AS, Saporito LR: Intermittent positive pressure ventilation via the mouth as an alternative to tracheostomy for 257 ventilator users. Chest 103:174–182, 1993.
14. Begin R, Bureau MA, Lupien L, Lemieux B: Control and modulation of respiration in Steinert's myotonic dystrophy. Am Rev Respir Dis 121:281–280, 1980.
15. Manni R, Zucca MR, Martinetti C, et al: Hypersomnia in dystrophia myotonica: A neurophysiological and immunogenetic study. Acta Neurol Scand 84:498–502, 1991.
16. Tejero G, Langevin B, Petitjean T, et al: Long-term home mechanical ventilation in myotonic dystrophy: Follow-up and compliance. Eighth Journees Internationales de Ventilation a Domicile, abstract 129, March 7, 2001, Hopital de la Croix-Rousse, Lyon, France.
17. Nugent AM, Smith IE, Shneerson JM: Domiciliary assisted ventilation in patients with myotonic dystrophy. Chest 121:459–464, 2002.
18. Bach JF, Alba A, Mosher R, Delaubier A: Intermittent positive pressure ventilation via nasal access in the management of respiratory insufficiency. Chest 92:168–170, 1987.
19. Putman MT, Wise RA: Myasthenia gravis and upper airway obstruction. Chest 109:400–404, 1996.
20. Bach JR, Alba AS, Bohatiuk G, et al: Mouth intermittent positive pressure ventilation in the management of post-polio respiratory insufficiency. Chest 91:859–864, 1987.
21. Bach JR, Penek J: Obstructive sleep apnea complicating negative pressure ventilatory support in patients with chronic paralytic/restrictive ventilatory dysfunction. Chest 99:1386–1393, 1991.
22. Ali NJ, Davies RJO, Fleetham JA, Stradling JR: The acute effects of continuous positive airway pressure and oxygen administration on blood pressure during obstructive sleep apnea. Chest 101:1526–1532, 1992.
23. Bach JR, Rajaraman R, Ballanger F, et al: Neuromuscular ventilatory insufficiency: the effect of home mechanical ventilator use vs. oxygen therapy on pneumonia and hospitalization rates. Am J Phys Med Rehabil 77:8–19, 1998.

24. Bach JR, Alba AS: Noninvasive options for ventilatory support of the traumatic high level quadriplegic. Chest 98:613–619, 1990.
25. Bach JR: New approaches in the rehabilitation of the traumatic high level quadriplegic. Am J Phys Med Rehabil 70:13–20, 1991.
26. Bach JR: Inappropriate weaning and late onset ventilatory failure of individuals with traumatic quadriplegia. Paraplegia 31:430–438, 1993.
27. Liistro G, Veriter C, Dury M, et al: Expiratory flow limitation in awake sleep-disordered breathing subjects. Eur Respir J 14:185–190, 1999.
28. Kang SW, Bach JR: Maximum insufflation capacity. Chest 118:61–65, 2000.
29. Hanayama K, Ishikawa Y, Bach JR: Amyotrophic lateral sclerosis: Successful treatment of mucus plugging by mechanical insufflation-exsufflation. Am J Phys Med Rehabil 76:338–339, 1997.
30. Buhr-Schinner H, Laier-Groeneveld G, Criee CP: Amyotrophic lateral sclerosis and intermittent self-ventilation therapy: Indications and follow up. Med Klin 90(Suppl 1):49–51, 1995.
31. Giess R, Naumann M, Werner E, et al: Injections of botulinum toxin A into the salivary glands improve sialorrhoea in amyotrophic lateral sclerosis. J Neurol Neurosurg Psychiatry 69:121–123, 2000.
32. Bach JR, Bach GA: Paradigm paralysis. In Respironics, Inc: Interventions. Murrysville, PA, Respironics, Inc., 1993, pp 3, 13.
33. Barker JL: Discovering the Future [video]. St. Paul-Minneapolis, MN, Infinity Limited, Inc., and Film Media, Inc.
34. Bach JR: A comparison of long-term ventilatory support alternatives from the perspective of the patient and care giver. Chest 104:1702–1706, 1993.
35. Bach JR, Intintola P, Alba AS, Holland I: The ventilator-assisted individual: Cost analysis of institutionalization versus rehabilitation and in-home management. Chest 101:26–30, 1992.
36. Celikel T, Sungur M, Ceyhan B, Karakurt S: Comparison of intermittent positive pressure ventilation with standard medical therapy in hypercapnic acute respiratory failure. Chest 114:1636–1642, 1998.
37. Benhamou D, Muir JF, Melen B: Mechanical ventilation in elderly patients. Monaldi Arch Chest Dis 53:547–551, 1998.
38. Guerin C, Girard R, Chemorin C, et al: Facial mask noninvasive mechanical ventilation reduces the incidence of nosocomial pneumonia: A prospective epidemiological survey from a single ICU. Intensive Care Med 10:1024–1032, 1997.
39. Navalesi P, Fanfulla F, Frigerio P, et al: Physiologic evaluation of noninvasive mechanical ventilation delivered with three types of masks in patients with chronic hypercapnic respiratory failure. Crit Care Med 28:1785–1790, 2000.
40. Baydur A, Gilgoff I, Prentice W, et al: Decline in respiratory function and experience with long-term assisted ventilation in advanced Duchenne's muscular dystrophy. Chest 97:884–889, 1990.
41. Gay PC, Patel AM, Viggiano RW, Hubmayr RD: Nocturnal nasal ventilation for treatment of patients with hypercapnic respiratory failure. Mayo Clin Proc 66:695–703, 1991.
42. Leger P, Jennequin J, Gerard M, Robert D: Home positive pressure ventilation via nasal mask for patients with neuromuscular weakness or restrictive lung or chest-wall disease. Respir Care 34:73–79, 1989.
43. Raphael J-C, Chevret S, Chastang C, Bouvet F: Randomised trial of preventive nasal ventilation in Duchenne muscular dystrophy. Lancet 343:1600–1604, 1994.
44. Colebatch HJH: Artificial coughing for patients with respiratory paralysis. Austr J Med 10:201–212, 1961.
45. McDermott I, Bach JR, Parker C, Sortor S: Custom fabricated interfaces for intermittent positive pressure ventilation. Int J Prosthodont 2:224–233, 1989.
46. Ishikawa Y, Ishikawa Y, Minami R: The effect of nasal IPPV on patients with respiratory failure during sleep due to Duchenne muscular dystrophy. Clin Neurol 33:856–861, 1993.
47. Stewart CA, Gilgoff I, Baydur A, et al: Gated radionuclide ventriculography in the evaluation of cardiac function in Duchenne's muscular dystrophy. Chest 94:1245–1248, 1988.

10 —— Noninvasive Ventilation in Children

JOHN R. BACH, M.D.
VIS NIRANJAN, M.D.

Is it worth the investment?
Is it worthy of your time?
What is the value of this one life?

Richard Clingman, Webmaster for DoctorBach.com

OUTCOMES OF CONVENTIONAL MECHANICAL VENTILATION IN CHILDREN

In the United States, 500,000 people (0.15% of the population) have neuromuscular disease (NMD); 1.5 million more, many of whom are children, suffer from spinal cord injury; and many others have thoracic wall restrictive lung disease and sleep-disordered breathing or obesity–hypoventilation. Neonatal ventilatory failure requiring ventilatory support is most common in NMDs, such as spinal muscular atrophy (SMA) type 1, but also occurs in certain congenital malformations such as Pierre Robin syndrome, congenital central hypoventilation, and bronchopulmonary dysplasia. It may result from subglottic stenosis due to damage from intubation or tracheostomy. Unless intubation is managed by the methods discussed in this book (see below for SMA type 1), pediatric survivors are ultimately discharged home with tracheostomy tubes. Ventilatory/respiratory failure also occurs in older children and adolescents with the diagnoses listed in Table 1 of Chapter 1 (see also Chapters 7–9).

Surveys of the United States, western Europe, and Japan indicate that the use of home mechanical ventilation is increasing rapidly among children.[2] Anne LeRoy, who represents ADEPT, the French organization that manages home mechanical ventilation, reported at the 11th International Symposium on Amyotrophic Lateral Sclerosis/Motor Neuron Disease in Arhus, Denmark, that as of December 2000 there were 6800 ventilator users in France, of whom 515 were children. About 500 of the 6800 patients had tracheostomies. The rest used noninvasive ventilation. A Swedish survey noted that 80% of 541 home mechanical ventilator users had neuromuscular ventilatory impairment and that the great majority used noninvasive ventilation.[3] Of 4500 people with NMD out of a population of 5.5 million in Finland, about 250 are ventilator users.[4] A survey in the United Kingdom noted that 141 children required long-term ventilatory assistance, of whom 33 used tracheostomy IPPV, 103 used nocturnal nasal IPPV, and 9 used negative-pressure body ventilators (NPBVs) (Fig. 1). Ninety-six of the children had primarily ventilatory

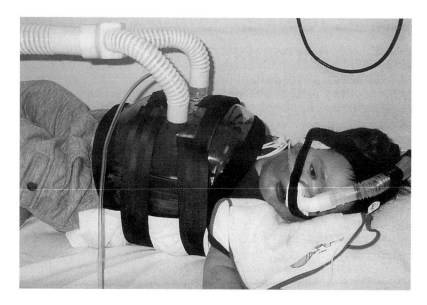

FIGURE 1. Child, now 7 years old, with spinal muscular atrophy type 1 who has required high-span nasal PIP + PEEP continuously since 5 months of age. He uses an Adam circuit (Mallincrodt-Puritan-Bennett) with small nasal pillows around the clock. CPAP prongs of an infant CPAP circuit (Hudson 15.0 French CPAP Nasal Prongs) were cut off and taped into the pillows. Chest-shell ventilator use was tried, but delivery of comparable volumes of air was not possible and application of the shell was considered by the parents to be inconvenient and by the patient to be less comfortable.

impairment, and the remainder had "other conditions." No reasons were given to explain the ventilatory assistance methods used by these children. Some children use more than one noninvasive ventilation method. Most children who appear to require more than nocturnal ventilator use, however, and children who have difficulty with weaning after intubation during chest infections generally undergo tracheotomy. When the tubes are not removed after the acute episode, the children usually remain on full-time ventilator dependence (see Chapter 5). Thus, conventional management for children resembles that for adults. Of interest, most of the children in the United Kingdom survey attended mainstream schools, but only one-half of the tracheostomy IPPV users resided in the community.

Although significant advances have been made in the management of respiratory failure in the pediatric intensive care unit (PICU), most of these entail ventilation and weaning strategies for managing the intubated child. Examples include high-frequency oscillatory ventilation, partial liquid ventilation, pressure-regulated volume control, pressure support ventilation, and volume support ventilation. This chapter reviews the current literature and the authors' own experience with noninvasive IPPV.

CONVENTIONAL INVASIVE MECHANICAL VENTILATION

Small children with weak expiratory muscles and inability to cooperate with noninvasive expiratory aids often undergo intubation during intercurrent chest infections. Although the use of noninvasive ventilation as an alternative to intubation has been extensively described for adults (see Chapters 8 and 11), there have been no comparable studies in children.

Before the development of the methods described in this book, intubated children had to undergo tracheotomy when they required ongoing ventilator use or when they could not effectively expectorate airway secretions. However, the trachea is much more easily damaged in young children than in adults; the most common complication is subglottic stenosis.[5] Thus, only uncuffed tracheostomy tubes should be used for children with primarily ventilatory impairment unless aspiration of upper airway secretions causes a continuous decrease in baseline SpO_2 below 95%. Cuffed tubes also should be avoided in children with primarily respiratory impairment unless decreased pulmonary compliance renders tracheostomy ventilation ineffective via uncuffed tubes. Excessive insufflation leakage usually can be managed by some combination of increasing the diameter of the tube, increasing air delivery volumes, or, if necessary, placing a tracheostomy tube with a cuff but leaving the cuff deflated.

After 10 years of age the shape of the larynx changes from conical to cylindrical, and the narrowest part of the airway and the trachea becomes more resilient to contact with the tube and cuff.[5] In patients with very narrow tubes and airways, silver tubes are often used because of their greater internal-to-external diameter ratio. The position and size of the tubes relative to the patient should be checked by radiograph at least every 6–12 months to optimize air delivery and minimize tracheal damage.

Although complications of intubation and tracheotomy described for adults (see Chapter 6) also occur in children, their incidence is less well known. The incidence of tracheostomy tube dislodgment in a 59-bed pediatric subacute facility was recently reported: 561 total dislodgments resulted in six emergency calls over 4.5 years. In addition, there were 5.4 dislodgments per 1000 days (total: 35,096 patient-days) in patients with tracheostomy tubes who were not using ventilators and 18.8 dislodgments per 1000 days (19,564 patient days) for patients using IPPV. Thus, dislodgments are more common with ventilator use.[6]

NONINVASIVE VENTILATION

Hillberg defined noninvasive ventilation as ventilatory support without establishing an endotracheal airway.[7] Although we agree that use of an interface makes the ventilation noninvasive, we believe that Hillberg's definition is not sufficiently limited. An ideal noninvasive interface comes in least contact with the mucosal surface. By the term *noninvasive interface* we imply the use of nasal, oronasal, and oral interfaces for the delivery of positive-pressure ventilation or the use of body ventilators that do not provoke the gag or cough reflex due to a direct mechanical stimulus. Thus, unlike Hillberg's definition, a nasopharyngeal airway or a laryngeal mask airway does not qualify as noninvasive despite the fact that no endotracheal airway is present. The noninvasive nature of the interface often necessitates a ventilator designed for noninvasive ventilation—most often volume- or pressure-limited machines that do not have expiratory volume alarms.

Whereas the adult patient plays the major role in choosing the interface, for infants the success of noninvasive ventilation depends on the clinician's appropriate choice of interface and ventilator. This choice is especially important because children have greater difficulties with synchronization to and triggering of the ventilator. There are also greater limitations in commercially available interfaces. The interface often has to be tailored to the size requirements and comfort of the child. One can often improvise its construction from supplies commonly available in the PICU.

Generic Positive-Pressure Interfaces

The simple Respironics (Murrysville, PA) 15-mm and 22-mm angled mouthpieces that are so commonly used for adults (see Fig. 19 of Chapter 7) also can be used from the age of 4 years by children who have good oromotor control. The air flow resistance or back pressure created by the 15-mm angled mouthpiece prevents the low-pressure alarm from sounding when it is set at its minimum level (2 cmH_2O). Thus, the alarms do not sound when the patient is eating or speaking or not taking a mouthpiece-assisted insufflation. The standard mouthpieces used for pulmonary function studies also can be used. However, they are straight and too wide for young children and do not prevent the low-pressure alarms from sounding.

For nocturnal use, IPPV is best delivered via a mouthpiece with lipseal phalange and cloth retention straps with Velcro closures (see Chapter 7). Unfortunately, the lipseal comes in a size only for adolescents and adults. The youngest child who has used the lipseal was 12 years of age.

There are now many manufactures of adult-size disposable nasal and oral interfaces and head gear of various sizes: large, medium wide, medium, medium small, small, and petite (see Table 1 of Chapter 7). The Mallincrodt Adam system (Mallincrodt, Pleasanton, CA) consists of a nasal shell (standard or narrow sizes) into which nasal pillows are inserted (small, medium, or large) and connected to a swivel adapter and headgear. An angle adapter is also available for more angled noses. Only the model with small pillows and narrow shell is useful for children (see Fig. 1). The Adam circuit is nondisposable and can be sterilized for repeat use. One advantage of this system is that it has no contact with the bridge of the nose. The seal is also easier and more comfortable when pressure requirements are high, although maintaining the seal can be difficult. Some patients experience nasal irritation or congestion when using this interface. For very small infants an option is to cut off the prongs of infant continuous positive airway pressure (CPAP) circuits (Hudson 15.0 French CPAP Nasal Prongs) and tape them into the prongs of the small adult Adam circuit (see Fig. 1). The larger prongs of the Adam circuit seal the child's nostrils, and the suspension system of the Adam circuit retains the interface.

Another option for infants below 1 year of age is to seal one end of the Hudson nasal prongs and connect the other end to the ventilation circuit using intervening tubing adapters (Fig. 2). The prongs themselves are passed through foamy material such as the nasal bridge cushions of a Respironics CPAP mask (Fig. 3) or the center of a Duoderm patch (Bristol Myers Squibb Co., New York) that adheres to the nostril linings and seals the nasal orifices. These prongs are designed for infants weighing 1500–2000 grams. Custom headgear is prepared to secure the interface. We have had success with these prongs in infants up to 2 years of age, at which time we often switch to the Respironics pediatric petite nasal interface (Fig. 4). This interface is generally effective for children from 6 months to 4 years of age and is the most widely used interface for children of this age.

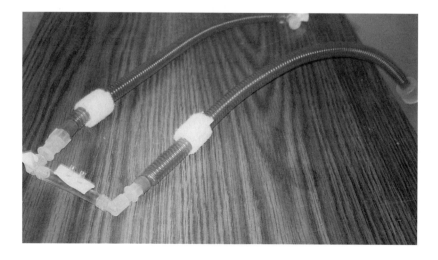

FIGURE 2. Hudson nasal prongs sealed at one end and connected to the ventilation circuit using intervening tubing adapters.

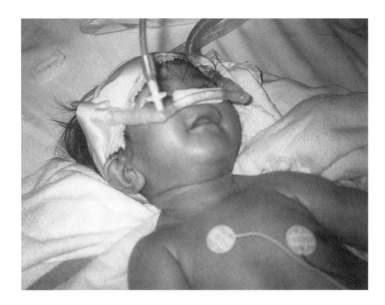

FIGURE 3. Infant with spinal muscular atrophy type 1 using CPAP prongs passed through the nasal bridge cushions of a Respironics CPAP mask that adheres to the nostril linings and seals the nasal orifices.

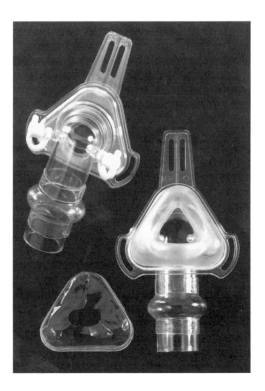

FIGURE 4. Respironics small-child mask/comfort flap, front and back views.

Respironics, Inc. (Murrysville, PA) makes nondisposable pediatric oral-nasal interfaces for children 6 months to 4 years of age and 2–8 years of age and a petite mask for older children. These inexpensive interfaces are adequate for the most children. The bridge of the nose is the most likely site of discomfort. Respironics also makes pediatric "bubble" nasal and oral-nasal interfaces. These interfaces include inner flaps that act like valves as ventilator-delivered air pushes them against the face. They are available in various sizes and shapes. Occasionally adult-size nasal interfaces can be used as oral-nasal interfaces for small children. Because of their wider surface area, it is much more difficult to eliminate air leaks when oral-nasal designs are used.

Nasal ventilation is the most practical means of noninvasive support in small children for several reasons: lipseals are not made for small children, they have no teeth, their lips are too weak to grab a mouthpiece, they may not be able to cooperate with the mouthpiece, pediatric exsufflation (IAPV) belts are difficult to procure, and infants are obligate nasal breathers. All patients are offered trials of various styles of interfaces, and the styles that are most comfortable and allow the least leakage are used. Occasionally, interfaces of different styles are alternated nightly and during the day, if they are needed around the clock.

No attempt is made to eliminate all insufflation leakage by tightening the interface straps. Ventilator volumes and pressures are adjusted to compensate for small air leakages. Lipseal IPPV is recommended for older children with signs of discomfort, skin irritation, or nasal congestion (e.g., during upper respiratory tract infections).

Complications of the Interface and Noninvasive Ventilation

The complications of the interface and noninvasive ventilation for children are the same as those for adults (see Chapter 7). In addition, because of the growth and greater plasticity of pediatric tissues, orthodontic deformities and facial flattening can be more severe in children. On the other hand, small children seem to be less susceptible to pressure discomfort and ulcers. There was one case report of a premature infant who developed cerebellar necrosis as a result of using ventilation via an oronasal interface.[8]

Intermittent Abdominal Pressure Ventilator

The Exsufflation Belt (Respironics, Inc.) is made in three sizes for adults. Intermittent abdominal pressure ventilators (IAPVs) also can be improvised from blood pressure cuffs (see Chapter 3). Adult and pediatric sizes are custom-made for children in France (Hôpital Gui de Chauliac, Montpelier).[9,10]

Negative-Pressure Body Ventilators

Although negative-pressure body ventilators (NPBVs; see Fig. 1) were the first methods of long-term ventilatory support for children as well as adults, there is little interest in them today because of the efficacy of noninvasive positive-pressure ventilation and the fact that NPBVs often cause obstructive sleep apneas. Nevertheless, occasional reports continue to suggest their utility in infants and other children.[11]

Ventilator Choice and Settings

In general, ventilator choice depends on age, vital capacity, lung and chest wall compliance, extent of gas exchange impairment, type of interface, and ability to cooperate. As for adults, pressure- and volume-limited portable ventilators are available for noninvasive ventilation. In general, pressure-limited ventilators have the advantage that they are triggered by flow-sensing. In intubated patients, flow-sensing ventilators significantly decrease the work of breathing in comparison with pressure-sensing ventilators. Flow-sensing also results in a shortened response time for ventilators and, therefore, can be effective even with the high respiratory rates of small children. Flow-sensing tends to prevent ventilator-patient dyssynchrony and increases patient tolerance. Use of pressure-limited ventilators may involve a smaller risk of causing barotrauma, but effectiveness is limited in patients with poor pulmonary compliance who may not receive adequate tidal volumes. Patient triggering is not always possible in very small and weak patients, for whom rate adjustment becomes very important. Such is typically the case for small patients who are extubated to nasal positive inspiratory pressure plus positive end-expiratory pressure (PIP + PEEP).

To facilitate patient-ventilator synchrony in patients unable to trigger the machine, the spontaneous time mode of pressure-cycled machines is used with a back-up rate set slightly higher than the spontaneous breathing rate of the infant. In general, back-up rates of 25–30 breaths/minute are required for infants, 15–20 breaths/minute for small children, and 10–12 breaths/minute for adolescents. Generally only high spans of inspiratory and expiratory positive airway pressure (IPAP and EPAP) are used, typically 15–18 cmH_2O IPAP and 2–3 cmH_2O EPAP. However, when high rates are required, as for infants immediately after extubation, lower IPAPs may need to be used so that the machine can deliver the air in the very brief inspiratory time. As the augmented assisted tidal volumes result in a decrease in the infant's spontaneous rate, the machine's back-up rate is decreased and IPAP is increased. This adjustment facilitates a slower breathing rate with more normal tidal volumes and minute ventilation. Particularly for small children, ventilator settings for noninvasive IPPV are initially adjusted to achieve good excursion of the chest wall and resolution of tachypnea and hypercapnia. The goal is to have the infant become accustomed to high-span nasal PIP + PEEP. Nocturnal ventilation usually remains adequate with mean nocturnal SpO_2 of at least 94%, resolution of pectus excavatum, chest expansion during insufflation, and relief of sleep disturbances and diaphoresis. Inspiratory times of 0.5–1 second and inspiratory-to-expiratory ratios of 1:1 to 1:2 are typically used. If the spontaneous rate is greater than the ventilator's highest set rate, a volume ventilator with highly sensitive triggering is used, such as the LTV-900 (Pulmonetics Systems, Inc., Colton, CA) or VIP (Innovative Product Technologies, Inc., Gainesville, FL). Once spontaneous rates decrease, the infant can continue to use the machine or be switched to much less expensive, simpler pressure-limited units.

In general, high-span nasal PIP + PEEP is used by children under 5 years of age with primarily ventilatory impairment, and low-span nasal PIP + PEEP is used by children of all ages with obstructive apneas or primarily respiratory insufficiency and adequate pulmonary compliance. Ventilator settings are tailored to the underlying disease condition. The EPAP replaces the normal PEEP generated by the larynx, especially during coughing, talking, and crying. Typically, EPAP levels of 2–3 cmH_2O should be adequate to maintain some expiratory airflow, thereby eliminating most rebreathing of carbon dioxide. EPAP levels may be increased in patients with severe hypoxemic insufficiency or air trapping to increase mean airway pressures, counter auto-PEEP, and thereby improve oxygenation. EPAP levels as high as 10 cmH_2O have been used safely in children.[12] Nasal PIP + PEEP is typically introduced while the child is asleep. IPAP levels are initially set at low levels (6–8 cmH_2O) to ensure patient acceptance and are quickly increased to the desired levels as tolerated. Soon children tolerate PIP + PEEP even when awake. When nasal PIP + PEEP is used for obstructive sleep apneas, EPAP levels of 5–6 cmH_2O are often most beneficial but should be titrated to optimize sleep SpO_2 and minimize polysomnographic evidence of obstructive apneas. Because the lesser respiratory rates of older children decrease the need for flow-sensing, pressure-limited ventilators and because older children need to air-stack (see Chapter 7), we switch children from pressure- to volume-limited ventilators after age 5 years.

HUMIDIFICATION

The need for humidification is individualized. Heated water humidifiers are usually needed during ventilation via tracheostomy tube and also in children under 3 years of age who autonomously breathe through a tracheostomy. Older autonomously breathing children may use a regenerative humidifier.

Nasal interface users do not generally require supplemental humidification. If, however, the patient has nasal congestion or sinusitis or expresses discomfort, a regenerative humidifier can be tried, although it is usually inadequate because most patients exhale from their mouth. The regenerative humidifier is connected to the tubing as close to the patient as possible. When it is inadequate, heated humidification is used. In a series of 15 patients, aged 4–21 years, using noninvasive nighttime support for up to 21 months, Padman et al. used no humidification.[12] Heated humidification is almost always required when oral interfaces are used for nocturnal, but not for daytime, noninvasive ventilation.

MECHANISMS FOR SECRETION CLEARANCE

In pediatric patients who are unable to cough adequately to eliminate secretions, chest physical therapy and assisted coughing are used as for adults (see Chapter 13). Chest percussion with postural drainage can help mobilize peripheral airway secretions but causes oxyhemoglobin desaturation and imposes respiratory work that can also fatigue respiratory muscles. These problems can be alleviated, at least for patients with cystic fibrosis, by the use of nasal PIP + PEEP. In a study of 16 patients with cystic fibrosis, aged 13 ± 4 years, who performed forced expiratory maneuvers, respiratory rate was significantly lower and tidal volumes, maximal inspiratory and expiratory pressures, and SpO_2 significantly higher during the sessions in which nasal PIP + PEEP was used. In addition, 15 patients reported feeling less tired, and 10 of 14 patients reported that expectoration was easier with nasal PIP + PEEP (two patients did not expectorate).[13]

Manually assisted coughing is avoided for the first 1.5 hours after a meal. If mechanically assisted coughing (MAC) is requested, it is done without a manual thrust. Mechanical insufflation-exsufflation (MI-E) with an exsufflation timed abdominal thrust (MAC) is used via an oral-nasal interface on manual mode to coincide insufflation and exsufflation with the infant's inspiration and expiration. Caregivers provide MI-E daily via oral-nasal interfaces to accustom 9- to 30-month-old infants to the procedure so that they will use it effectively during chest infections. Some infants as young as 11 months old relax and successfully use MI-E via oronasal interfaces to bring up airway secretions. Although timing MI-E to an infant's breathing may be helpful, when the patient does not cooperate, MI-E can be optimally effective only when used via a translaryngeal or tracheostomy tube with the cuff inflated. Relative contraindications for the insufflation phases of MI-E include a history of recent pneumothoraces or other documented evidence of barotrauma. There are no known contraindications for using the exsufflation phases.

Settings of + 30 to – 30 cmH$_2$O are used initially and advanced quickly, as tolerated, to the more effective settings of + 40 to – 40 cmH$_2$O. These pressures are used via oral-nasal interfaces, but higher pressures must be used via translaryngeal or tracheostomy tubes. The magnitude of the pressures reaching the airways after the drop-off across the narrow pediatric tubes is only now being studied (see Chapter 7).

No large case series examine the use of MI-E in children. Our recommendations for 35- to 40-cmH$_2$O pressures are based on observed clinical efficacy; these are the pressures that patients almost invariably want to use. It also has been found that these pressures are optimal for maximizing deflation volumes and flows in Rhesus monkeys.[14] A pressure of 35–40 cmH$_2$O also happens to be the standard pressure pop-off for the manual resuscitators used in cardiopulmonary resuscitation. We recently reported the use of MI-E with no untoward effects in series of pediatric patients.[15,16] We routinely use MI-E via the translaryngeal tubes of infants as young as 4 months old.

SURVEY OF CONVENTIONAL MANAGEMENT

Outcomes must be considered for home mechanical ventilation via tracheostomy as well as via noninvasive interfaces. Outcomes for older children with spinal cord injury, myopathies, and the milder neuropathies who use tracheostomy IPPV are discussed in Chapter 6. Conventional outcomes for patients with infantile SMA are discussed below. A few studies have reported long-term tracheostomy ventilation outcomes for a variety of conditions. In one study of 54 children with primarily ventilatory impairment, including 17 with spinal cord injury, 33 used tracheostomy ventilation and 21 used NPBVs. The 1-year survival rate was 84%, and the 5-year survival rate was only 65%. The patients averaged almost 1 hospitalization per year. Six patients eventually weaned from ventilatory support, but 17 died over a 20-year period. Three deaths were due to accidental tube disconnection, one to power failure during use of an iron lung, five to probable hypotension or arrhythmia, seven to cardiomyopathy, and one to trauma from falling out of a wheelchair.[17] Thus, 9 of the 16 patients may well have died from causes related to the methods by which they were ventilated. Mortality rates probably would have been quite different if patients had used noninvasive IPPV and learned glossopharyngeal breathing (GPB). In an earlier study of 55 patients by the same group, 22 with chronic lung disease and 33 with primarily ventilatory impairment,[17] the survival rate was 93% at 21.3 months, and the prognosis was similar for all three groups.[18] No direct comparisons can be made with children who suffer primarily from respiratory impairment and are managed over the long term by noninvasive means because few, if any, such children have been reported. Nonetheless, these results are clearly poor in comparison with the results in children who suffer primarily from ventilatory impairment and are managed noninvasively. The patients with lung disease had a significantly higher incidence of tracheobronchomalacia and also tended to wean from ventilator use. Hospitalization rates were similar.[19]

A number of clinical investigators have reported the pediatric use of nasal PIP + PEEP in the intensive care setting. Pope et al. reported success in using nasal PIP + PEEP during anesthesia with fentanyl and propofol for five gastrointestinal endoscopic procedures in patients with DMD.[20] Birnkrant et al. used nasal IPPV for 22 patients with neuromuscular weakness.[21] Pope and Birnkrant recently reported facilitation of successful extubation for 22 of 25 patients, including 10 with NMD and a mean age of 15 years, with the use of post-extubation nasal PIP + PEEP.[22] Padman et al. used nasal PIP + PEEP to treat acute respiratory failure in 15 patients, aged 4–21 years, including 4 patients with cystic fibrosis and 11 with chronic neuromuscular weakness and ventilatory failure. All patients were managed outside of intensive care with reduced hospital stays or until lung transplantation (for patients with cystic fibrosis). Only one 4-year-old girl with a myopathy underwent intubation for secretion clearance.[12] In a later study, Padman et al. treated 34 patients with nasal PIP + PEEP for 35 episodes of ventilatory/respiratory failure in the PICU. Exclusion criteria were absent cough or gag, multiple organ system failure, vocal cord paralysis, and lack of cooperation with a nasal interface. The children showed significant improvements in heart rate, respiratory rate, dyspnea, serum bicarbonate concentrations, and carbon dioxide during unassisted breathing. Intubation was avoided in all but three patients.[23] Simonds et al. delivered nasal or facemask ventilation to 38 children with ventilatory insufficiency due to skeletal or congenital NMD and nasal CPAP to 2 children with frequent chest infections associated with sleep-disordered breathing (age: 9 months to 16 years) for a mean of 30 months (range: 1–105 months). Of the children with ventilatory insufficiency, 18 had symptomatic nocturnal hypoventilation, 17 had diurnal hypercapnia, and three were referred for weaning. In general, nasal PIP + PEEP spans of only 10 cmH$_2$O were used. Thirty-eight of the 40 patients tolerated the treatments over the long term and had significantly improved PaO$_2$, PaCO$_2$, and nocturnal transcutaneous carbon dioxide.[24] One patient did not tolerate the treatment, did not return for follow-up, and died 21 months later. Two children with SMA died at 7 and 26 months of age when intubation and tracheotomy were not done. None of these investigators noted the use of mouthpiece IPPV, maximal insuffla-tions, or MAC.

In a study using nasal ventilation in 4 infants with SMA type 1, all died as a result of failed extubations or after the parents were encouraged to avoid repeat intubation or tra-cheostomy.[25] The use of nasal ventilation was reported to have failed to prolong life.[25] However, in this attempt, as in the others, the low nasal PIP + PEEP spans may not have been adequate, and supplemental oxygen was used. All four patients died from inadequate ventilatory assistance or failure to intubate or use expiratory aids during chest infections once the parents were resigned to let their children die.[25]

PRACTICE AND OUTCOMES IN DIAGNOSIS-SPECIFIC PEDIATRIC POPULATIONS

For young patients with NMD, about 90% of episodes of acute respiratory failure result from inability to eliminate effectively airway secretions and mucus during otherwise benign intercurrent chest infections.[26] As for adults, children with primarily ventilatory impairment (see Table 1 in Chapter 1) can benefit from the use of the oximetry feedback-respiratory muscle aid protocol (see Chapter 8) to avoid hospitalization, intubation, and tracheostomy.[27]

Infants and Small Children

Spinal Muscular Atrophy Type 1 and Extubation

Members of pediatric sections of national medical societies, including 75 intensivists, 61 physiatrists, and 51 neurologists, responded to a survey asking what treatment they would recommend for an infant with SMA type 1 in respiratory distress. Noninvasive ven-tilation would be offered by 70% of the respondents but recommended by only 23% and neither offered nor recommended by 7%. Intubation would be offered and recommended by 38%, offered but not recommended by 48%, and neither offered nor recommended by 14%. Tracheotomy would be offered and recommended by 29%, offered but not recom-mended by 47%, and neither offered nor recommended by 24%.[28] Ninety percent of in-fants with SMA type 1 who do not benefit from respiratory interventions die by 1 year of age.[29] Thus, it is not surprising that physicians almost invariably tell parents that infants with SMA are not likely to survive for 2 years.

Infants with SMA are evaluated for vital capacity during crying[30] (or vital capacity after the age of 2 years), the presence and extent of paradoxical breathing and pectus excava-tum, and SpO_2; occasionally, carbon dioxide is measured noninvasively. Although espe-cially helpful in older children and adults, end-tidal carbon dioxide is less accurate than transcutaneous carbon dioxide monitoring in infants and toddlers.[31] SpO_2 tends to decrease when infants cry and while they are asleep during periods of diaphoresis and frequent arousals associated with inspiratory muscle weakness.

The simplest and perhaps best differentiation of children with SMA type 1 is based on two levels of severity. About 10% of children are most severely affected and develop chronic respiratory muscle failure and require ongoing continuous ventilatory support before 6 months of age, whether or not the respiratory failure is triggered by a respiratory infection. Some of these children may develop such severe weakness from poor nutritional support during an intercurrent chest infection or after surgery (see Chapter 14) that they become ventilator-dependent. Such children conventionally either undergo tracheotomy for full-time IPPV or are left to die.

Most children with SMA type 1 have less severe involvement. They develop respiratory failure only during intercurrent chest infections because of inability to cough effectively. When conventionally treated, they require intubation and then undergo tracheotomy because of inability to wean from ventilator use or because the clinician is uneasy with extubation because of anticipated difficulties with clearing airway secretions. However, when a new protocol (Table 1) that includes extubation to high-span nasal PIP + PEEP is followed,[32] they wean to nocturnal-only nasal PIP + PEEP and require daytime aid only during inter-current chest infections. In addition, they develop normal speech. About 20% of patients fall between the severe and milder types. Their speech is moderately dysarthric, and they require varying periods of daytime noninvasive ventilatory assistance.

All children with SMA type 1 demonstrate paradoxical thoracic retraction during inspiration by 1 year of age.[32] The great majority have paradoxical retractions from birth. If untreated, this condition results in severe pectus excavatum and severe lung and chest wall

---

TABLE 1. Conventional vs. Protocol Management of Intubated Patients with SMA Type 1

Conventional management
1. Oxygen is administrated arbitrarily in concentrations that maintain SpO_2 well above 95%.
2. Frequent airway suctioning via the tube.
3. Supplemental oxygen is increased when desaturations occur.
4. Ventilator weaning is attempted at the expense of hypercapnia.
5. Extubation is not attempted unless the patient appears to be ventilator-weaned.
6. Extubation to CPAP or low-span bilevel positive airway pressure and continued oxygen therapy.
7. Deep airway suctioning by catheterizing the upper airway along with postural drainage and chest physical therapy.
8. With increasing CO_2 retention or hypoxia, supplemental oxygen is increased and ultimately the patient is reintubated.
9. After reintubation, tracheostomy is thought to be the only long-term option; after successful extubation bronchodilators and ongoing routine chest physical therapy are used.
10. Eventually discharged home with a tracheostomy, often after a prolonged rehabilitation stay for family training.

Protocol management
1. Oxygen administration is limited to approach 95% SaO_2.
2. Mechanical insufflation-exsufflation is used via the tube at pressures from 25–70 cmH_2O to – 25 to –70 cmH_2O as often as every few minutes (as needed) to reverse oxyhemoglobin desaturations due to airway mucus accumulation and when ascultatory evidence indicates secretion accumulation. Abdominal thrusts are applied during exsufflation. Tube and upper airway are suctioned after use of expiratory aids as needed. Pressures are titrated to achieve rapid chest expansion and rapid lung emptying (1.5–2 sec).
3. Expiratory aids are used when desaturations occur.
4. Ventilator weaning is attempted without permitting hypercapnia.
5. Extubation is attempted whether or not the patient is ventilator weaned when the following criteria are met:
   • Afebrile
   • No supplemental oxygen requirement to maintain SaO_2 >94%
   • Chest radiograph abnormalities cleared or clearing
   • Any respiratory depressants discontinued
   • Airway suctioning required less than 1–2 times/8 hours
   • Coryza diminished sufficiently so that suctioning of the nasal orifices is required less than once every 6 hours (important to facilitate use of nasal prongs/mask for postextubation nasal ventilation)
6. Extubation to continuous high-span PIP + PEEP with no supplemental oxygen.
7. Oximetry feedback is used to guide the use of expiratory aids, postural drainage, and chest physical therapy for reversal of any desaturations due to airway mucus accumulation.
8. With CO_2 retention or ventilator synchronization difficulties, nasal interface leaks are eliminated, pressure support and ventilator rate are increased, or the patient is switched from BiPAP-ST to a volume-limited ventilator. Persistent oxyhemoglobin desaturation despite eucapnia and aggressive use of expiratory aids indicates impending respiratory distress and need to reintubate.
9. After reintubation, the protocol is used for a second trial of extubation to high-span nasal PIP + PEEP, or after successful extubation bronchodilators and chest physical therapy are discontinued and the patient is weaned to sleep high-span nasal PIP + PEEP.
10. Discharge home after the SpO_2 remains within normal limits for 2 days and when assisted coughing is needed less than 4 times per day.

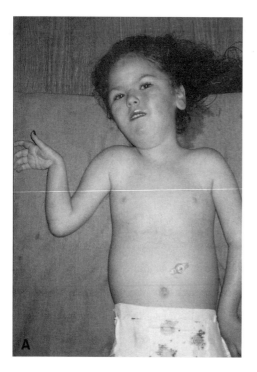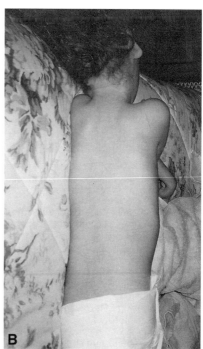

FIGURES 5. *A* and *B*, Six-year-old girl with spinal muscular atrophy type 1 shows good chest development and no sign of the pectus excavatum that was present before she began nocturnal high-span nasal PIP + PEEP at 9 months of age.

undergrowth and pulmonary restriction. Usually, after a period of sleeping comfortably without noticeable arousals, the child begins to awaken every hour or two and is diaphoretic. Episodes of diaphoresis can be associated with bradycardias. Nocturnal high-span PIP + PEEP alleviates diaphoresis, permits more restful sleep, and prevents or reverses pectus deformity and promotes lung growth (Fig. 5). It is indicated for all patients with SMA type 1. Nocturnal high-span PIP + PEEP also normalizes nocturnal SpO_2 and end-tidal carbon dioxide when either is abnormal. IPAPs of 15–20 cmH_2O are used with minimal EPAP (about 2 cmH_2O).

At least 5% of infants with SMA type 1 have symptomatic bradycardias. Bradycardia may result from sudden, severe oxyhemoglobin desaturation, or, in some cases, the SpO_2 decreases only after bradycardia has lasted for a minute or so. Bradycardia may result from autonomic instability. Episodes of respiratory distress, such as those caused by airway mucus accumulation, usually result in sinus tachycardia, not bradycardia. Although bradycardia can be triggered by airway suctioning or tracheal stimulation, it also can occur without apparent warning, most often during sleep. Bradycardia or other arrhythmias may be responsible for some sudden deaths—generally, those that occur after tracheotomy in infants with SMA. During periods of stress (e.g., intercurrent respiratory tract infections or after surgery), severe bradycardia can cause skin blanching and loss of consciousness as well as diaphoresis and may be confused with seizure activity. Most episodes of bradycardia that precede decreases in SpO_2 resolve spontaneously or with stimulation of the child. Bradycardia that is associated with loss of consciousness and refractory to stimulation, however, should be managed with atropine and, occasionally, cardiac resuscitation efforts. Cardiac pacemakers also may be a therapeutic option. Diaphoresis and bradycardia that result from decreases in SpO_2 are alleviated by effective high-span PIP + PEEP and airway secretion management. These episodes appear to become less frequent after the child's second birthday.

Other than from our center, there have been no reports of 2-year survival of conventionally managed children with SMA type 1 who do not undergo tracheotomy. In one study of infants with NMD, a 57% mortality rate was reported for 7 children with NMD supported by invasive ventilation after an intubation before age 2 years.[33] Two children had SMA; two had nemaline myopathy; and one each had congenital myotonic dystrophy, congenital muscular dystrophy, and fiber type disproportion. Three of the children died from pneumonia and one from aspiration after ventilator use was discontinued. Total duration of mechanical ventilation was an average of 23 months, of which 19 were spent in hospitals. Two of the four children who were discharged home, all with professional nursing support, died. All seven patients had recurrent atelectasis and pneumonia. Three of the four who died had autopsy evidence of cor pulmonale.

Despite the above study, long-term survival of tracheostomy IPPV users is possible. Our center is managing 16 tracheostomy IPPV users with SMA type 1. Although 15 of the 16 have no breathing tolerance, they have a mean age of 74 ± 57 months. All of the 15 children lost the ability to breathe without ventilatory support immediately after tracheotomy for the reasons stated in Chapter 5 as well as because of severe inspiratory muscle weakness and hypoplastic lungs and chest walls. Once tracheostomy tubes were placed, hospitalization rates were 0.58 per year from birth to the third birthday and 0.21 per year from 3 to 19 years of age. One child died within 3 months of tracheotomy because of lung collapse. Respiratory infections, hemorrhage, other tube-related complications, and cardiac arrhythmias were also associated with tracheostomy. Only 1 of the 16 children developed the ability to speak. In addition, there are two male patients with SMA type 1, 20 and 14 years of age, in Japan (both are continuous tracheostomy IPPV users), a 10-year-old patient with SMA type 1 in Hong Kong, and a 19-year-old male patient with SMA type 1, who has been a full-time tracheostomy IPPV user since 2 months of age, in Pennsylvania. All four patients have severe cases of SMA type 1; they are averbal but communicate by a Morse code system of grunting as well as by computer-driven voice synthesizers. One patient has used a highly sophisticated combination of guttural sounds in a Morse code–like system developed with his mother to communicate needs and even to spell out letters of the alphabet since 3 years of age. All four patients are straight A students, including the two patients in college. The 19-year-old boy from Pennsylvania graduated third in his high school class.

Of our 34 patients with SMA type 1 who use nocturnal high-span nasal PIP + PEEP, two died suddenly at 6 and 13 months of age. The other 32 are now 41.8 ± 26.0 months old, and one child is 8 years and 2 months old. Fourteen children are over age 4 years; 8 are over age 5 years. Although hospitalization rates are 1.52 per year until the third birthday, they decrease to 0.20 per year from 3 to 9 years of age, and no child has been hospitalized after the fifth birthday in 17 patient-years. Twenty-eight of the 32 noninvasively managed children have developed the ability to speak, and only three require continuous high-span nasal PIP + PEEP. Thus, even children with severe SMA type 1 who become continuously ventilator-dependent during the first 6 months of life often can be managed noninvasively, and the great majority of children with SMA type 1 require only nocturnal PIP + PEEP and develop the ability to speak. These children usually do not develop respiratory difficulties until 4 months to 2 years of age, and the difficulties almost always result from a chest cold. Even at 20 years of age, patients lose none of the facial and finger muscle function that they have had since infancy.

Besides the nocturnal use of PIP + PEEP to promote more normal lung growth, rest inspiratory muscles, and reverse pectus excavatum, noninvasively managed children also may benefit from delivery of 10–15 maximal insufflations 2 or 3 times/day via a manual resuscitator or a Cough-Assist (J. H. Emerson Co., Cambridge, MA) timed to their inspirations.

Although no data support this approach, periodic maximal insufflations may complement nocturnal PIP + PEEP. Barois has treated over 100 infants with SMA, 9 months and older, with regular deep insufflation therapy and later provided them with mouthpieces or nasal interfaces for nocturnal aid. She reported that this treatment ameliorated restrictive pulmonary syndrome.[34,35] She also used an abdominal binder so that the insufflated air entered the upper and middle thorax rather than ventilated only the lower lobes. We support the use of this maximal insufflation technique in children from the age of 9 months but recommend using the palm of the hand to restrict abdominal expansion rather than an abdominal binder. Because of daily use, several children as young as 11 months have been able to use MI-E successfully. These mobilization "exercises" familiarize and help accustom the child to MI-E. Nocturnal use of PIP + PEEP and perhaps daytime lung and chest wall range of motion are the only respiratory interventions needed between chest infections.

At times auscultatory evidence of airway mucus is confused with the wheezing of reversible bronchospasm. Family physicians often prescribe ongoing oxygen supplementation, bronchodilators, nebulizer treatments, and chest physical therapy even when the children are well. Without a history of asthma or bronchospasm, such treatments are unnecessary and waste care provider time for the healthy child between chest infections. Oxygen therapy also can be harmful (see Chapter 2).

Until the child is old enough (usually 2.5–4.5 years of age) to cooperate fully with the oximetry protocol (see Chapter 8), most chest infections necessitate hospitalization and intubation. Most treating physicians are reluctant to intubate out of fear that the children may permanently lose breathing tolerance, whether from the correction of compensatory metabolic alkalosis that accompanies normalization of arterial carbon dioxide tensions or from exacerbation of weakness due to acute illness and undernutrition. Tracheotomy is often recommended but refused by parents during these episodes, especially if they learn about noninvasive alternatives.

Because parents have refused tracheotomy when we and others have recommended it, we have been forced to modify the noninvasive approaches that we use successfully for older children and adults. As a result, we discovered that children can survive without tracheostomy tubes. Because most children with typical SMA type 1 develop effective articulation and communication capabilities, they usually also retain enough oromotor control to avoid severe aspiration of upper airway secretions that otherwise would cause a decrease in baseline SpO_2 below 95% and recurrent aspiration pneumonias. Even our children with severe, averbal SMA type 1 usually do not aspirate oral secretions to the extent of causing a decrease in SpO_2 baseline or pneumonia.

From the time of diagnosis an oximeter is prescribed along with a manual resuscitator and nocturnal high-span nasal PIP + PEEP. The family is told to use the oximeter at the first sign of oxyhemoglobin desaturation, particularly during colds, to guide the use of manually assisted coughing and MAC chest physical therapy, and to initiate postural drainage to maintain or return SpO_2 levels to normal (oximetry protocol—see Chapter 8). MAC is ideally timed to the infant's own coughing attempts. In addition to carefully timed manually assisted coughing, coughs can be facilitated by holding the child against the shoulder and gently squeezing his or her belly against the shoulder as he or she coughs. This position not only assists the cough but also is less likely to result in reflux of stomach contents and aspiration.

If infants with SMA type 1 use manual resuscitators or the positive pressure of MI-E for regular daily maximal insufflations, if they use nasal PIP + PEEP nightly, and especially if they have had frequent episodes of respiratory failure and intubation and have experienced MI-E via invasive tubes, they tend to cooperate with MI-E via oral-nasal interfaces at a very early age. They simply relax, keep the airways open, and let MI-E bring up the airway secretions, sometimes at as early as 11 months of age. Other children, often those who have had fewer respiratory complications and have not been using these methods daily, may not cooperate with MAC until 2.5–6 years of age. Full cooperation with the oximetry protocol is vital to avoid pneumonia and hospitalizations. With bouts of dehydration, high fever, or a steady decrease in SpO_2 baseline below 95%, the child is evaluated by the physician for hospitalization and, possibly, intubation. Supplemental oxygen is avoided unless SpO_2 baseline is less than 94%, in which case patients often need to be intubated anyway.

Intubated infants receive MI-E at 35- to 50-cmH$_2$O insufflation and exsufflation via the tube along with concomitant abdominal thrusts applied during the exsufflation cycle (MAC), just as for adults. Whether via a tube or the upper airway, children neither show discomfort nor develop evidence of barotrauma. Antibiotics and hydration are used according to convention in patients with pneumonia, gross atelectasis, or lung collapse. Hypercapnia is avoided. If aggressive airway secretion management and MI-E via the tube fail to maintain normal SpO_2, oxygen supplementation is provided to increase SpO_2 to 93–95% but no greater. This limit is set because hospital personnel tend to treat oxyhemoglobin desaturation by increasing oxygen administration rather than by clearing airway debris, the principal cause of pneumonia and lung collapse.

Once the SpO_2 is normal on room air, one should attempt to wean the patient from ventilatory support before extubation. If, despite maintaining normal SpO_2 on room air and having four or fewer interventions (suctioning or MI-E) to clear the airways of secretions during a 24-hour period, the child still has not weaned from ventilator use, extubation should not be delayed more than a few days for weaning efforts.

Criteria for extubation are similar to but more restrictive than those for older children and adults (see Chapter 8). The patient is not extubated until no supplemental oxygen is required to maintain SpO_2 greater than 94% for at least 1 or 2 days, chest radiograph abnormalities are cleared or clearing, respiratory depressants are discontinued, endotracheal tube secretions are diminished to a minimum or to the point of necessitating minimal use of suctioning and expiratory aid, and coryza is diminished sufficiently to facilitate use of nasal prongs/mask for transition to nasal ventilation. Even continuously ventilator-dependent children can be safely extubated and effectively ventilated after extubation by immediately placing them on high-span nasal PIP + PEEP at rates slightly greater than the autonomous breathing rate. For small children who may not be able to trigger PIP + PEEP delivery, see "Ventilator Choice and Settings" above. Because children with SMA type 1 should have been using nasal PIP + PEEP nightly before hospitalization, transition from tube to nasal ventilation is usually smooth. We have never had to keep children with SMA type 1 intubated for more than 10 days. They must not be extubated prematurely.

Because it is difficult, if not impossible, to expect intensive care nurses and respiratory therapists to use manually assisted coughing and MI-E every few minutes or so while the patient is awake, we rely heavily on the child's parents or primary care providers. Because MI-E is associated with no sequelae in this population, we let family members apply MI-E via oral-nasal interfaces and even via translaryngeal tubes in the intensive care unit. Certainly, after extubation the family is given the responsibility of providing essentially all of the airway secretion management and is trained in respiratory resuscitation, including manual resuscitation with oxygen supplementation. The family needs this knowledge to avoid future hospitalizations.

After extubation, airway secretions continue to be removed by some combination of chest physical therapy, postural drainage, and MAC for a few days until the airways "dry up" and are clear on auscultation. Transmitted sounds from throat and pharyngeal secretions are not a reason to continue chest physical therapy. Thus, chest physical therapy and postural drainage are discontinued, the premorbid routine of nocturnal nasal PIP + PEEP and daytime insufflations is continued, and the patient is discharged home, with or without the ability to breathe autonomously. Many children wean from full-time to nocturnal-only ventilator use 1 or 2 weeks after hospital discharge.[32] If such children had undergone tracheotomy, lifetime 24-hour ventilator dependence would have resulted (see Chapter 5). A recent study of extubation of 28 pediatric patients to noninvasive IPPV strongly supports this approach.[36] It appears that such children can be managed predominantly and indefinitely by nocturnal noninvasive IPPV.[32] Most children do well until the next chest infection.

For children with SMA who undergo tracheotomy, the use of MI-E via the tracheostomy tube is a more comfortable and effective alternative to deep tracheal suctioning. In addition, as in other patients, oxygen supplementation must be avoided in favor of aggressive airway secretion management and the maintenance of SpO_2 greater than 94% by use of MAC and assisted ventilation, when necessary.

In a recent study we attempted to manage children with SMA type 1 without resort to tracheotomy and compared our extubation outcomes using the oximetry feedback-respiratory muscle aid protocol with conventional management (see Table 1). Eleven children with SMA type 1 were studied during episodes of respiratory failure. Nine children required multiple intubations. Along with standard treatments, they received manually and mechanically assisted coughing to reverse airway mucus-associated oxyhemoglobin desaturation, and extubation was not attempted until our criteria were met. After extubation all patients received high-span nasal PIP + PEEP. Successful extubation was defined as no need to reintubate during the current hospitalization. The nine children were successfully extubated by our protocol on 23 of 28 occasions. The same children managed conventionally were successfully extubated on 2 of 20 occasions ($p < 0.001$). Thus, although intercurrent chest infections necessitate periods of hospitalization and intubation until children are old enough to cooperate with the oximetry protocol, tracheotomy can be avoided for about 5 of 6 children with SMA type 1.[32]

In a follow-up of this study, 56 infants with SMA type 1 were intubated a total of 116 times for respiratory failure. Twenty-six of 31 extubations performed in our center and according to our protocol were successful. Fourteen of 22 other extubations to high-span PIP + PEEP were also successful. Only three of 47 conventional extubations without postextubation PIP + PEEP were successful. The other 16 extubations were done after tracheotomy.

A chief concern in caring for chronic respirator-dependent children in hospitals has been the enormous financial and psychosocial burden.[37,38] Kettrick reported a mean stay in the intensive care unit of over 200 days for children with NMD receiving invasive mechanical ventilation.[39] Because patients with SMA type 1 who undergo tracheostomy usually remain ventilator-dependent and hospitalized for extensive periods and avoidance of tracheostomy usually results in avoidance of continuous ventilator dependence, the benefits in cost and quality of life are obvious. It is much easier to avoid invasive ventilation in the first place than it is to decannulate children because of their tendency to be fearful and to develop tracheal damage from placement of the tube.

Spinal Muscular Atrophy Type 2

SMA type 2 has a wide range of severity. Some children may be able to maintain the sitting position for only a minute or so, whereas others may almost be able to walk. Children with SMA type 2 may initially recover from chest infections without hospitalization. Depending on severity, they usually first develop pneumonia and respiratory failure at some time from late infancy to early adolescence. Such children are managed like children with SMA type 1 with hospitalization and intubation, when needed, until they are old enough to cooperate with the oximetry protocol. They should rarely if ever require tracheostomy tubes. Often the vital capacity continues to increase into early adulthood and plateaus at more than 50% of predicted normal. As patients become older, they can make highly effective use of respiratory muscle aids to avert hospitalizations and tracheostomy.[40]

Nocturnal nasal ventilation is used for the 30–50% of children with SMA type 2 who have paradoxical thoracic movement with decreased upper thoracic volumes during inspiration[41] or symptoms of hypoventilation. They, too, awaken frequently from sleep with diaphoresis. Nocturnal oximetry, end-tidal carbon dioxide monitoring, and even polysomnography or plethysmography may be helpful in deciding whether to introduce nocturnal nasal ventilation. Some children with SMA type 2 do not benefit from ongoing nocturnal nasal IPPV until late adulthood. Many patients with SMA type 2 require gastrostomy tubes.

Spinal Muscular Atrophy Types 3–5

Patients with SMA types 3–5 can walk at least temporarily. They should never require tracheostomy tubes and, until late in life, usually require noninvasive IPPV and expiratory aids only during severe chest infections. Concomitant scoliosis, obesity, or other factors that hamper lung or respiratory muscle functioning, combined with underlying respiratory muscle weakness and the effect of aging on muscles and senescent loss of anterior horn cells, result in the need for nighttime and even full-time noninvasive IPPV in later life.

In a study of 12 ventilator users with infantile or adult-type SMA who had survived 9.7 + 8.3 years, six patients had received IPPV via oral and/or nasal interfaces for 5.5 + 6.1 years, and the others (a total of 7 patients in all, including one who used both methods) had used tracheostomy IPPV. The tracheostomy IPPV users had significantly more pulmonary complications than the noninvasive IPPV users. The noninvasive IPPV users had access to MI-E to clear airway secretions. All patients could communicate verbally and take nutrition by mouth. Five of the seven tracheostomy IPPV users but none of the six noninvasive IPPV users remained institutionalized. Except for the two ventilator users with SMA type 1, all patients remained socially active and four were gainfully employed. Thus, noninvasive IPPV methods are effective and practical alternatives to tracheostomy for patients with SMA of all ages.[42] Patients with milder NMDs who typically live into adulthood using noninvasive IPPV are discussed in Chapters 7–9.

NONINVASIVE VENTILATION FOR CHILDREN WHO DO NOT REQUIRE EXPIRATORY AID

Children with congenital central hypoventilation or congenital diaphragmatic hernia are often excellent candidates for nocturnal noninvasive ventilation because their cough and bulbar muscles are generally intact. A 75% survival rate was reported with the use of noninvasive ventilation and delayed surgical repair of congenital diaphragmatic hernia.[43] Thus, nocturnal noninvasive IPPV or PIP + PEEP may be all that is required to avoid tracheotomy. A number of centers have reported success with noninvasive management of such patients from infancy (see Table 1 in Chapter 1). Caution should be used, however, to optimize assisted ventilation by avoiding delivery of inappropriately low volumes or spans.

HYPOXEMIC INSUFFICIENCY

Patients with hypoxemic respiratory insufficiency may benefit from noninvasive IPPV along with oxygen therapy. The early institution of noninvasive ventilation may defer or avoid respiratory muscle fatigue and overt respiratory failure both in acute and chronic care settings. The maximal fractional concentration of oxygen in inspired gas (FiO_2) that can be achieved with most pressure-cycled ventilators is about 40%. With supplemental oxygen, great caution must be taken to avoid increasing insufflation leakage and hypercapnia.

Fortenberry et al. demonstrated significant improvements in respiratory rate, PCO_2, PO_2, pH, SpO_2, alveolar-arterial oxygen gradient, and PaO_2-to-FiO_2 ratios with the use of nasal PIP + PEEP in 28 pediatric patients with acute hypoxemic respiratory insufficiency.[36] Intubation or reintubation was prevented in 25 of the patients. We also have observed that patients with hypoxemic respiratory failure from causes such as interstitial pneumonia, reactive airways, and sickle cell chest syndrome benefit from noninvasive ventilation.

Endotracheal intubation of acute asthmatics increases airway resistance and is associated with a high rate of complications. CPAP decreases airway resistance but does not improve gas exchange. Increasing evidence indicates that in patients with bronchial asthma the use of nasal PIP + PEEP can successfully avert intubation[44] and be of use in the postoperative management of severe reactive airway disease.[45] Bronchodilators can be administered successfully during the use of nasal PIP + PEEP.[46] In a recent report, intubation was avoided during 15 of 17 episodes of status asthmaticus largely by the use of PIP + PEEP via an oral-nasal interface for 16 ± 21 hours.[47] Settings of 14 ± 5 cmH_2O with PEEP of 4 ± 2 cmH_2O were adjusted to reduce respiratory rate below 25 breaths/minute. Blood pH, $PaCO_2$, and respiratory rate were essentially normalized and PaO_2 fraction of inspired oxygen increased from 315 to 472. The initial peak inspiratory pressure to ventilate was 18 ± 5 cmH_2O and always less than 25 cmH_2O. There were no complications or difficulties with expectoration. Full liquid oral intake was preserved. Sedation was required for only two patients. Noninvasive ventilation also was reported to be successful for avoiding intubation in patients with status asthmaticus at least two other centers.[48,49]

PIP + PEEP may have a role in infants with bronchiolitis, although the high respiratory rates may make ventilator dyssynchrony a problem. Some evidence already supports the role of CPAP in the management of bronchiolitis.[50,51] Soong et al. successfully extubated patients with bronchiolitis to CPAP.

PATIENTS WITH MIXED OXYGENATION/VENTILATION IMPAIRMENT

Occasional patients present with a combination of oxygenation and ventilation impairment, although one of the two dominates the clinical picture. For example, an obese, asthmatic 8-year-old girl developed a chest cold and presented in severe respiratory distress with bilateral pneumonitis and reactive airways. She received intravenous theophylline, high-dose methylprednisolone, and continuous albuterol aerosol and had trials of intravenous magnesium, aerosolized anticholinergics, furosemide, isoproterenol, and CPAP without relief of dyspnea and hypoxemic respiratory failure. Nasal PIP + PEEP was begun at an IPAP of 12 and an EPAP of 5 cmH_2O in spontaneous mode. The patient immediately improved sufficiently to decrease FiO_2 from 100% to 50% and had a marked improvement in dyspnea, degree of reactive airway disease, heart rate, respiratory rate, and SpO_2. It was believed that she would have required intubation without use of nasal PIP + PEEP.[52] Noninvasive ventilation also was reported to facilitate successful extubation of 25- and 22-month-old children with tracheal edema and pulmonary dysfunction after laryngotracheal reconstruction for subglottic stenosis. The children developed respiratory failure after extubation and avoided reintubation by using noninvasive ventilation, which provided airway stenting and ventilatory support while the edema and dysfunction were resolving.[53]

Thus, there is an important role for the use of noninvasive ventilation in the PICU for the management of ventilatory insufficiency, and it has an increasing role in the management of the pediatric patient with hypoxemic insufficiency.

Cada uno es hijo de sus obras.
(Everyone is the son of his works.)

Miguel de Cervantes, *Don Quijote de La Mancha*

REFERENCES

1. Devereauz K: Bridging the information gap. RRTC/NMD Program Overview 1998–2003. National Institute on Disability and Rehabilitation Research: Rehabilitaiton Research and Training Center in Neuromuscular Diseases at the University of California, Davis: http://www.rehabinfo.net/Clearinghouse/Virtual Library/Index.html.
2. Jardine E, O'Toole M, Paton JY, Wallis C: Current status of long term ventilation of children in the United Kingdom: Questionnaire survey. Br Med J 318:295–298, 1999.
3. Midgren B, Olofson J, Harlid R, et al: Home mechanical ventilation in Sweden, with reference to Danish experiences. Respir Med 94:135–138, 2000.
4. Pirttimaa-Kaitanen R, Luft M: Home mechanical ventilation in Finland. IVUN News 14:3, 2000.
5. Shneerson JM: Home mechanical ventilation in children: Techniques, outcomes and ethics. Monaldi Arch Chest Dis 51:426–430, 1996.
6. Payton P, Padgett D, van Stralen D, Newsom H: Incidence of tracheostomy dislodgments in a pediatric subacute facility. Eighth Journées Internationales de Ventilation à Domicile, abstract 111, March 7, 2001, Hôpital de la Croix-Rousse, Lyon, France.
7. Hillberg RE, Johnson DC: Noninvasive ventilation. N Engl J Med 337:1746–1752, 1997.
8. de Lemos RA: Management of pediatric acute hypoxemic respiratory insufficiency with bilevel positive pressure nasal mask ventilation. Chest 108:894–895, 1995.
9. Milane J, Bertrand P, Montredon C, et al: Intérèt de l'assistance ventilatoire abdomino-diaphragmatique dans la réadaptation des grands handicapés respiratoires. In Simon L (ed.): Actualites en Rééducation Fonctionel et Réadaptation, vol. Paris, Masson, 1990.
10. Milane J, Bertrand A: Indications de la ventilation par prothee extra-thoracique. Bull Eur Physiopathol Respir 22:37–40, 1986.
11. Klonin H, Bowman B, Peters M, et al: Negative pressure ventilation via chest cuirass to decrease ventilator-associated complications in infants with acute respiratory failure: A case series. Respir Care 45:486–490, 2000.
12. Padman R, Lawless S, von Nessen S: Use of bilevel positive airway pressure by nasal mask in the treatment of respiratory insufficiency in pediatric patients: Preliminary investigation. Pediatr Pulmonol 17:119–123, 1994.
13. Fauroux B, Boule M, Lofaso F, et al: Chest physiotherapy in cystic fibrosis: Improved tolerance with nasal pressure support ventilation. Pediatrics 103:E32, 1999.
14. Newth CJL, Asmler B, Anderson GP, Morley J: The effects of varying inflation and deflation pressures on the maximal expiratory deflation flow-volume relationship in anesthetized Rhesus monkeys. Am Rev Respir Dis 144:807–813, 1991.
15. Bach JR, Ishikawa Y, Kim H: Prevention of pulmonary morbidity for patients with Duchenne muscular dystrophy. Chest 112:1024–1028, 1997.
16. Niranjan V, Bach JR: Noninvasive management of pediatric neuromuscular ventilatory failure. Crit Care Med 26:2061–2065, 1998.
17. Frates RC, Splaingard ML, Smith EO, Harrison GM: Outcome of home mechanical ventilation in children. J Pediatr 106:850–856, 1985.
18. Splaingard ML, Frates RC, Harrison GM, et al: Home positive pressure ventilation: Twenty years experience. Chest 84:376–382, 1983.
19. Wheeler WB, Maguire EL, Kurachek SC, et al: Chronic respiratory failure of infancy and childhood: clinical outcomes based on underlying etiology. Pediatr Pulmonol 17:1–5, 1994.
20. Pope JF, Birnkrant DJ, Martin JE, Repucci AH: Noninvasive ventilation during percutaneous gastrostomy placenment in Duchenne muscular dystrophy. Pediatr Pulmonol 23:468–471, 1997.
21. Birnkrant DJ, Pope JF, Eiben RM: Pediatric noninvasive nasal ventilation. J Child Neurol 12:231–236, 1997.
22. Pope JF, Birnkrant DJ: Noninvasive ventilation to facilitate extubation in a pediatric intensive care unit. J Intens Care Med 15:99–103, 2000.
23. Padman R, Lawless ST, Kettrick RG: Noninvasive ventilation via bilevel positive airway pressure support in pediatric practice. Crit Care Med 26:169–173, 1998.
24. Simonds AK, Ward S, Heather S, et al: Outcome of paediatric domiciliary mask ventilation in neuromuscular and skeletal disease. Eur Respir J 16:476–481, 2000.
25. Birnkrant DJ, Pope JF, Martin JE, et al: Treatment of type 1 spinal muscular atrophy with noninvasive ventilation and gastrostomy feeding. Pediatr Neurol 18:407–410, 1998.
26. Bach JR, Rajaraman R, Ballanger F, et al: Neuromuscular ventilatory insufficiency: The effect of home mechanical ventilator use vs. oxygen therapy on pneumonia and hospitalization rates. Am J Phys Med Rehabil 77:8–19, 1998.
27. Niranjan V, Bach JR: Noninvasive management of pediatric neuromuscular ventilatory failure. Crit Care Med 26:2061–2065, 1998.
28. Moynihan Hardart K, Burns J, Truog RD: Variation in approaches to respiratory support in spinal muscular atrophy-type 1 [abstract]. Crit Care Med 28:(Suppl)A110, 2000.
29. Dubowitz V: Very severe spinal muscular atrophy (SMA type 0): An expanding clinical phenotype. Eur J Paediatr Neurol 3:49–51, 1999.

30. Chiswick ML, Milner RD: Crying vital capacity: Measurement of neonatal lung function. Arch Dis Child 51:22–27, 1976.

31. Tobias JD, Meyer DJ: Noninvasive monitoring of carbon dioxide during respiratory failure in toddlers and infants: End-tidal versus transcutaneous carbon dioxide. Anesth Anag 85:55–58, 1997.

32. Bach JR, Niranjan V: Spinal muscular atrophy type 1: A noninvasive respiratory management approach. Chest 117:1100–1105, 2000.

33. Iannaccone ST, Guilfoile T: Long-term mechanical ventilation in infants with neuromuscular disease. J Child Neurol 3:30–32, 1988.

34. Barois A, Bataille J, Estournet B: La ventilation à domicile par voie buccale chez l'enfant dans les maladies neuromusculaires. Agressologie 26:645–649, 1985.

35. Barois A, Estournet B, Duval-Beaupere G, et al: Amyotrophie spinale infantile. Rev Neurol (Paris) 145:299–304, 1989.

36. Fortenberry JD, DelToro J, Jefferson LS, et al: Management of pediatric acute hypoxemic respiratory insufficiency with bilevel positive pressure nasal mask ventilation. Chest 108:1059–1064, 1995.

37. Goldberg AI: The Illinois plan: Report of the Surgeon General's workshop, DHHS Publ PHS-83-50194. Washington, D.C., Department of Health and Human Services, 1983, p 20.

38. Burr BH, Guyer B, Todres ID, et al: Home care for children on respirators. N Engl J Med 309:1319–1323, 1983.

39. Kettrick RG: The Pennsylvania program: Report of the Surgeon General's workshop, DHHS Publ PHS-83-50194. Washington, D.C., Department of Health and Human Services, 1983.

40. Wang TG, Bach JR, Avilez C, et al: Survival of individuals with spinal muscular atrophy on ventilatory support. Am J Phys Med Rehabil 73:207–211, 1994.

41. Lissoni A, Aliverti A, Molteni F, Bach JR: Spinal muscular atrophy: Kinematic breathing analysis. Am J Phys Med Rehabil 75:332–339, 1996.

42. Bach JR, Wang TG: Noninvasive long-term ventilatory support for individuals with spinal muscular atrophy and functional bulbar musculature. Arch Phys Med Rehabil 76:213–217, 1995.

43. Chu SM, Hsieh WS, Lin JN, et al: Treatment and outcome of congenital diaphragmatic hernia. J Formos Med Assoc 99:844–847, 2000.

44. Wetzel RC: Pressure support ventilation in children with severe asthma. Crit Care Med 24:1603–1605, 1996.

45. Groudine B, Lumb PD: Pressure support ventilation with the laryngeal mask airway: a method to manage severe reactive airway disease postoperatively. Can J Anesth 42:341–343, 1995.

46. Pollack CV, Fleisch KB, Dowsey K: Treatment of acute bronchospasm with beta adrenergic agonist aerososls delivered by a nasal bilevel airway positive pressure circuit. Ann Emerg Med 26:552–557, 1995.

47. Meduri GU, Cook TR, Turner RE, et al: Noninvasive positive pressure ventilation in status asthmaticus. Chest 110:767–774, 1996.

48. Patrick W, Webster K, Ludwig L, et al: Noninvasive positive-pressure ventilation in acute respiratory distress without prior chronic respiratory failure. Am J Respir Crit Care Med 153:1005–1011, 1996.

49. Smyth RJ: Ventilatory care in status asthmaticus. Can Respir J 5:485–490, 1998.

50. Soong WJ, Hwang B, Tang RB: Coninuous positive airway pressure by nasal prongs in bronchiolitis. Pediatr Pulmonol 16:163–166, 1993.

51. Cahill J, Moore KP, Wren WS: Nasopharyngeal continuous positive airway pressure in the management of bronchiolitis. Irish Med J 76:191–192, 1983.

52. Padman R, Nadkarni VM: Noninvasive nasal mask positive pressure ventilation in a pediatric patient with acute hypoxic respiratory failure. Pediatr Emerg Care 12:44–47, 1996.

53. Hertzog JH, Siegel LB, Hauser GJ, Dalton HJ: Noninvasive positive-pressure ventilation facilitates tracheal extubation after laryngotracheal reconstruction in children. Chest 116:260–263, 1999.

11 —— Noninvasive Ventilation in the Acute Care Setting

JOHN J. MARINI, M.D.
JOHN R. HOTCHKISS, M.D.
JOHN R. BACH, M.D.

Noninvasive positive-pressure ventilation (NPPV) with or without positive end-expiratory pressure (PEEP) provides ventilatory support without endotracheal intubation. After the successful application of NPPV in the chronic care setting and the success of continuous positive airway pressure (CPAP) in the treatment of certain subsets of patients with acute hypoxemic respiratory failure, NPPV is now extensively used in a variety of settings. The application of these techniques to emergency medicine and critical care has been the subject of numerous commentaries, case studies, physiologic investigations, and controlled clinical trials[1–45] and is the focus of this chapter.

INVASIVE VS. NONINVASIVE POSITIVE-PRESSURE VENTILATION

Despite concerns about the potential consequences of endotracheal intubation and the deleterious effects of invasive mechanical ventilation, both are generally considered effective, safe, and the established standard of care in life-threatening respiratory failure. Accordingly, deviations from this traditional practice must be based on firm evidence of the therapeutic effectiveness of the alternative technique, in this case, NPPV. NPPV should offer additional benefit over endotracheal intubation, such as improved survival, fewer complications, increased comfort, or decreased cost.[32] Many putative advantages of NPPV center on the avoidance of the complications of endotracheal intubation. Indeed, an accumulating body of evidence suggests that NPPV is associated with fewer hazards (Fig. 1). Sedation requirements are lower, and infection occurs less frequently. Mortality advantages are more difficult to document. In many published studies, NPPV has been compared with no ventilation, with the need for intubation considered as the primary adverse outcome, and with conventional mechanical ventilation as a salvage intervention.[27,29,33]

Endotracheal intubation followed by mechanical ventilation is associated with well-defined hazards and costs. Appropriate placement of the endotracheal tube is not always easy, and misplacement may have severe or fatal consequences.[46–48] In appropriate patients, NPPV avoids these potential pitfalls; however, this advantage comes at the cost of losing control of the airway. In patients who are unable to cooperate with noninvasive methods or require airway access for removal of retained secretions and in most patients with altered mental status or significant airway edema, the invasive nature of endotracheal intubation is outweighed by the airway control that it affords.

An endotracheal tube may have deleterious physiologic consequences. It not only narrows the central airway by its physical presence but also may incite constriction of the distal airways.[46,49,50] In the setting of coronary artery disease, the physical distress accompanying

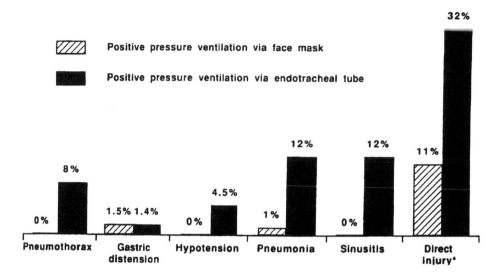

FIGURE 1. A comparison of complications resulting from 203 patients treated by noninvasive ventilation *(cross-hatched bars)* in one institution vs. ventilation delivered via endotracheal tube from a variety of studies. (From Meduri GU: Noninvasive ventilation in acute respiratory failure. In Marini JJ, Slutsky AS (eds): Physiologic Basis of Ventilatory Support. New York, Marcel Dekker, 1998, with permission.)

the intubation procedure may increase adrenergic tone and thereby worsen ischemia.[46,51] Endotracheal intubation attempted without a neuroprotective induction agent (e.g., etomidate) may increase intracranial pressure.[52]

Inherent to the nature of endotracheal intubation is the potential for pulmonary infection due to the presence of the tube. There is heightened risk of gastric aspiration during the process of intubation; 4–8% of patients experience clinically evident aspiration during intubation.[47,48] In addition to the unavoidable interruption of the mucociliary elevator, the region of the airway immediately above the endotracheal tube cuff pools oropharyngeal secretions, is cut off from natural mechanisms of airway clearance, and is shielded from routine suctioning. This region can become a reservoir for bacterial growth. Subsequent microaspiration of high-density bacterial inocula around the perimeter of the endotracheal tube cuff can contaminate the lower airway and lead to pneumonia. Ventilator associated pneumonia is a common problem in the intensive care unit. Its incidence increases nearly linearly with duration of intubation and ventilation. Tube-related infection is accompanied by a high attributable mortality rate.[53] By avoiding compromise of native defenses, NPPV may mitigate this problem. In fact, the four-fold lower incidence of ventilator-associated pneumonia in patients using NPPV vs. intubation strongly suggests such a benefit.[54,55] Maintenance of normal airway barriers and defenses is an unquestioned benefit of NPPV, although the generally shorter duration of NPPV use in the ICU confounds interpretation of this finding.

Orotracheal and nasotracheal intubation are uncomfortable and preclude expectoration, eating, and speech. Many patients require pharmacologically induced coma to overcome its attendant pain and frustration, further impeding communication. This sedation requirement renders an already ill patient even more dependent on ventilatory support, may prolong the weaning process, and sometimes makes the physical examination for intercurrent problems difficult. Furthermore, attempts to limit sedation may precipitate discomfort, agitation, patient-ventilator dyssynchrony, and sympathetic overactivity. Once connected and accommodated to NPPV, alert patients find it to be more comfortable and less frustrating.

The invasive nature of endotracheal intubation may make the physician reluctant to intubate patients (see Chapter 10). Many caregivers prefer to wait as long as possible, hoping that the patient will respond to medical therapies. While this approach may seem reasonable given the level of care and risks to which endotracheal intubation commits the patient, it may not be physiologically optimal. A protracted period of labored breathing may induce muscular fatigue and necessitate a longer period of respiratory muscle recovery if ventilatory assistance is eventually required.[56] Another important advantage is that NPPV can be applied and removed frequently, essentially without adverse consequence, encouraging its use early in the patient's course.

For appropriately selected patients, the important shortcomings of NPPV are relatively few. Airway access and protection are foregone in the decision to implement NPPV for patients with primarily respiratory impairment, but these deficiencies must be weighed against the concerns raised about endotracheal intubation. The level of support attainable by using NPPV in the intensive care unit does not generally equal the level of support possible with endotracheal intubation and mechanical ventilation. The reasons are obvious: mask leaks can become prohibitively large, and gastric insufflation may become excessive at the high pressures sometimes needed (peak airway pressures may exceed 40 cmH_2O) for patients with primarily respiratory impairment or severe restrictive lung disease. Although the initial period of NPPV clearly requires more nursing and respiratory therapist support than mechanical ventilation and endotracheal intubation, subsequent care is less effort-intensive. Contrary to earlier concerns, recent studies have not found NPPV to be significantly more expensive than conventional treatment.[16,37,38]

PHYSIOLOGIC EFFECTS OF NONINVASIVE VENTILATION

Well-adjusted NPPV usually assumes much of the work required for adequate ventilation. When the waveform of applied flow or pressure is appropriately matched to patient needs, the patient's breathing workload significantly decreases. This benefit has been demonstrated with particular clarity in the setting of chronic obstructive pulmonary disease (COPD).[1,5,26] Numerous studies have confirmed its efficacy in COPD, many through use of surrogate indicators of patient stress, such as respiratory frequency and heart rate.

Applying positive pressure to the airway can confer benefits beyond those arising from reduced ventilatory effort. Relief of respiratory distress and agitation can alter cardiac loading and dramatically diminish cardiac oxygen demands and adrenergic discharge. The lessened workload can help to restore balance between systemic oxygen delivery and demand, improving mixed venous PO_2 and often causing arterial PO_2 to rise as a consequence. The positive airway pressure applied during inspiration (IPAP) will increase mean airway pressure, an effect accentuated by maintaining a lower level of positive pressure during expiration (EPAP). Elevating mean airway pressure tends to improve oxygen transfer across the lung in patients with acute parenchymal diseases. This effect was most clearly documented in the older literature pertaining to the use of mask CPAP in pulmonary edema[43] and confirmed by the use of CPAP in patients with acute parenchymal lung injury.[44] Improved oxygenation is usually attributed to better recruitment of collapsed lung units together with beneficial redistribution of lung water and attenuation of the work of breathing. On the other hand, excessive elevations of mean airway pressure have the potential to decrease venous return, cardiac output, and blood pressure, but such adverse results occur less commonly during patient-triggered ventilation than during passive inflation.[57,58] Furthermore, in the presence of a focal consolidation of the lung resistant to recruitment, increased alveolar pressure in the uninvolved lung regions may divert blood flow to the consolidated zones. Pulmonary shunt fraction would then increase as blood flow is directed away from overdistended aerated regions to low ventilation/perfusion regions or to airless zones of consolidation or atelectasis.

TECHNIQUES FOR APPLYING NONINVASIVE POSITIVE-PRESSURE VENTILATION

With NPPV, respiratory support results from the cyclic application of an airway pressure or flow. Most commonly in the intensive care setting, a pressure rather than volume inspiratory target is selected to compensate for intermittent leaks, provide flow sufficient to meet patient demands, and avoid overpressurizing of the airway. In traditional pressure-limited NPPV, the ventilator cycles between a clinician-selected IPAP (the sum of CPAP and the pressure excursion during the inspiratory phase) and a set lower EPAP or CPAP. Although the terminology differs, the airway pressure profile in NPPV with pressure-limiting resembles that of pressure support added to CPAP in intubated patients. The respiratory rate may either be fixed or variable as the patient triggers breaths above a set back-up rate. The ventilation achieved from a set airway pressure varies with patient effort and the mechanical characteristics of the patient's respiratory system, such as compliance, resistance, and the presence or absence of auto-PEEP. Inspiratory flow terminates when IPAP cycles to EPAP. Depressurization can occur purely as a function of time, or the ventilator may have an algorithm for terminating inspiration when inspiratory flow, which declines through the inspiratory cycle as a consequence of lung filling or muscular effort, reaches a preselected level. This is a point of some importance, because prolonging the inspiratory phase beyond the point at which the patient ceases to inspire can impede expiration with resultant increases in patient work and discomfort.

An interesting variant of this problem occurs when the patient-ventilator interface develops a large leakage of air during the attempted delivery of a pressure-limited, flow-cycled volume. In this situation, the ventilator prolongs inspiration because it does not sense the drop in flow required to terminate inspiration. Such cycle-length dyssynchrony can be at least partially obviated by limiting the duration of the machine's inspiratory cycle, a feature incorporated on most modern pressure generators. Peak inspiratory flow also must satisfy patient demand. If the patient is dyspneic and strong, the ventilator may not generate sufficient flow to maintain adequate inspiratory pressure. Not only does the patient work harder than intended, but if the discrepancy is large enough, the patient also "pulls" against the ventilator circuitry, actually increasing the work of breathing. In contrast, a subset of patients experience discomfort when exposed to an inspiratory flow exceeding demand (perhaps as a reflex to prevent overdistention). Under these conditions, achieving synchrony can require adjustment of the ventilator to attain peak inspiratory pressure more slowly.

An interesting alternative to conventional pressure-limiting is proportional assist ventilation (PAV). PAV affords the patient maximal control over the timing and power assistance received from the ventilator. Because PAV scales pressure output to patient demand, its applied pressure profile closely matches that of patient effort.[21] Although this technique has been applied successfully in a number of clinical settings, experience with PAV is restricted to a few centers. Published experience with PAV is insufficient to allow conclusions about its relative merits, but on a theoretical basis it seems especially promising as a means of providing adequate support and comfort.

In volume-limited NPPV, the ventilator applies a set flow to the patient's airway for a timed interval at a specified frequency or in response to an inspiratory effort. The ventilator terminates flow when a preset gas volume has been delivered, cycling to a clinician-set value for expiratory airway pressure. Because leakage at the patient-ventilator interface markedly diminishes effective gas delivery, volume-limited NPPV must be used with extreme caution in acutely ill patients when the leak is variable or the interface insecure. Accordingly, pressure-limited NPPV may be preferable in acute settings such as the emergency department and intensive care unit, although both pressure- and volume-limited modes of NPPV have been used successfully in both venues. A recent comparative study found that the level of support attained during volume-limited NPPV, as indicated by decreased work of breathing, was greater than that achieved with pressure-limited NPPV.[26] However, patients reported that they were more comfortable using the pressure-limited mode. Close attention to patient comfort and response and a willingness to alter therapy appear more important than the initial technique chosen.

A related consideration is the choice between devices designed specifically for NPPV and traditional full-capacity ventilators capable of providing a broad spectrum of support and monitoring of intubated patients. Although the pressure-flow characteristics of many purposefully designed noninvasive ventilators are excellent, a recent study found that at least one of them was inferior to a traditional ventilator in terms of reducing patient work-load.[30] Older devices specifically designed for NPPV generally lack the precise oxygen titration capabilities, extensive adjustability of inspiratory waveform, and sophisticated alarm systems found on modern intensive care ventilators. These deficiencies suggest that more tenuous patients with primarily respiratory impairment may benefit more from conventional invasive ventilation.

Ventilatory Interface

Unlike endotracheal intubation and mechanical ventilation, NPPV requires the patient to be alert and cooperative. The nature of the interface between patient and ventilator, a crucial issue in NPPV, also has received considerable attention. In the acute setting the choice is generally between nasal and oronasal interfaces. Although both routes have been used effectively, higher levels of support are attained more readily with oronasal interfaces, which allow better control of the insufflated volume. With nasal IPPV, the ability to pressurize the airway requires minimization of volume loss. If air leaks out of the mouth, the airway depressurizes with a corresponding loss of ventilatory support.[59] Moreover, pressure-limited NPPV may be less effective in the presence of nasal congestion or structural abnormality of the nasopharynx because of increased flow resistance.

For patients with primarily respiratory impairment who have lower assisted ventilation requirements, nasal IPPV offers several advantages over NPPV via oronasal interfaces. Nasal IPPV may be more comfortable and better tolerated by patients with claustrophobia. Eating, drinking, and expectoration are possible with only brief interruptions of ventilatory support. Furthermore, if the patient vomits, there is an open path of egress. A tightly sealed pressurized face mask increases the risk of gastric aspiration. Fortunately, vomiting has not been reported and seems to occur rarely during NPPV. Fit and comfort are critical; accordingly, several types and sizes of nasal and full-face interfaces should be readily available when NPPV is initiated. Finally, specialized padding and skin protection may improve sealing effectiveness. Although simple mouthpieces and lipseals have been used as interfaces for full ventilatory support in both chronic and acute care settings in patients with primarily ventilatory impairment, their use in patients with primarily respiratory impairment remains anecdotal in the medical literature (see Case 19 in Chapter 15).

PRACTICAL APPLICATION OF NONINVASIVE VENTILATION

The success or failure of NPPV often depends on the specific manner in which it is implemented (Table 1). A simplified protocol for the application of NPPV, described by Meduri and colleagues, was applied to a large number of patients with either primarily ventilatory or primarily respiratory failure.[19] In their study, a conventional intensive care ventilator operating in the pressure-support mode was used in conjunction with a full-face interface. Patients were maintained in a semi-upright position. A skin patch (Duoderm, Bristol-Myers Squibb, Princeton, NJ) was applied over the bridge of the nose to prevent erosion, and tincture of benzoin was applied to the skin to obtain a better interface-facial seal. The interface was initially held manually to the patient's face, without attachments, to facilitate familiarization. After a brief accommodation period, the mask was secured

TABLE 1.   Keys to Successful Noninvasive Ventilation in Acute Respiratory Failure

Appropriate patient selection with:
  • Symptoms and signs of acute respiratory distress
  • $PaCO_2 > 45$ mmHg, pH < 7.35, or $PaO_2/FiO_2 < 200$

Early intervention

Experienced, dedicated respiratory therapists and nurses

Physician involvement

Sufficient pressure support

Patient comfort

with rubber straps. While the interface was held against the patient's face, the connected ventilator was set to a pressure support of 10 cmH$_2$O and a CPAP of 0 cmH$_2$O. Patrick et al. accustomed patients to NPPV by initially having them breathe through a cardboard mouthpiece attached to ventilator circuitry until they were comfortable with interface application.[21] After interface placement, Meduri et al. increased set CPAP to 5 cmH$_2$O. The inspiratory pressure (Pset, equivalent to IPAP) was titrated upward to obtain an exhaled tidal volume greater than 7 ml/kg, a respiratory rate less than 25 breaths/minute, and "patient comfort." This last goal often required more than 12 cmH$_2$O IPAP, and the pressure threshold separating discomfort from comfort was often quite sharply defined. Fractional inspired oxygen concentration (FiO$_2$) was adjusted to maintain SpO$_2$ greater than 90%. For patients with hypoxemic respiratory failure, CPAP was titrated in increments of 2–3 cmH$_2$O until the required FiO$_2$ was less than 0.6.[19] Patients were monitored for gastric distention, arrhythmia, and oxyhemoglobin desaturation. After an initial period of continuous support, patients were allowed "rest" periods of 15–30 minutes without NPPV. If interface leakage proved problematic, the patient was converted to synchronized intermittent mandatory ventilation. This protocol avoided endotracheal intubation in 65% of supported patients, including most etiologies of acute respiratory failure, and represented a simple, practical approach to the institution of NPPV for patients with respiratory impairment. The success rate for avoiding intubation has been duplicated in a number of centers (see below).

Indications for Noninvasive Positive-Pressure Ventilation

NPPV is appropriate for any patient with mild-to-moderate respiratory insufficiency who does not have a clear contraindication to its use. However, certain applications are of particular interest because they occur commonly in the acute care setting: exacerbated COPD, acute asthma, severe community-acquired pneumonia, pulmonary edema, and respiratory failure of any origin in patients for whom endotracheal intubation and mechanical ventilation are not a desirable alternative (e.g., patients who have expressed the wish not to be intubated), and patients experiencing respiratory difficulty after extubation. As the supporting evidence for effective acute application of NPPV is strongest in COPD, a common diagnosis, it is discussed below in greater detail.

Contraindications to Noninvasive Positive-Pressure Ventilation

There are few absolute contraindications to NPPV, the majority of which assume that endotracheal intubation is an immediate option (Table 2). The need for a secure airway contraindicates use of NPPV, as do severe facial trauma or burns and an ongoing need to clear airway secretions that cannot be cleared by noninvasive means. Altered mental status not due to carbon dioxide retention is a commonly cited contraindication, as are nausea and vomiting, which are of particular relevance with the use of oronasal or lipseal IPPV. Most studies have excluded patients with significant hypotension and/or recent gastric surgery (within 1 week). An uncooperative or combative patient is unlikely to benefit from NPPV. Light sedation or analgesia may aid in the control of such patients.

TABLE 2. Contraindications to Noninvasive Positive-pressure Ventilation

Uncooperative, intolerant, agitated patient
Inability to protect airway
Respiratory arrest, coma, or obtundation*
Hemodynamic instability
Need for controlled ventilation
Acute abdominal process
Facial trauma, burns, or surgery, or anatomic abnormalities interfering with mask fit

* Certain patients obtunded secondary to carbon dioxide retention may qualify as candidates for noninvasive IPPV (see Chapters 7–9).

The exclusion of patients with acute apnea, active cardiac ischemia, or ongoing arrhythmia seems reasonable.

Complications of Noninvasive Positive-Pressure Ventilation

Relatively few serious complications relate solely to the application of NPPV.[35] Facial skin necrosis due to mechanical trauma is relatively common, usually clears with an interface change or cessation of NPPV, and may be avoidable if the skin, particularly the bridge of the nose (with the commonly used interfaces), is protected by a synthetic covering. Clinically significant gastric insufflation is apparently unusual, perhaps because the resting tone of the normal esophageal sphincter (usually 25 cmH$_2$O) retains its seal against the pressures used in NPPV, which are generally less than 25 cmH$_2$O. Nonetheless, patients with known esophageal reflux may be at increased risk. Conjunctivitis resulting from interface leaks is easily treatable and potentially avoidable by changing interface styles. Sinus complaints have been noted, but they respond to topical decongestants, corticosteroids, and antibiotics. Drying and thickening of oral secretions and nasal congestion are an annoying consequence of protracted mouth-breathing with unhumidified gas. Inadequate humidification also can result in an increase in upper airway resistance to airflow (see Chapter 13). Inadvertent removal of the interface is a significant and even life-threatening hazard in patients who are oxygen- or PEEP-dependent, but this risk should be largely offset in closely monitored emergency and intensive care settings by direct observation and adequate monitoring. As already noted, aspiration from emesis while the patient is wearing a pressurized face mask is a feared complication with a low incidence in patients without underlying abdominal disorders. Barotrauma seldom occurs with NPPV, probably because relatively low (less than 25 cmH$_2$O) peak pressures are typically used in the intensive care unit and because overdistention activates native (Hering-Breuer) stretch reflexes.

USE OF NONINVASIVE POSITIVE-PRESSURE VENTILATION IN SPECIFIC SETTINGS

Exacerbated Chronic Obstructive Pulmonary Disease

As the subject of numerous case series, physiologic studies, and randomized, controlled trials, exacerbated COPD has been the most intensively studied indication for NPPV in acute care. Reported experiences have generally been positive. Every randomized study and the majority of those not randomized demonstrated reduced rates of intubation in patients receiving NPPV.[4,6,16]

Bott et al. conducted a randomized, controlled trial of volume-limited nasal IPPV added to conventional medical therapy vs. conventional medical therapy alone for 60 patients with COPD in acute respiratory failure.[6] Patients randomized to NPPV experienced less breathlessness, pH change, and PaCO$_2$ compared with the control group. Significant blood gas improvements were observed within 1 hour. Four of 30 patients randomized to NPPV did not actually use it. One of 26 patients treated with NPPV and three of the 30 patients randomized to NPPV died, whereas 9 of the 30 control patients died. The mortality difference statistically favored the NPPV-treated group (p < 0.05). When analyzed on an intention-to-treat basis, the data revealed a suggestive trend toward statistical significance (p = 0.1). Although there were no rigidly defined criteria for intubating control patients, the rate of intubation was not used as a primary outcome measure.

Kramer et al. included 23 patients with COPD in a larger randomized, controlled trial of pressure-limited nasal IPPV vs. conventional therapy in acute respiratory failure.[16] Inclusion criteria were broad; exclusion criteria were reasonable; and explicit intubation guidelines were followed. The NPPV group experienced a substantially lower incidence of intubation than controls with COPD (1/11 vs. 8/12). Although specific results for patients with COPD were not reported, the NPPV group experienced relative declines in heart rate, respiratory rate, and dyspnea score and relative increases in PaO_2 and maximal inspiratory pressure (a measure of respiratory muscle strength). Hospital mortality, length of hospital stay, and nursing and respiratory therapist time demands did not differ between NPPV and control patients. Complications specific to NPPV were mild.

Following up on an initial encouraging experience,[5] Brochard et al. carried out a randomized, controlled trial of pressure-limited NPPV via full-face interface in 85 patients with COPD and acute respiratory failure of moderate severity.[4] Because of tight entry criteria, less than 40% of patients with exacerbated COPD proved eligible for the study. Strict criteria for intubation also were set. Patients were treated with NPPV and medical therapy or with medical therapy alone. The NPPV group required intubation less frequently (26% vs. 74%), experienced fewer complications (particularly pneumonia and complicated intubation), and exhibited a lower mortality rate (9% vs. 29%). Most patients who failed NPPV required intubation within the first 12 hours of its application. Of particular interest, patients who failed NPPV and required endotracheal intubation and mechanical ventilation experienced a similar mortality rate as those intubated without prior NPPV. This equivalence suggests that no increase in mortality attended the delay in initiating intubation.

Angus reported that none of the 9 patients with COPD in acute respiratory failure who used nasal NPPV required intubation compared with 3 of 8 controls who did.[60] Likewise, Celikel avoided intubation in 14 of 15 NPPV users but in only 9 of 15 controls,[61] and for Plant the figures were 100 of 118 users and 86 of 118 controls.[62] In a prospective study with historical controls, Servera et al. reported significant improvements in gas exchange using NPPV.[63] Barbe, on the other hand, intubated 10 of 14 NPPV users and 0 of 10 controls.[64] Overall, in the seven randomized, controlled studies, the success rate for avoiding intubation was 83% using NPPV and 61% without it. Only the Barbe study and one other randomized study of 49 patients by Ambrosino et al., in which volume-limited ventilation was used,[65] failed to find significant benefits from the use of NPPV. In these studies, however, the patients had more normal arterial blood gases and blood pH than in the successful studies, suggesting that success is more likely to be appreciated in more severely affected groups. Ambrosino and his group subsequently reported successful use of NPPV with oronasal interfaces and pressure-limited ventilation to avoid intubation in patients with more severe exacerbations of COPD.[9] In a prospective, controlled study of 30 exacerbations of COPD, Bardi et al. reported significantly improved blood gases and reductions in in-hospital mortality, need for intubation, mean length of hospitalization and repeat hospitalizations, and mortality rate for up to 1 year.[66] Other randomized, prospective trials of NPPV that have included patients with COPD in acute respiratory failure also demonstrated significantly lower intubation rates.[67] Three studies also found that postacute respiratory failure, hospitalization, and survival rates were better for up to 1 year in patients treated by NPPV than in patients treated with conventional management.[7,8,66] In addition to the randomized, controlled trials, other published reports indicated successful experiences using NPPV to manage exacerbations of COPD.[1,3,10,20,26,68] The NPPV success rates (defined as avoidance of intubation) of these studies ranged from 50% to more than 90%,[69] and a meta-analysis of controlled studies supported the effectiveness of NPPV in treating acute exacerbations.[39]

Predictors of Success

Several recent studies have sought to identify the patient characteristics associated with success or failure of NPPV in the acute setting. Soo Hoo et al. prospectively evaluated 14 episodes of acute respiratory failure due to COPD in 12 patients treated with volume-limited nasal IPPV.[3] Nasal IPPV initiated after failure of conventional medical therapy permitted the avoidance of intubation in 50% of acute respiratory failure episodes. The authors suggested that patients with pneumonia, severe illness, failure to improve rapidly, ongoing mouth leaks, and secretion retention are less likely to benefit from nasal IPPV. The entry precondition of failed conventional medical therapy may help to explain the low success rate in this study. Ambrosino et al. retrospectively evaluated 59 episodes of acute respiratory failure due to COPD for predictors of NPPV success or failure.[2] The authors reported an overall success rate of 78%, but strict criteria for intubation were not stated. Pneumonia, impaired neurologic status, higher APACHE II scores, severity of initial blood gas abnormalities (pH and PCO_2), and failure to improve rapidly on NPPV seemed to be associated with greater risk of treatment failure. However, only initial pH (7.28 vs. 7.22) was found to have a statistically significant correlation with success or failure. Consensus groups have suggested the following as predictors of success for acute applications of NPPV[70]: younger age, lower acuity of illness, ability to cooperate and coordinate breathing with a ventilator, less air leaking, intact dentition, hypercarbia (but > 92 mmHg), acidemia (but pH > 7.100), and improvements in gas exchange and heart and respiratory rates within the first two hours.[71] In addition, pulmonary hyperinflation should not be exacerbated by excessively high levels of PEEP to avoid counteracting the beneficial effect of removing intrinsic PEEP by decreasing respiratory muscle length and force.[72] Thus, application of PEEP in patients with COPD requires close monitoring of the end-expiratory lung volume (e.g., by inspection of flow-volume loops).

Severe Asthma

NPPV presents a theoretically attractive option for asthma treatment because acute asthmatic exacerbations often reverse more rapidly than those of COPD. In contrast to the extensive experience with COPD, however, no randomized controlled trials and few other studies have evaluated the use of NPPV in acute severe exacerbations of asthma. Meduri et al. reported the use of pressure-limited NPPV to treat 17 asthmatic episodes refractory to medical management.[24] Only two patients required intubation: one at 30 minutes and one 4 days later in the treatment course. No complications occurred in either patients as a result of delaying intubation. NPPV corrected hypercarbia for 15 patients, but one subsequently worsened required intubation 4 days later. There were no complications of NPPV; sedative use was minimal (2/17); and the average durations of mechanical support and hospital stay were shorter than for patients undergoing endotracheal intubation and mechanical ventilation (16 vs. 208 hours and 5 vs. 12 days, respectively). NPPV was reported to improve rapidly both respiratory rate and pH. Patients with previous experience with endotracheal intubation and mechanical ventilation described NPPV as more comfortable. While the patients undergoing endotracheal intubation and mechanical ventilation may have been more ill (pH 7.07 vs. 7.25), this study suggests that NPPV can be a treatment option. Pollack et al. included six patients in status asthmaticus in a larger series of patients treated with pressure-limited NPPV.[17] Overall, the NPPV users had an 86% success rate, and treatment results were reported as similar in all disease categories. Patrick et al. described the successful use of PAV by two patients with status asthmaticus.[21] Although the reported clinical experience is small and a randomized, controlled trial for patients with asthma is lacking, these results suggest that NPPV may be a reasonable alternative to endotracheal intubation and mechanical ventilation for selected asthmatic patients who are both alert and treated early in their course. It must be remembered, however, that endotracheal intubation and mechanical ventilation are relatively safe, effective, and time-tested for treating asthma when care is taken to avoid excessive alveolar pressures.[73]

Patients Who Are Not Candidates for Intubation

NPPV is of value in supporting the patient with respiratory failure of treatable cause who is not a candidate for intubation, either because of a prior directive or poor prognosis related to an underlying disease. In this setting, a patient with acute respiratory compromise may be supported with NPPV while efforts are undertaken to reverse the acute process or gather further information about patient preferences in relation to life closure. Benhamou et al. applied volume-limited NPPV to 30 elderly patients in whom endotracheal intubation and mechanical ventilation was either contraindicated or deferred.[14] All but one patient had congestive heart failure, COPD, or restrictive lung disease. Precipitants of acute respiratory failure were varied (70% infection, 13% congestive heart failure, 6% bronchospasm, 3% pulmonary embolism, 3% trauma, 3% unknown). All patients were in severe respiratory distress. Approximately half of the patients survived to be discharged home on levels of respiratory support that varied from no support to nocturnal NPPV. Although one-fourth of the patients did not tolerate the intervention, few complications related directly to NPPV. Benhamou et al. subsequently reported similar benefits in 243 elderly NPPV users, citing less discomfort, fewer complications, and better short-term results than with endotracheal intubation and mechanical ventilation.[74] Similar results have been reported by others.[25] It appears, therefore, that NPPV offers an effective approach when endotracheal intubation and mechanical ventilation are not an option. Understandably, concerns have been voiced that such results will lead to the inappropriate application of NPPV to otherwise terminally ill patients, thereby increasing the costs of medical care.

Pneumonia and Hypoxemic Respiratory Failure

The experience with NPPV is less well documented in the treatment of pneumonia than in the treatment of COPD, and supportive evidence for its use is less compelling.[75] The majority of data concerning NPPV and pneumonia must be culled from studies in which pneumonia, with or without antecedent lung disease, is included among a mix of other causes of acute respiratory failure. In one randomized, controlled trial of NPPV for 56 patients with community-acquired pneumonia and acute respiratory failure,[76] NPPV users had a significant reduction in respiratory rate, need for endotracheal intubation (21% vs. 50%, p = 0.03), and duration of ICU stay (1.8 ± 1.7 vs. 6.0 ± 1.8 days, p = 0.04). The two groups had a similar intensity of nursing care workload, time interval from study entry to intubation, duration of hospitalization, and hospital mortality. The NPPV users with COPD had a lower intensity of nursing care workload and improved 2-month survival (89% vs. 38%, p < 0.05). Thus, NPPV was associated with a significant reduction in the rate of intubation and duration of stay in the intensive care unit.

Wysocki et al. conducted a randomized, controlled trial of NPPV in the treatment of acute hypoxemic respiratory failure due to several non-COPD causes. Sixteen patients had pneumonia as a primary cause of respiratory distress.[13] None of the seven patients with pneumonia who were randomized to receive NPPV eluded intubation. However, only 36% of these patients were hypercapnic. Intubation in the NPPV group as a whole was delayed 17 hours from study entry (no different from controls), and overall mortality was no different between the groups. The authors detailed the potential reasons for the lack of success with NPPV, suggesting that secretions, high ventilatory requirements, reduced lung compliance, and focal consolidation can render NPPV ineffective.

By contrast, the previously discussed case series of Benhamou et al.[14] suggested some utility for NPPV in the treatment of acute pneumonia. Of the 10 patients in that series who had acute respiratory failure due to pneumonia, six avoided intubation. Meduri and colleagues reported a series that included the use of NPPV in three subsets of patients with pneumonia.[19] Fifty-nine percent of the 27 patients avoided endotracheal intubation. Seventy-one percent of NPPV-treated patients with severe community-acquired pneumonia and 82% of NPPV-treated patients with AIDS and opportunistic pneumonia did not require endotracheal intubation.[77] Pollack et al. included 10 patients with pneumonia in their series of patients with acute respiratory failure.[17] Although important specifics about subgroup analysis were not detailed, the great majority of acute respiratory failure episodes were successfully treated with NPPV in the emergency department, and no differences in likelihood of response were identified between the groups.

Given the fact that PEEP, elevating mean airway pressure, and relieving ventilatory workload improve oxygenation, there is a clear rationale for using NPPV in this setting. However, considering the greatly varied nature of pneumonia and of the population of patients it affects, the limitations of NPPV for patients with lung disease, the potentially focal nature of the pneumonic process, the important role of secretions in acute respiratory failure due to pneumonia, and the general lack of consistency among investigators in selecting patients for and applying this methodology, perhaps it is not surprising that observed results are contradictory. Lack of consistency among investigators is obviously crucial to interpreting such work. NPPV will appear uniformly successful in avoiding intubation if none of the selected patients actually requires such support.

In the treatment of adult respiratory distress syndrome, Rocker et al. retrospectively reported that intubation was avoided in 6 of 12 episodes among 10 patients with an average initial PaO_2/FiO_2 of 102 with the use of NPPV.[78] They concluded that NPPV was highly successful and should be considered for patients who are hemodynamically stable in the early phase of acute lung injury or adult respiratory distress syndrome. Beltrame retrospectively reported a 72% success rate for 46 trauma patients with respiratory insufficiency treated with NPPV.[79] Eliminating patients who had more than two organ system failures or who responded poorly to antineoplastic therapy, Conti et al. avoided intubation in 15 of 16 patients with acute respiratory failure complicating hematologic malignancies.[80] Antonelli et al. randomized 40 patients with acute respiratory failure after solid organ transplantation to NPPV or conventional management. The NPPV users required fewer intubations and had a lower mortality rate, about 20 vs. 50% for both, as well as fewer complications.[81] A randomized, controlled trial of 61 patients in acute respiratory failure for a variety of reasons, found a significantly reduced intubation rate (7.5 vs. 22.6 intubations per 100 days in the intensive care unit) when patients were treated with NPPV rather than conventional management.[67]

In another controlled trial of 64 hypoxemic patients in respiratory failure who were randomized to NPPV or intubation, only 31% of the NPPV users required endotracheal intubation; blood gas improvements were similar in both groups; and the NPPV users had less mortality and length of stay and significantly fewer episodes of sepsis, sinusitis, and pneumonia.[82] A prospective survey of 42 intensive care units revealed that 581 patients were treated with endotracheal intubation and mechanical ventilation and 108 others with NPPV. NPPV was used for 14% of patients with hypoxemic acute respiratory failure, in 27% with pulmonary edema, and in 50% of those with hypercapnic respiratory failure. Forty percent of the NPPV users were ultimately intubated. However, the incidence of nosocomial pneumonia and mortality was lower for the NPPV users.[83]

Pulmonary Edema

Patients with acute pulmonary edema often benefit from CPAP and ventilatory assistance for several reasons: reduced work of breathing, reduced oxygen consumption, improved mixed venous oxygen content, (possibly) decreased sympathetic tone, and increased alveolar recruitment with improved oxygenation. Like exacerbated asthma, episodes of acute pulmonary edema are often brief. However, despite its potential advantages, NPPV has not been systematically evaluated. There is a relative lack of randomized, controlled trials focused specifically on this problem. This lack contrasts with the well-documented efficacy of mask CPAP for pulmonary edema, including a review of four randomized, prospective trials and one large prospective series that demonstrated significant improvements in vital signs and gas exchange and a significant reduction in endotracheal intubation rates with CPAP.[71] Moreover, whereas most reports compare NPPV that usually includes high PEEP levels with no mechanical support, comparison of NPPV with CPAP by mask provides a more appropriate control.

Mehta et al. recently reported the results of a randomized, controlled trial of NPPV vs. CPAP in 27 patients suffering from cardiogenic pulmonary edema.[23] The NPPV group had a lower mean $PaCO_2$ at 30 minutes (36 vs. 47 mmHg) as well as a lower mean arterial pressure (92 vs. 107 mmHg). One patient in each group required intubation. Despite improved ventilation, the NPPV group experienced a larger mean rise in peak creatine phosphokinase (400 vs. 135; p = 0.023) and a higher incidence of myocardial infarction (10 vs. 4 infarctions in the CPAP group; p = 0.02). The authors speculated that the lower arterial pressure in the NPPV group may have contributed to these disturbing results.

Some of the reported experience of NPPV in congestive heart failure is more encouraging. Sacchetti et al. reported a retrospective case series of NPPV in 22 patients presenting to the emergency department with acute congestive heart failure.[12] The duration of therapy was short, and no technical difficulties were encountered. Nine percent of patients required endotracheal intubation, and the mortality rate was 14%. The case series of Pollack et al. included 19 patients with either congestive heart failure[16] or congestive heart failure and COPD.[3,17] Only 7 of 50 patients in the total study population required endotracheal intubation, suggesting a success rate of at least 63% in patients with isolated congestive heart failure or congestive heart failure and COPD. Numerous other studies have included small numbers of patients with pulmonary edema. Success rates in avoiding intubation ranged from 50% to 100%.[15,33] Thus, considerable evidence suggests the usefulness of NPPV in pulmonary edema. However, given the anecdotal nature of much of this evidence and the disturbing report of Mehta,[23] large randomized, controlled trials of NPPV (vs. CPAP) are urgently needed. Despite the excellent physiologic rationale for its use in this setting, until more data are available, caution is warranted.

NONINVASIVE VENTILATION AS A BRIDGE TO SPONTANEOUS BREATHING

Delayed extubation failure, expressed as the need for reintubation, may occur in as many as 23% of patients judged ready for extubation/decannulation. These failures often occur because of upper airway obstruction, muscle fatigue, and congestive heart failure, conditions that are often aided by temporary use of positive airway pressure and ventilatory support. In 1992, Uwadia and colleagues reported that NPPV provided a useful bridge across an unstable postextubation period for patients otherwise too tenuous to wean from ventilatory support.[41] In 1993 Restrick et al. reported successful extubation or decannulation of 13 of 14 patients to NPPV, some of whom had failed extubation.[84] Gregoretti et al. reported extubating 22 trauma patients to NPPV before they met standard extubation criteria.[85] Nava and colleagues demonstrated that NPPV may be effectively used as a deliberate technique to shorten the duration of intubation in exacerbated COPD.[42] Patients failing a T-piece trial were extubated to NPPV after an initial stabilization and rest period of 2–3 days on full endotracheal intubation and mechanical ventilation. This strategy appeared to reduce complications and to shorten the duration of ventilation and intensive care (Fig. 2). Hilbert et al. found that patients with COPD and postextubation hypercapnic respiratory

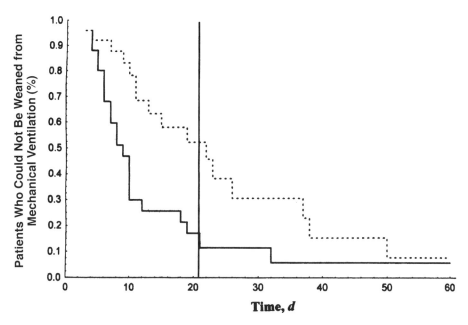

FIGURE 2. Kaplan-Meier plots of ventilator dependence for patients with exacerbated COPD treated conventionally *(dashed line)* and for patients deliberately extubated after 48 hours and ventilated noninvasively by facemask *(solid line)*. At 21 days, a time point often used to distinguish "weanable" from "unweanable" patients, many fewer patients receiving early extubation and noninvasive positive pressure ventilation required continued ventilatory support. (From Nava S, Ambrosino N, Clini E, et al: Noninvasive mechanical ventilation in the weaning of patients with respiratory failure due to chronic obstructive pulmonary disease. A randomized, controlled trial. Ann Intern Med 128:721–728, 1998, with permission.)

failure who used NPPV required reintubation less often (20 vs. 67%) than historically matched controls.[86] Kilger et al. reported improved pulmonary gas exchange and breathing pattern, decreased intrapulmonary shunt fraction, and reduced work of breathing in 15 non-COPD patients after early extubation with acute respiratory insufficiency with the use of 5 cmH$_2$O of CPAP or 15 cmH$_2$O of pressure-support ventilation. Only two patients required reintubation.[87] Girault et al. reported use of NPPV as a systematic extubation and weaning technique in acute-on-chronic respiratory failure in 33 patients who failed a 2-hour T-piece weaning trial. NPPV permitted earlier extubation and resulted in reduced duration of daily ventilatory support without increasing the risk of weaning failures. The authors concluded that NPPV should be used systematically for difficult-to-wean patients.[88] Kuhlen and Rossaint also reported that extubation can be performed very early in the course of acute respiratory failure by extubating patients to NPPV,[89] and others have concurred.[90] However, Jiang et al. randomized nonselected extubated patients to NPPV or conventional therapy and found lower reintubation rates with conventional therapy, suggesting that nondiscriminant use of NPPV for patients who will breathe spontaneously in any case is fruitless.[91] Thus, an aggressive noninvasive approach can be an effective strategy in managing patients extubated after acute respiratory failure, as it has been in patients with ventilatory failure (see Chapter 8).

Postoperative Noninvasive Ventilation

NPPV has been reported to be more effective than CPAP or chest physiotherapy in improving lung mechanics and oxygenation after coronary artery bypass surgery.[92] It was subsequently reported that both CPAP and PIP + PEEP reduce extravascular lung water after cardiac surgery.[93] Aguilo et al. randomized 19 patients to either NPPV or routine care after extubation for lung resection. Oxygenation was improved in the NPPV group without adverse effects.[94] Pennock et al. used nasal PIP + PEEP to avoid reintubation in 73% of 22 patients in respiratory distress more than 36 hours after various types of surgery.[22] Varon et al. reported that PIP + PEEP decreased the need for intubation of postoperative cancer patients.[95] Joris et al. found that PIP + PEEP reduced pulmonary dysfunction after gastroplasty compared with oxygen supplementation alone among morbidly obese patients.[96] Patients with obesity-hypoventilation, however, suffer primarily from ventilation impairment and would be expected to be excellent candidates for NPPV. Indeed, because their vital capacity is significantly diminished, we have had success in treating them with volume-limited mouthpiece and nasal IPPV as alternatives to endotracheal intubation or tracheotomy. Volume-cycle ventilation permits such patients to air-stack to expand their lungs and to improve alveolar ventilation.

CONCLUSION

Although NPPV is not suitable for the most critically ill subset of patients, it often can be effective for ventilatory support in the emergency[45] and intensive care setting. In general, these are conditions in which pulmonary compliance is not severely diminished, the patient is alert and cooperative, and the acute disease process reverses within a few days. When successful, NPPV avoids the need for intubation and its attendant complications. Early intervention and appropriate patient selection are the keys to its success. To date, the evidence supporting in-hospital use is clearly strongest for exacerbated COPD, for which randomized controlled trials have been conducted. The utility of NPPV for many acute patients who are not candidates for or refuse intubation is clear. The use of NPPV as a bridge to spontaneous breathing or as a "salvage" intervention for patients experiencing difficulty after extubation is an exciting concept with encouraging early data. In acute respiratory failure of other causes, however, the role of NPPV is less well established, either because of conflicting study results or because the published experience includes relatively few patients or provides uncontrolled, anecdotal evidence.

Although NPPV has been used successfully in pneumonia, results have been less compelling than in obstructive airways disease. This difference may be due to patient heterogeneity, the role of secretions, the often focal nature of the disease, and the frequent need for uninterrupted ventilation and oxygenation support. The type of support needed by a patient with acute lung injury or pneumonia also may differ from the type of support needed in diffuse obstructive lung disease. Maintenance of lung volume and intrapulmonary shunt reduction may be the most pressing needs in the former as opposed to reduction of patient work in the setting of hyperinflation. Whereas the role of CPAP is well established in the care of patients with cardiogenic pulmonary edema, the use of NPPV, although theoretically attractive and anecdotally effective, remains less secure.

The relative paucity of data supporting the use of NPPV in acute care settings other than exacerbated COPD, however, must be weighed against its low morbidity. Little evidence suggests that carefully monitored NPPV is a risky undertaking in carefully chosen patients. Furthermore, in a large majority of studies, patients destined to improve with NPPV responded rapidly to its institution, usually within the first 30–60 minutes. Delaying intubation to allow a trial of NPPV has not increased patient complications or mortality in patients who fail to respond. Most studies have excluded patients in need of "immediate intubation," implying inadequate time for a therapeutic trial of NPPV. Appropriate candidates for this intervention can avoid the problems and discomfort associated with endotracheal intubation until they improve or deteriorate on NPPV and eventually require endotracheal intubation. Given the potential benefits of NPPV and the apparently low risks associated with its use, an individualized therapeutic trial may be more appropriate than rigid guidelines for patient selection and management. The important decision, then, may be choosing which patients can tolerate the failure of a trial of NPPV rather than which patients are likely to tolerate NPPV and improve with the therapy.

ACKNOWLEDGMENT

The work reported in this chapter was supported in part by grants from the National Institutes of Health (NIH SCOR 50152), the Health Partners Research Foundation, and the American Heart Association (SDG 9930184N).

REFERENCES

1. Diaz O, Iglesia R, Ferrer M, et al: Effects of noninvasive ventilation on pulmonary gas exchange and hemodynamics during acute hypercapnic exacerbations of chronic obstructive pulmonary disease. Am J Respir Crit Care Med 156:1840–1845, 1997.
2. Ambrosino N, Foglio K, Rubini F, et al: Non-invasive mechanical ventilation in acute respiratory failure due to chronic obstructive pulmonary disease: Correlates for success. Thorax 50:755–757, 1995.
3. Soo Hoo G, Santiago S, Williams AJ: Nasal mechanical ventilation for hypercapnic respiratory failure in chronic obstructive pulmonary disease: Determinants of success and failure. Crit Care Med 22:1253–1261, 1994.
4. Brochard L, Mancebo J, Wysocki M, et al: Noninvasive ventilation for acute exacerbations of chronic obstructive pulmonary disease. N Engl J Med 333:817–822, 1995.
5. Brochard L, Isabey D, Piquet J, et al: Reversal of acute exacerbations of chronic obstructive lung disease by inspiratory assistance with a face mask. N Engl J Med 323:1523–1530,1990.
6. Bott J, Carroll MP, Conway JH, et al: Randomized controlled trial of nasal ventilation in acute ventilatory failure due to chronic obstructive airways disease. Lancet 341:1555–1557, 1993.
7. Confalonieri M, Parigi P, Scartabellati A, et al: Noninvasive mechanical ventilation improves the immediate and long-term outcome of COPD patients with acute respiratory failure. Eur Resp J 9:422–430, 1996.
8. Vitacca M, Clini E, Rubini F, et al: Non-invasive mechanical ventilation in severe chronic obstructive lung disease and acute respiratory failure: Short- and long-term prognosis. Intens Care Med 22:94–100, 1996.
9. Vitacca M, Rubini F, Foglio K, et al: Non-invasive modalities of positive pressure ventilation improve the outcome of acute exacerbations in COLD patients. Intens Care Med 19:450–455, 1993.
10. Fernandez R, Blanch LI, Vailes J, et al: Pressure support ventilation via face mask in acute respiratory failure in hypercapnic COPD patients. Intens Care Med 19:456–461, 1993.
11. Newberry DL, Noblett KE, Kolhouse L: Noninvasive bi-level positive pressure ventilation in severe acute pulmonary edema. Am J Emerg Med 13:479–482, 1995.
12. Sacchetti AD, Harris RH, Paston C, Hernandez Z: Bi-level positive airway pressure support system use in acute congestive heart failure: Preliminary case series. Acad Emerg Med 2:714–718, 1995.
13. Wysocki M, Tric L, Wolff MA, et al: Noninvasive pressure support ventilation in patients with acute respiratory failure. Chest 107:761–768, 1995.
14. Benhamou D, Girault C, Faure C, et al: Nasal mask ventilation in acute respiratory failure: Experience in elderly patients. Chest 102:912–917, 1992.
15. Lapinsky SE, Mount DB, Mackey D, Grossman RF: Management of acute respiratory failure due to pulmonary edema with nasal positive pressure support. Chest 105:229–231, 1994.
16. Kramer N, Meyer TJ, Meharg J, et al: Randomized, prospective trial of noninvasive positive pressure ventilation in acute respiratory failure. Am J Respir Crit Care Med 151:1799–1806, 1995.
17. Pollack CV, Torres MT, Alexander L: Feasibility study of the use of bi-level positive airway pressure for respiratory support in the emergency department. Ann Emerg Med 27:189–192, 1996.
18. Meduri GU, Conoscenti CC, Menashe P, Nair S: Noninvasive face mask ventilation in patients with acute respiratory failure. Chest 95:865–870, 1989.
19. Meduri GU, Turner RE, Abou-Shala N, et al: Noninvasive positive pressure ventilation via face mask-first line intervention in patients with acute hypercapnic and hypoxemic respiratory failure. Chest 109:179–193, 1996.
20. Meduri GU, Abou-Shala N, Fox RC, et al: Noninvasive face mask mechanical ventilation in patients with acute hypercapnic respiratory failure. Chest 100:445–454, 1991.
21. Patrick W, Webster K, Ludwig L, et al: Noninvasive positive-pressure ventilation in acute respiratory distress without prior chronic respiratory failure. Am J Respir Crit Care Med 153:1005–1011, 1996.
22. Pennock BE, Kaplan PD, Carlin BW, et al: Pressure support ventilation with a simplified ventilatory support system administered with a nasal mask in patients with respiratory failure. Chest 100:1371–1376, 1991.
23. Mehta S, Jay GD, Woolard RH, et al: Randomized, prospective trial of bi-level versus continuous positive airway pressure in acute pulmonary edema. Crit Care Med 25:620–628, 1997.
24. Meduri GU, Cook TR, Turner RE, et al: Noninvasive positive pressure ventilation in status asthmaticus. Chest 110:767–774, 1996.

25. Meduri GU, Fox RC, Abou-Shala N, et al: Noninvasive mechanical ventilation via face mask in patients with acute respiratory failure who refused endotracheal intubation. Crit Care Med 22:1584–1590, 1994.
26. Girault C, Richard J-C, Chevron V, et al: Comparative physiologic effects of noninvasive assist-control and pressure support ventilation in acute hypercapnic respiratory failure. Chest 111:1639–1648, 1997.
27. Hill NS: Noninvasive ventilation: Does it work, for whom, and how? Am Rev Respir Dis 147:1050–1055, 1993.
28. Abou-Shala N, Meduri GU: Noninvasive mechanical ventilation in patients with acute respiratory failure. Crit Care Med 24:705–715, 1996.
29. Jasmer RM, Luce JM, Matthay MA: Noninvasive positive pressure ventilation for acute respiratory failure: Underutilized or overrated? Chest 111:1672–1678, 1997.
30. Lofaso F, Brochard L, Hang T, et al: Home versus intensive care pressure support devices: Experimental and clinical comparison. Am J Respir Crit Care Med 153:1591–1599, 1996.
31. Hill NS, Mehta S, Carlisle CC, McCool FD: Evaluation of the Puritan Bennett 335 portable pressure support ventilator: Comparison with the Respironics BiPAP S/T. Respir Care 41:885–894, 1996.
32. Rubenfeld GD: Study design in the evaluation of noninvasive positive pressure ventilation. Consensus Conference: Noninvasive positive pressure ventilation. Respir Care 42:443–449, 1997.
33. Hess D: Noninvasive positive pressure ventilation: Predictors of success and failure for adult acute care applications. Consensus Conference: Noninvasive positive pressure ventilation. Respir Care 42:424–431, 1997.
34. Kacmarek RM: Characteristics of pressure-targeted ventilators used for noninvasive positive pressure ventilation. Consensus Conference: Noninvasive positive pressure ventilation. Respir Care 42:380–388, 1997.
35. Hill NS: Complications of noninvasive positive pressure ventilation. Consensus Conference: Noninvasive positive pressure ventilation. Respir Care 42:432–442, 1997.
36. Brochard L: Noninvasive ventilation: Practical issues. Intens Care Med 19:431–432, 1993.
37. Chevrolet J-C, Jolliet P, Abajo B, et al: Nasal positive pressure ventilation in patients with acute respiratory failure: A difficult and time consuming procedure for nurses. Chest 100:775–782, 1991.
38. Nava S, Evangelisti I, Rampulla C, et al: Human and financial costs of noninvasive mechanical ventilation in patients affected by COPD and acute respiratory failure. Chest 111:1631–1638, 1997.
39. Keenan SP, Kernerman PD, Cook DJ, et al: Effect of noninvasive positive pressure ventilation on mortality in patients admitted with acute respiratory failure: A meta-analysis. Crit Care Med 25:1685–1692, 1997.
40. Appendini L, Patessio A, Zanaboni S, et al: Physiologic effects of positive end-expiratory pressure and mask pressure support during exacerbations of chronic obstructive pulmonary disease. Am J Respir Crit Care Med 149:1069–1076, 1994.
41. Udwadia ZF, Santis GK, Steven MH, Simonds AK: Nasal ventilation to facilitate weaning in patients with chronic respiratory insufficiency. Thorax 47:715–718, 1992.
42. Nava S, Ambrosino N, Clini E, et al: Noninvasive mechanical ventilation in the weaning of patients with respiratory failure due to chronic obstructive pulmonary disease. A randomized, controlled trial. Ann Intern Med 128:721–728, 1998.
43. Bersten AD, Holt AW, Vedig AE, et al: Treatment of severe cardiogenic pulmonary edema with continuous positive airway pressure delivered by face mask. N Eng J Med 325:1825–1830, 1991.
44. Crimi G, Conti G, Candiani A, et al: Clinical use of differential continuous positive airway pressure in the treatment of unilateral acute lung injury. Intens Care Med 13:416–418, 1987.
45. Hotchkiss JR, Marini JJ: Noninvasive ventilation: An emerging supportive technique for the emergency department. Ann Emerg Med 32:470–479, 1998.
46. Kaplan JD, Schuster DP: Physiologic consequences of tracheal intubation. Clin Chest Med 12:425–432, 1991.
47. Schwartz DE, Matthay MA, Cohen NH: Death and other complications of emergency airway management in critically ill adults. Anesthesiology 82:367–376, 1996.
48. Stauffer JL, Olson DE, Petty TL: Complications and consequences of endotracheal intubation and tracheotomy: A prospective study of 150 critically ill adult patients. Am J Med 70:65–76, 1981.
49. Gal TJ, Suratt PM: Resistance to breathing in healthy subjects following endotracheal intubation under topical anesthesia. Anesth Analg 59:270–274, 1980.
50. Gal TJ: Pulmonary mechanics in normal subjects following endotracheal intubation. Anesthesiology 52:27–35, 1980.
51. Stoelting RK: Circulatory changes during direct laryngoscopy and tracheal intubation: Influence of duration of laryngoscopy with or without prior lidocaine. Anesthesiology 47:381–384, 1977.
52. Akbar AN, Lopatka CW, Ebert TJ: Neurocirculatory responses to intubation with either an endotracheal tube or laryngeal mask airway in humans. J Clin Anesth 8:194–197, 1996.
53. Fagon J-Y, Chastre J, Domart Y, et al: Nosocomial pneumonia in patients receiving continuous mechanical ventilation. Am Rev Respir Dis 139:877–884, 1989.
54. Guerin C, Girard R, Chemorin C, et al: Facial mask noninvasive ventilation reduces the incidence of nosocomial pneumonia: A prospective epidemiological study from a single ICU. Intensive Care Med 23:1024–1032, 1997.
55. Nourdine K, Combes P, Carton MJ, et al: Does noninvasive ventilation reduce the ICU nosocomial infection risk? A prospective clinical survey. Intens Care Med 25:567–573, 1999.

56. Laghi F, D'Alfonso N, Tobin MJ: Pattern of recovery from diaphragmatic fatigue over 24 hours. J Appl Physiol 79:539–546, 1995.
57. Marini JJ, Ravenscraft SA: Mean airway pressure: physiologic determinants and clinical importance. Part 1: Physiologic determinants and measurements. Crit Care Med 20:1461–1472, 1992.
58. Marini JJ, Ravenscraft SA: Mean airway pressure: Physiologic determinants and clinical importance. Part 2: Clinical implications. Crit Care Med 20:1604–1016, 1992.
59. Carrey Z, Gottfried SB, Levy RD: Ventilatory muscle support in respiratory failure with nasal positive pressure ventilation. Chest 97:150–158, 1990.
60. Angus RM, Ahmed AA, Fenwick LJ, Peacock AJ: Comparison of the acute effects on gas exchange of nasal ventilation and doxapram in exacerbations of chronic obstructive pulmonary disease. Thorax 51:1048–1050, 1996.
61. Celikel T, Sungur M, Ceyhan B, Karakurt S: Comparison of noninvasive positive pressure ventilation with standard medical therapy in hypercapnic acute respiratory failure. Chest 114:1636–1642, 1998.
62. Plant PK, Owen JL, Elliott MW: Early use of noninvasive ventilation for acute exacerbations of chronic obstructive pulmonary disease on general respiratory wards: A multicenter randomized controlled trial. Lancet 355:1931–3195, 2000.
63. Servera E, Perez M, Marin J, et al: Noninvasive nasal mask ventilation beyond the ICU for an exacerbation of chronic respiratory insufficiency. Chest 108:1572–1576, 1995.
64. Barbe F, Togores B, Rubi M, et al: Noninvasive ventilatory support does not facilitate recovery from acute respiratory failure in chronic obstructive pulmonary disease. Eur Respir J 9:1240–1245, 1996.
65. Foglio C, Vitacca M, Quadri A, et al: Acute exacerbations in severe COPD patients: Treatment using positive pressure ventilation by nasal mask. Chest 101:1533–1538, 1992.
66. Bardi G, Pierotello R, Desideri M, et al: Nasal ventilation in COPD exacerbations: Early and late results of a prospective, controlled study. Eur Respir J 15:98–104, 2000.
67. Martin TJ, Hovis JD, Constantino JP, et al: A randomized prospective evaluation of noninvasive ventilation for acute respiratory failure. Am J Respir Crit Care Med 161:807–813, 2000.
68. Guell AA, Gomez J, Serrano J, et al: Predicting the result of noninvasive ventilation in severe acute exacerbations of patients with chronic airflow limitation. Chest 117:828–833, 2000.
69. Ambrosino N: Noninvasive mechanical ventilation in acute respiratory failure. Eur Respir J 9:795–807, 1996.
70. American Respiratory Care Foundation: Consensus Conference: Non-invasive positive pressure ventilation. Respir Care 42:364–369, 1997.
71. Mehta S, Hill NS: Noninvasive ventilation. Am J Respir Crit Care Med 163:540–577, 2001.
72. Rossi A, Brandolese R, Milic-Emili J, Gottfried SB: The role of PEEP in patients with chronic obstructive pulmonary disease during assisted ventilation. Eur Respir J 3:818–822, 1990.
73. Darioli R, Perret C: Mechanical controlled hypoventilation in status asthmaticus. Am Rev Resp Dis 129:385–387, 1984.
74. Benhamou D, Muir JF, Melen B: Mechanical ventilation in elderly patients. Monaldi Arch Chest Dis 53:547–551, 1998.
75. Karg O, Bullemer F, Heindl S: Limitations of noninvasive mask ventilation in acute hypoxemic gas exchange disorders. Pneumologie 53:S95–S97, 1999.
76. Confalonieri M, Potena A, Carbone G, et al: Acute respiratory failure in patients with severe community-acquired pneumonia: a prospective randomized evaluation of noninvasive ventilation. Am J Respir Crit Care Med 160:1585–1591, 1999.
77. Girou E, Schortgen F, Delclaux C, et al: Association of noninvasive ventilation with nosocomial infections and survival in critically ill patients. JAMA 284:2361–2367, 2000.
78. Rocker GM, Mackensie M-G, Williams B, Logan PM: Noninvasive positive pressure ventilation: successful outcome in patients with acute lung injury/ARDS. Chest 115:173–177, 1999.
79. Beltrame F, Lucangelo U, Gregori D, Gregoretti C: Noninvasive positive presure ventilation in trauma patients with acute respiratory failure. Monaldi Arch Chest Dis 54:109–114, 1999.
80. Conti G, Marino P, Cogliati A, et al: Noninvasive ventilation for the treatment of acute respiratory failure in patients with hematologic malignancies: A pilot study. Intens Care Med 24:1283–1288, 1998.
81. Antonelli M, Conti C, Bufi M, et al: Noninvasive ventialtion for treatment of acute respiratory failure in patients undergoing solid organ transplantation JAMA 283:235–241, 2000.
82. Antonelli M, Conti G, Rocco M, et al: A comparison of noninvasive positive-pressure ventilation and conventional mechanical ventilation in patients with acute respiratory failure. N Engl J Med 339:429–435, 1998.
83. Carlucci A, Richard J-C, Wysocki M, et al: Noninvasive versus conventional mechanical ventilation: An epidemiologic survey. Am J Respir Crit Care Med 163:874–880, 2001.
84. Restrick LJ, Scott AD, Ward EM, et al: Nasal intermittent positive pressure ventilation in weaning intubated patients with chronic respiratory disease from assisted intermittent positive pressure ventilation. Respir Med 87:199–204, 1993.
85. Gregoretti C, Beltrame F, Lucangelo U, et al: Physiologic evaluation of noninvasive pressure support ventilation in trauma patients with acute respiratory failure. Intens Care Med 24:785–790, 1998.

86. Hilbert G, Gruson D, Portel L, et al: Noninvasive pressure support ventilation in COPD patients with post-extubation hypercapnic respiratory insufficiency. Eur Respir J 11:1349–1353, 1998.
87. Kilger E, Briegel J, Haller M, et al: Effects of noninvasive positive pressure ventilatory support in non-COPD patients with acute respiratory insufficiency after early extubation. Intens Care Med 25:1374–1380, 1999.
88. Girault C, Daudenthun I, Chevron V, et al: Noninvasive ventilation as a systematic extubation and weaning technique in acute-on-chronic respiratory failure. Am J Respir Crit Care Med 160:86–92, 1999.
89. Kuhlen R, Rossaint R: Noninvasive positive pressure ventilation for weaning from invasive mechanical ventilation. Intens Care Med 25:1355–1356, 1999.
90. Chiang AA, Lee KC: Use of noninvasive positive pressure ventilation via nasal mask in patients with respiratory distress after extubation. Chung Hua I Hsueh Tsa Chih 56:94–101, 1995.
91. Jiang JS, Kao SJ, Wang SN: Effect of early application of biphasic positive airway pressure on the outcome of extubation in ventilator weaning. Respirology 4:161–165, 1999.
92. Matte P, Jacquet L, Van Dyck M, Goenen M: Effects of conventional physiotherapy, continuous positive airway pressure and non-invasive ventilatory support with bilevel positive airway pressure after coronary artery bypass grafting. Acta Anaesthesiol Scand 44:75–81, 2000.
93. Gust R, Gottschalk A, Schmidt H, et al: Effects of continuous and bi-level positive airway pressure on extravascular lung water after extubation of the trachea in patients following coronary artery bypass grafting. Intens Care Med 22:1345–1350, 1996.
94. Aguilo R, Togores B, Pons S, et al: Noninvasive ventilatory support after lung resectional surgery. Chest 112:117–121, 1997.
95. Varon J, Walsh G, Fromm RE Jr: Feasibility of noninvasive mechanical ventilation in the treatment of acute respiratory failure in postoperative cancer patients. J Crit Care 13:55–57, 1998.
96. Joris JL, Sottiaux TM, Chiche JD, et al: Effect of bi-level positive airway pressure nasal ventilation on the postperative pulmonary restrictive syndrome in obese patients undergoing gastroplasty. Chest 111:665–670, 1997.

12 —— Home Noninvasive Ventilation in Patients with Lung Disease

NICHOLAS S. HILL, M.D.

Over the past decade, use of noninvasive ventilation in the home has proliferated rapidly. Most of the increase has been among patients with restrictive thoracic disorders or central hypoventilation, whose lungs are essentially normal. For such patients, the use of noninvasive ventilation to restore ventilatory mechanics or enhance central drive is widely accepted, as discussed in other chapters in this volume. Noninvasive ventilation also has increased in patients with parenchymal lung disease. Its use has generated more controversy among these patients than among patients with thoracic cage abnormalities, partly because the rationale is not so strong and the data are more conflicting. This chapter considers the types of parenchymal lung diseases for which noninvasive positive-pressure ventilation (NPPV) has been used, discusses the rationale and physiologic bases for use of NPPV, critically appraises the pertinent literature examining these applications, and assembles tentative guidelines for appropriate applications. In addition, suggestions are presented for future work in the area.

TYPES OF PARENCHYMAL LUNG DISEASES AMENABLE TO THERAPY WITH NPPV

As shown in Table 1, parenchymal lung diseases can be classified broadly into obstructive, restrictive, and combined defects. Pulmonary vascular disorders also may be classified under this rubric, but little rationale and no evidence suggests that they are amenable to therapy with noninvasive ventilation. The most common forms of obstructive lung disease in which NPPV may be used are emphysema and chronic bronchitis, which lead to severe airway obstruction in long-term cigarette smokers.[1]

Other forms of chronic airway obstruction that are amenable to therapy with NPPV include cystic fibrosis and diffuse bronchiectasis. Both affect younger people than smoking- or pollution-related chronic obstructive pulmonary disease (COPD) and may involve pediatric age groups. Both are considerably less common than emphysema, but cystic fibrosis is a relatively common autosomal recessive genetic disorder.

Restrictive lung diseases have rarely been treated with noninvasive ventilation. They must be distinguished from restrictive thoracic disorders, such as those due to neuromuscular weakness or chest-wall deformity, which respond well to noninvasive ventilation. Restrictive lung diseases result from decreased compliance of the lung parenchyma, as occurs with idiopathic pulmonary fibrosis. Fibrotic lung diseases often cause severe hypoxemia, but carbon dioxide retention is generally a manifestation of the terminal stage. Because chronic ventilatory failure is unusual in restrictive lung disease, noninvasive ventilation has little, if any, role in its treatment.

TABLE 1. Types of Parenchymal Lung Diseases Considered for Noninvasive Ventilation

Obstructive
Chronic obstructive pulmonary disease (COPD): emphysema and chronic bronchitis
Cystic fibrosis
Diffuse bronchiectasis
Restrictive
Pulmonary fibrosis
Combined
Obstructive with restrictive thoracic movement: sequelae of tuberculosis

Noninvasive ventilation has been used successfully in patients with combined restrictive and obstructive defects. Patients with sequelae of tuberculosis develop chronic hypoventilation and are amenable to therapy with noninvasive ventilation. Such patients often have parenchymal damage with bronchiectasis, cystic changes, scarring, and chest-wall restriction related to therapy. Patients were treated with thoracoplasties, recurrent pneumothoraces, and other therapies that reduce chest-wall compliance and predispose to the development of chronic respiratory failure.

POTENTIAL MECHANISMS OF ACTION OF NONINVASIVE VENTILATION

Respiratory Muscle Rest

The concept that NPPV may be beneficial for patients with severe COPD arose from physiologic studies of respiratory muscle function.[2] Such studies demonstrated that the hyperinflation in patients with emphysema places the respiratory muscles at a mechanical disadvantage. Flattening of the diaphragm shortens average sarcomere length and diminishes the capability to generate a maximal force. The greater radius of diaphragmatic curvature increases muscle tension, according to the law of LaPlace, as well as impedance to blood flow. The zone of apposition between the diaphragm and chest wall is reduced, limiting the bucket-handle action of the diaphragm on the ribs that augments chest-wall expansion during inspiration. The recruitment of accessory inspiratory muscles necessitated by the hyperinflation increases the oxygen cost of breathing, which, in combination with increased impedance to blood flow, predisposes to supply-demand imbalances.

Another factor that contributes to ventilatory muscle inefficiency in patients with severe COPD is the phenomenon of auto (or intrinsic) positive end-expiratory pressure (auto-PEEP).[3] This term refers to positive intrapulmonary pressure at end-expiration due to incomplete emptying of the lungs. Inspiratory muscles are forced to perform additional work to lower intrapulmonary pressure below atmospheric pressure to initiate the next inspiration. The above factors that contribute to respiratory muscle dysfunction in severe COPD are summarized in Figure 1.

These physiologic observations lead to the hypothesis that noninvasive ventilation would be of value in patients with severe COPD by unloading overtaxed respiratory muscles, providing rest, and alleviating chronic muscle fatigue (see Chapter 4).[4] Periods of intermittent rest would permit recovery of muscle function, increase muscle strength, and improve pulmonary function and gas exchange. These improvements would translate into less dyspnea, enhanced sense of well-being, and improved overall function. Such goals would be accomplished not only by providing ventilatory assistance during inspiration, but also by using extrinsic PEEP to counterbalance auto-PEEP, if present. Extrinsic PEEP reduces work by eliminating the need to lower intrapulmonary pressure to subatmospheric levels before the next inspiration. Patients with restrictive lung diseases are less likely to

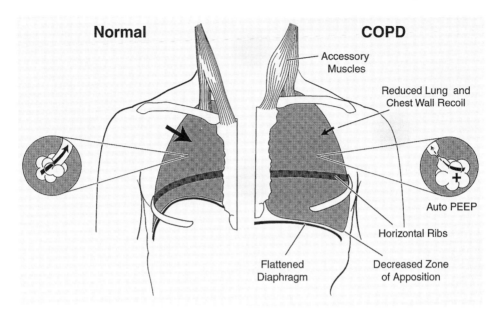

FIGURE 1. Mechanical dysfunction in patients with severe COPD. Hyperinflation leads to flattened diaphragm, decreased zone of apposition between the diaphragm and chest wall, and horizontal positioning of the ribs, all of which decrease muscular efficiency. The need to use accessory muscles adds to the energy cost of breathing. Flow limitation results from decreased elastic recoil and collapse of small airways during exhalation, which contribute to auto-PEEP.

benefit from noninvasive ventilatory assistance because the inspiratory muscles are not placed at a mechanical disadvantage, auto-PEEP is absent, and lung stiffness necessitates inflation pressures that are difficult to achieve with noninvasive ventilation.

Improved Nocturnal Gas Exchange and Sleep Quality

Patients with severe COPD have a high prevalence of sleep-disordered breathing. Obstructive sleep apnea is estimated to occur in 10–15% of patients with COPD—a substantially higher prevalence than the 3–4% estimated for the general population.[5] In addition, patients with COPD have frequent, sometimes profound episodes of oxyhemoglobin desaturation unassociated with apneas, most apt to occur during rapid-eye-movement (REM) sleep. Such episodes are predicted by low PaO_2 in the awake state and are at least partly explained by hypoventilation because of reported increases in transcutaneous $PaCO_2$. Ventilation-perfusion mismatching is also thought to contribute to some of these episodes, not all of which are explainable by hypoventilation.[5] Nocturnal gas exchange disturbances are thought to contribute to arousals and sleep fragmentation in patients with COPD, who have poor sleep quality with less REM sleep and shorter total sleep times than the normal population.[6]

Such observations raise the question of whether nocturnal use of noninvasive ventilation may prevent episodes of sleep-disordered breathing and hypoventilation, thereby reducing associated arousals and improving the quality of sleep. By ameliorating nocturnal hypoventilation, noninvasive ventilation during sleep also may permit a downward resetting of the respiratory center sensitivity for carbon dioxide. As a consequence of the above effects, noninvasive ventilation would improve daytime gas exchange and sleep quality in patients with severe obstructive lung disease, translating into enhanced daytime function and quality of life.

Other Potential Mechanisms

The muscle-resting and improved sleep hypotheses are not mutually exclusive, and both may apply to greater or lesser degrees, depending on the patient. Other investigators have hypothesized that NPPV reverses micro-atelectasis, improving respiratory compliance and enhancing ventilatory efficiency by reducing work of breathing. This mechanism is more apt to apply in patients with restrictive lung disease, but substantiating evidence is scanty. Another potential benefit in patients with COPD is reduced hospitalization. Patients adapted to the use of noninvasive ventilation may feel more comfortable treating exacerbations at home by increasing hours of noninvasive ventilation use and alleviating dyspnea. This approach is similar to the practice at centers that manage respiratory infections in patients with neuromuscular disease without hospitalization.[7] Only patients with severe exacerbations would require hospitalization, hospital stays may be shortened, and management of COPD would thereby become more convenient for patients as well as less costly.

EVIDENCE OF EFFICACY

Negative-pressure Body Ventilation for Severe Stable COPD

During the 1980s, there was considerable interest in negative-pressure body ventilation (NPBV) of the tank or "wrap" type to provide intermittent respiratory muscle rest in patients with severe COPD (see Chapter 3).

Braun and Marino[4] were the first to demonstrate a favorable effect of long-term NPBV on patients with severe COPD. They provided 5 hours of daily wrap ventilation to 16 patients with COPD. After 5 months, vital capacity, maximal inspiratory and expiratory pressures, and daytime $PaCO_2$ were improved, whereas forced expiratory volume in one second (FEV_1) was unchanged. Although the study suggested that intermittent respiratory muscle rest may be beneficial, it was uncontrolled and could not exclude the possibility that other aspects of a rehabilitation program or even passage of time may have been responsible for the observed improvements. Nonetheless, it generated much interest and stimulated further studies (Table 2). Another favorable long-term trial by Gutierrez et al.[8] used one 8-hour period of wrap ventilation weekly for 4 months and showed benefits similar to those observed by Braun and Marino. The other three favorable trials were controlled but of short duration, ranging from 3 to 7 days.[9–11] Like the study of Braun and Marino, they showed improvements in daytime $PaCO_2$ as well as maximal inspiratory

TABLE 2. Negative-pressure Ventilation for COPD

Author	Year	Hr/24 Hr	Duration	n	$PaCO_2$ (mmHg) Before	After	MIP (cmH$_2$O) Before	After
Favorable studies								
Braun	1984	5	5 mo	16	54	45	36	58
Cropp	1987*	3–6	3 days	8	50	42	67	77
Gutierrez	1988	8 hr/wk	4 mo	5	60	52	45	62
Scano	1990*	4	7 days	6	61	51	41	45
Ambrosino	1990*	6	5 days	10	56	51	34	42
Average					56	48	45	57
Unfavorable studies								
Zibrak	1988*	4	3 mo	9	47	50	30	30
Celli	1989*	5	13 days	9	45	42	51	48
Shapiro	1992*	5	3 mo	184	44	44	42	41
Average					45	45	41	40

$PaCO_2$ = partial pressure of carbon dioxide in arterial blood, MIP = maximal inspiratory pressure.
* Controlled trial.

pressure, but their short duration limits their applicability to the use of long-term ventilatory support in patients with COPD.

Studies that found no benefit from NPBV are also listed in Table 2. All of these were controlled and ranged in duration from 3 weeks to 6 months. Zibrak et al.[12] used a 3- to 6-month crossover design and found no improvement in daytime gas exchange, inspiratory muscle strength, or treadmill walking time compared with conventional therapy. They also found that patients with COPD tolerated the "wrap" ventilator poorly. Celli et al.[13] randomized 16 inpatients to receive pulmonary rehabilitation alone or rehabilitation plus wrap ventilation for 3 weeks. Both groups showed improvements in daytime gas exchange, but the improvements were equivalent and no benefits were attributable to use of the wrap ventilator. Shapiro et al.[14] performed the largest study, which consisted of 184 patients randomized to don wrap ventilators to receive either assisted or sham ventilation for 12 weeks. No improvements in 6-minute walking distance, dyspnea scores, quality of life, or daytime gas exchange were observed. Patients tolerated the ventilators poorly and used them for less time than recommended.

The favorable controlled studies listed in Table 2 suggest that NPBV benefits muscles, but the studies do not prove the presence of chronic respiratory muscle fatigue in patients with COPD. Indeed, the improvement in inspiratory muscle strength may be related to the reduction in $PaCO_2$ rather than to alleviation of fatigue per se. Some investigators have even questioned the existence of chronic respiratory muscle fatigue in patients with severe but clinically stable COPD, based on the finding that, in fact, indices of inspiratory muscle strength may be slightly greater in patients with COPD than in the normal population at equivalent lung volumes.[15] Although the conflicting results of the above studies cast doubt on the efficacy of NPBV in treating patients with severe stable COPD, it is notable that the average baseline $PaCO_2$ was 10 mmHg higher in the favorable studies (57 mmHg) than in the unfavorable studies (47 mmHg).

Noninvasive Positive-Pressure Ventilation in Severe Stable COPD

The poor tolerance of patients with severe COPD for receiving long-term NPBV led investigators to try NPPV. Favorable studies of its use for severe COPD are listed in Table 3. Elliott et al.[16] treated 8 patients with severe COPD with nocturnal nasal ventilation using a portable volume-limited ventilator for 6 months. Six of the patients had a reduction in daytime $PaCO_2$. Ventilatory responsiveness to carbon dioxide, total sleep time, and sleep efficiency also were improved. In the only controlled trial to show significant favorable effects of NPPV in patients with severe COPD, Meecham-Jones et al.[17] enrolled 18 patients (14 of whom completed the study) in a 3-month crossover trial. Patients received nasal ventilation

TABLE 3. Noninvasive Positive-pressure Ventilation for Stable COPD: Favorable Studies

Author	Year	n*	Hr/24 Hr	Duration	Vent	PaCO₂ Before	PaCO₂ After	
Elliot	1991	8	6–20	6 mo	Volume	58	51	
Meecham-Jones†	1995	18 (14)	7	3 mo	BiPAP S (18/2)	56	53	↑ TST
Sivasothy	1998	26	8	18 mo	Various	62	52	↑ QOL
Clini	1998	28 (21)	9	32 mo	PSV	54	47	↑ 6 MW
Jones	1998	11	6.5	3 yr	PSV	61	48	↓ HOSP
Average						58	50	

Vent = ventilation mode, BiPAP = BiPAP pressure support ventilator (Respironics, Inc., Murrysville, PA), S = spontaneous (inspiratory/expiratory pressures in cmH₂O), PSV = pressures support ventilation, TST = total sleep time, QOL = quality of life, 6 MW = 6-minute walk test, HOSP = hospitalization.
* Number in parentheses indicates number of patients completing the trial.
† Crossover study.

using the BiPAP (Respironics, Inc., Murrysville, PA) ventilator set in the spontaneous mode at inspiratory and expiratory pressures of 18 and 2 cmH_2O, respectively. Patients receiving NPPV had significant reductions in daytime $PaCO_2$ (56 vs. 53 mmHg), increased total sleep time, and improvements in quality-of-life scores. In addition, the frequent episodes of oxyhemoglobin desaturation and hypoventilation that occurred during control nights were ameliorated by NPPV. The authors concluded that NPPV improved sleep quality and nocturnal gas exchange and thus enhanced quality of life. In support of this conclusion, Krachman et al.[18] recently demonstrated that six hypercapnic patients with COPD had longer total sleep times (from 205 to 262 min, $p < 0.05$) and improved sleep efficiency (from 63 to 81%, $p < 0.05$) during periods of nocturnal NPPV use, although gas exchange was not improved.

Three other uncontrolled studies also provided favorable results. Jones et al.[19] used NPPV therapy in 11 patients with severe COPD who had symptomatic hypercapnia when treated with oxygen therapy alone. They observed a sustained improvement in gas exchange, good compliance with the therapy, and a reduction in the number of days of hospitalization per patient per year from 16 to 7 after initiation of NPPV ($p < 0.05$). In a retrospective study of 26 patients with COPD who developed worsening hypercapnia with oxygen supplementation, Sivasothy et al.[20] reported that nocturnal NPPV reduced daytime and nocturnal carbon dioxide tensions and improved daytime and nocturnal oxygenation, even in patients for whom oxygen supplementation was discontinued. NPPV use also was associated with enhanced quality of life and a substantially improved survival rate compared with historical controls. In a prospective trial that compared 28 patients who tolerated NPPV with 21 nonrandomized controls who were intolerant, Clini et al.[21] found similar survival rates. However, intensive care admissions were fewer (1 vs. 0.2/year, $p < 0.05$), and the distance walked in 6 minutes increased more (245 to 291 meters, $p < 0.05$) in the NPPV group compared with controls.

Studies using NPPV for severe COPD that found minimal or no benefit are listed in Table 4. Strumpf et al.[22] used the BiPAP in the timed mode at an inspiratory positive airway pressure (IPAP) of 15 cmH_2O and an expiratory positive airway pressure (EPAP) of 2 cmH_2O in a 3-month crossover trial involving 19 patients with severe COPD. Only seven patients completed the trial; most patients withdrew because of mask intolerance or various medical reasons. Nocturnal nasal ventilation failed to improve daytime gas exchange, indices of respiratory muscle strength, exercise endurance, or symptom scores, and duration of sleep tended to be decreased during NPPV. The only significant improvement was in indices of neuropsychological function; this improvement was not explainable in physiologic terms.

TABLE 4. Noninvasive Negative-pressure Ventilation for Severe Stable COPD: Unfavorable Studies

Author	Year	n*	Hr/24 Hr	Duration	BiPAP†	$PaCO_2$ (mmHg) Before	After	MIP (cmH_2O) Before	After
Strumpf	1992	19 (7)	6.7	3 mo	T (15/2)	45	50	3.8	3.2
Gay	1996	13 (4)	5.1	3 mo	S/T (10/2)	54	58	5.0	4.6
Lin	1996	12 (10)	4.3	2 wk	S (12/2)	51	50	4.3	3.5
Casanova	2000	52 (44)	6.2	1 yr	S (12/4)	53	51		
Average						51	52	4.4	3.8

$PaCO_2$ = partial pressure of carbon dioxide in arterial blood, MIP = maximal inspiratory pressure, BiPAP = BiPAP pressure support ventilator (Respironics, Inc., Murrysville, PA), T = timed mode, S = spontaneous mode, S/T = spontaenous/timed mode.
* Number in parentheses indicates number of patients completing the trial.
† Numbers in parentheses indicate inspiratory/expiratory pressures in cmH_2O.

In another randomized trial, Gay et al.[23] attempted to study only patients with hypercarbia ($PaCO_2 > 45$ mmHg). They screened 85 hypercarbic patients, but 72 were eliminated for various reasons, including psychiatric disturbances, complicating medical conditions, and refusal to participate. The remaining 13 patients were randomized to receive nasal bilevel positive airway pressure in the spontaneous/timed mode at IPAP of 10 cmH_2O and EPAP of 2 cmH_2O or sham ventilation. Of the seven patients randomized to NPPV, only four completed the 3-month study. No significant improvements were observed in the NPPV group; only one patient had a substantial drop in daytime $PaCO_2$ (from 50 to 42 mmHg). All sham-ventilated patients completed the trial.

A third controlled trial by Lin et al.[24] enrolled 12 patients with COPD and an average initial $PaCO_2$ of 51 mmHg. Ten patients completed an 8-week inpatient protocol consisting of four randomized 2-week periods. Controls fell into one of three categories: neither oxygen supplementation nor NPPV; either oxygen supplementation or NPPV alone; or both oxygen supplementation and NPPV. NPPV was provided using the BiPAP in the spontaneous/timed mode with an average IPAP of 12 cmH_2O and an average EPAP of 2 cmH_2O. As anticipated, use of oxygen significantly improved oxygenation, but no benefits were attributable to the use of NPPV. In fact, NPPV caused a significant decrease in total sleep time.

In a recent controlled trial, Casanova et al.[25] randomized 52 patients to receive nasal bilevel positive airway pressure or standard therapy. After 1 year of therapy, patients experienced no reduction in $PaCO_2$, mortality, or need for hospital admission, but there was a significant improvement in the Borg dyspnea score and one measure of neuropsychologic function. The authors concluded that NPPV was of marginal benefit.

These unfavorable studies have been criticized for a number of methodologic deficiencies. The high drop-out rate in the Strumpf study has been attributed to the lack of initial inpatient hospitalization, although initial hospitalization has not been proved to improve compliance rates. The Gay study used relatively low inspiratory pressures that may have been insufficient to achieve benefit. The Lin study used 2-week periods that may have been insufficient for successful patient adaptation. The Casanova study was larger than the others but still underpowered to assess survival and did not examine sleep- or health-related quality of life. Despite such shortcomings, these studies have raised doubts about the efficacy of NPPV for treatment of severe stable COPD, at least in patients without substantial carbon dioxide retention.

Two additional randomized long-term trials have been reported only in abstract form and have yielded mixed results.[26,27] Both trials selected patients with $PaCO_2$ exceeding 50 mmHg and randomized them to receive nocturnal nasal ventilation plus conventional therapy or conventional therapy alone. The multicenter European trial that began in 1992 randomized 122 patients with an average $PaCO_2$ of 56 mmHg. Until this point, only NPPV users over 65 years of age had shown a significant improvement in survival rate, although overall there was a 16% advantage in the 3-year survival rate in favor of NPPV (80% vs. 64%, p = 0.12).[26] The second trial was performed at multiple sites in Italy and has shown no significant survival advantage in patients using NPPV compared with conventionally treated controls. There was, however, a significant reduction in the number of hospital days per patient per year in the NPPV group. Furthermore, the Italian study had only 42 patients per group; a total of 18 patients (21%) dropped out during the first year. Once again, although the results have been disappointing, both studies were underpowered to demonstrate a significant difference in survival.

Noninvasive Ventilation for Cystic Fibrosis

No controlled studies of the use of noninvasive ventilation in patients with cystic fibrosis have been published, but the uncontrolled studies are encouraging. NPPV has been shown to effect acute physiologic improvements in patients with severe, stable cystic fibrosis, including increased tidal volumes, lower respiratory rates, better oxygenation, and reduced carbon dioxide tensions.[28] Hodson et al.[29] and Piper et al.[30] reported four patients with cystic

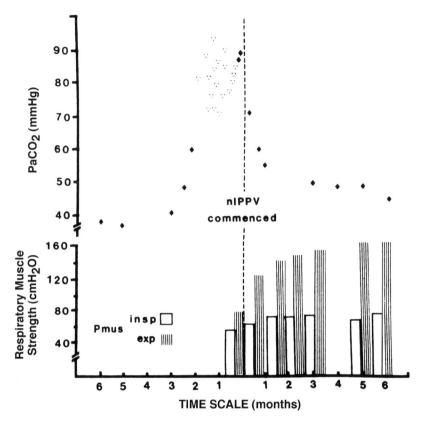

FIGURE 2. Response of patient with cystic fibrosis to nasal intermittent positive-pressure ventilation (IPPV). Top graph shows a prompt drop in $PaCO_2$ after commencement of IPPV, and bottom graph shows increases in maximal inspiratory (insp) and expiratory (exp) pressures (Pmus). (From Piper AJ, Parker S, Torzillo PJ, et al: Nocturnal nasal IPPV stabilizes patients with cystic fibrosis and hypercapnic respiratory failure. Chest 102:846–850, 1992, with permission.)

fibrosis and severe carbon dioxide retention who were stabilized by nasal ventilation (Fig. 2). In the series of seven patients awaiting lung transplantation reported by Padman et al.,[31] average $PaCO_2$ decreased from 68 to 51 mmHg during the first 72 hours of nearly continuous assisted ventilation. Dyspnea scores, accessory muscle use, and daytime $PaCO_2$ also decreased and remained improved for periods ranging from 3 weeks to 15 months of nocturnal nasal ventilation use. Five patients eventually underwent transplantation; two patients died while awaiting transplantation. The authors concluded that NPPV is an effective therapy for bridging patients to transplantation. Piper et al.[30] speculated that the mechanism for symptomatic improvement was related to resting of the respiratory muscles, improvement of sleep quality, and lowering of the "CO_2 stat" so that carbon dioxide retention was alleviated—possible mechanisms similar to those described for COPD.

Gozal recently compared NPPV plus oxygen supplementation with oxygen supplementation alone in six patients with cystic fibrosis.[32] Although improvements in oxygenation and sleep quality were similar in the two groups, patients treated with nasal bilevel positive airway pressure had less hypercapnia during sleep. However, when asked to state their preference for oxygen vs. NPPV after the study, four of the six patients chose oxygen supplementation alone.

These studies strongly support the idea that NPPV improves and stabilizes gas exchange in patients with cystic fibrosis and severe hypercapnia, but controlled studies are needed to compare the relative effectiveness of oxygen supplementation, continuous positive airway pressure (CPAP), and NPPV. As a consequence of these benefits, a major application in patients with cystic fibrosis currently is to maintain stability as they await availability of donor lungs for transplantation. In this sense, NPPV is seen as a bridge to transplantation.[33]

Noninvasive Ventilation for Diffuse Bronchiectasis

Reports of the use of NPPV for diffuse bronchiectasis consist of uncontrolled case series. Benhamou et al.[34] observed improvements in functional scores, mean daytime $PaCO_2$ (from 57 to 52 mmHg), and PaO_2 after initiation of nocturnal nasal volume-limited ventilation in 14 patients with severe airway obstruction caused by diffuse bronchiectasis. Average days of hospitalization decreased from 46 for the year before to 21 for the year after initiation. However, in comparison with historically matched controls treated with oxygen supplementation alone, patients treated with NPPV had similar declines in oxygenation and survival rates. These results indicate that NPPV is an effective therapy for improving gas exchange and symptoms in patients with diffuse bronchiectasis, but further controlled studies are needed to delineate effects on survival.

Noninvasive Ventilation for Restrictive Lung Disease

Few data are available about the use of NPPV in restrictive lung diseases in contrast to restrictive thoracic disorders. Leger et al.[35] reported that seven patients with sequelae of tuberculosis had favorable responses to nocturnal nasal ventilation. Although the severity of parenchymal involvement was not characterized, the patients generally had various combinations of chest-wall, pleural and parenchymal involvement that led to severe restriction (average vital capacity: 866 ml or 34% of predicted). After a year of NPPV, daytime $PaCO_2$ fell from 55 to 40 mmHg and symptoms of morning headache, somnolence, and daytime fatigue were improved.

The author has treated five patients with combined restrictive chest-wall and parenchymal disease. As shown in Table 5, these patients had severe restriction and carbon dioxide retention before initiating NPPV. Symptoms and carbon dioxide retention improved after nocturnal use of NPPV in all patients, at least initially. Two patients died after four years of successful use. One had pneumonia, whereas the other had worsening respiratory failure despite increases in insufflation pressures. In both patients daytime $PaCO_2$ increased preterminally, and both patients declined endotracheal intubation. In the author's experience, patients with combined chest-wall and parenchymal disease are more difficult to ventilate than patients with restrictive thoracic disease alone. Higher inspiratory pressures are usually necessary, and it is more difficult to decrease daytime $PaCO_2$.

TABLE 5.   Patients with Mixed Restrictive Thoracic Obstruction Lung Disease

Patient	Age (yr)*	Diagnosis	FVC (c)	FEV_1 (c)	TLC (c)	Pre ABG[†]	Post ABG[†]	Duration[‡]
1	56	Old TB	1.31 (45%)	0.66 (28%)	2.43 (52%)	7.34/70/54	7.43/57/57	3.4 yr
2	75	KS/COPD	0.98 (38%)	0.59 (30%)	2.18 (47%)	7.38/56/68	7.44/58/55	2.8 yr
3	67	Old TB	0.95 (29%)	0.85 (33%)	1.76 (32%)	7.35/63/52	7.36/55/64	8.5 yr
4	66[§]	Old TB	0.56 (21%)	0.37 (21%)	1.28 (29%)	7.35/71/55	7.36/71/61	4.0 yr
5	63[§]	Old TB	0.88 (33%)	0.56 (26%)	1.77 (37%)	7.36/80/54	7.40/77/60	4.0 yr

FVC = forced vital capacity, FEV_1 = forced expiratory volume in one second, TLC = total lung capacity, ABG = arterial blood gases, old TB = tuberculosis during the pre-chemotherapy era complicated by extensive parenchymal destruction, KS = kyphoscoliosis, COPD = chronic obstructive pulmonary disease.
* Current or at death.
[†] Values are pH/PCO_2 (mmHg)/PO_2 (mmHg). All were assesssed in the sitting position with the patient breathing spontaneously. All patients except number 3 were receiving oxygen supplementation.
[‡] Duration refers to length of time using nasal ventilator.
[§] Patient expired.

Long-term Studies of NPPV in Chronic Respiratory Failure

Large retrospective analyses have examined outcomes of patients treated with NPPV.[35,36] These studies included patients with all varieties of chronic respiratory failure. The major outcome variable was likelihood of continuing NPPV rather than survival per se, although this parameter was deemed a close approximation of survival.[35] Patients with COPD were less apt to continue NPPV than patients with neuromuscular disorders or chest-wall deformities, but the average duration of continuation for patients with COPD was still 3–5 years. In the Leger study, patients with diffuse bronchiectasis had less favorable responses, with average continuation rates of only 1 year. Other outcomes improved by NPPV for patients with COPD included daytime gas exchange (from 55 to 46 mmHg) and days of hospitalization (49 days for the year before initiation to 17 days for the following year).[35] Whether the reduction in days of hospitalization was related to a decrease in the incidence of exacerbations, enhanced ability to treat exacerbations at home, or some combination could not be determined. Future studies should examine utilization of health care resources in a prospective fashion because of the obvious implications for cost reduction.

Continuation curves for NPPV in patients with severe COPD were similar to survival curves obtained from an earlier study of patients with COPD who were treated with tracheostomy positive-pressure ventilation[37] (Fig. 3). In addition, continuation of NPPV among patients with COPD was comparable to survival curves for patients treated with continuous long-term oxygen therapy, as reported in a nocturnal oxygen therapy trial.[36] Thus, the use of long-term NPPV by patients with severe COPD did not appear to affect survival outcomes in any major way compared with tracheostomy ventilation or long-term oxygen therapy alone. However, the retrospective and uncontrolled nature of the NPPV continuation trials greatly weakens any conclusions that can be drawn.

NPPV to Enhance Training during Rehabilitation

Another application of NPPV for patients with parenchymal lung disease may be to augment exercise tolerance. This application is based on the notion that the training effect

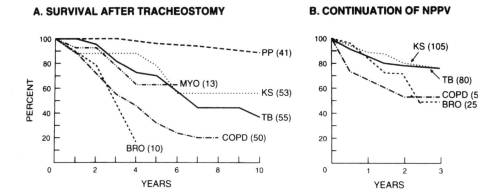

FIGURE 3. Graph on left shows survival curves for patients receiving tracheostomy ventilation at home in France. On the right the curves represent the likelihood of continuing noninvasive positive-pressure ventilation (NPPV). BRO = diffuse bronchiectasis; COPD = chronic obstructive pulmonary disease; DMD = Duchenne muscular dystrophy; MYO = myopathies, including muscular dystrophies; KS = kyphoscoliosis; PP = postpoliomyelitis; TB = old tuberculosis. (Graph on left from Robert D, Gerard M, Leger P, et al: La ventilation mechanique à domicile definitive par tracheostomie de l'insuffisant respiratoire chronique. Rev Fr Mal Resp 11:923–936, 1983, with permission. Graph on right from Leger P, Bedicam JM, Cornette A, et al: Nasal intermittent positive pressure: Long-term follow-up in patients with severe chronic respiratory insufficiency. Chest 105:100–105, 1994, with permission.)

of exercise is partly determined by the exercise intensity achieved during training sessions. Thus, the exercise limitation posed by a severe ventilatory defect may interfere with the effectiveness of training. Accordingly, if ventilation is assisted during training sessions, exercise intensity and duration may be increased and training effect enhanced.[38]

This hypothesis was tested in patients with COPD but also may apply to patients with other parenchymal processes. Merely applying CPAP by facemask has been shown to reduce inspiratory effort and dyspnea in hypercapnic patients with COPD who used a cycle ergometer,[39] presumably by counterbalancing the auto-PEEP that is increased in obstructive patients during exercise. Likewise, pressure support ventilation reduces the sensation of dyspnea and diaphragmatic pressure-time product and increases exercise tolerance in patients with severe stable COPD.[40,41]

Proportional assist ventilation (PAV), a new mode that responds instantaneously to alterations in inspiratory airflow demands, also has been reported to increase exercise tolerance in patients with severe stable COPD.[38] In a recent study, CPAP, pressure support ventilation, and PAV were administered via a nasal interface to 15 patients with stable severe COPD (mean baseline $PaCO_2$: 52 mmHg). All three modes were associated with increased exercise duration on a cycle ergometer and a significantly lower Borg dyspnea score.[42] PAV was reported to increase exercise duration more than the other modes. However, the authors pointed out that, because different methods were used to titrate the various modes, conclusions about relative effectiveness could not be drawn. In another recent study, use of an average of slightly over 2 hours of nasal ventilation per day was associated with an increase in the shuttle walk distance for patients with severe, stable COPD.[43]

These studies demonstrate that NPPV, used either during exercise or in conjunction with rehabilitation but not during exercise per se, can increase the intensity or prolong exercise for patients with severe COPD. Whether these gains can be reproduced for patients with other parenchymal lung disorders or translate into improved overall function remains to be seen. As ventilators become more compact, ventilatory assistance will be able to benefit patients with severe lung disease not only within the confines of a rehabilitation program, but also during everyday activities such as walking or shopping.[44]

SELECTION OF PATIENTS WITH PARENCHYMAL LUNG DISEASE FOR HOME NONINVASIVE VENTILATION

Evaluation

Patients with parenchymal lung disease who are candidates for NPPV should undergo a thorough evaluation to characterize the severity and nature of their symptoms and physiologic defects. Unlike many patients with neuromuscular disease whose exertional capacity is more limited by skeletal muscle weakness than by respiratory muscle weakness, patients with severe parenchymal lung disease complain foremost of exertional dyspnea. Scales such as the New York Heart Association classification for functional incapacity are helpful in grading severity of exertional dyspnea. Other symptoms that should be sought include those associated with nocturnal hypoventilation and sleep disturbance (see Chapter 7).

On the physical examination, evidence of airway obstruction should be sought. Airway obstruction may manifest during auscultation as expiratory wheezing or prolongation of the expiratory phase of breathing. Evidence of accessory muscle use or diminished diaphragm excursion may be seen along with hyperinflation. A blood screen is also indicated to identify possible factors that may contribute to fatigue or hypoventilation, such as electrolyte disturbances or hypothyroidism.

Pulmonary function studies are the most useful part of the evaluation to characterize parenchymal lung disease. Pulmonary function, lung volumes, and diffusion capacity are reduced in patients with parenchymal destruction, such as that due to emphysema or interstitial lung disease. Arterial blood gases can be essential for establishing the presence of hypoventilation. Noninvasive measures of pCO_2 determination, such as end-tidal or transcutaneous techniques, are not sufficiently precise for patients with impaired diffusion or when dead-space ratios change, as may occur in patients with severe COPD. Even trending data using end-tidal carbon dioxide measurements may be misleading.

The need for a routine sleep study in patients with severe parenchymal lung disease is debatable. Patients with features that suggest obstructive sleep apnea, such as snoring, obesity, systemic hypertension, and daytime hypersomnolence, should be referred for full polysomnography. Sleep studies in patients without these features may be useful as well, considering the prevalence of sleep-disordered breathing and nocturnal gas exchange disturbances in this population,[5] but the expense of routine polysomnography in all patients with COPD considered for NPPV is hard to justify. As a compromise, nocturnal oximetry may be performed initially, followed by more sophisticated monitoring if unexplained abnormalities are detected.

Optimization of Supportive Therapy

Before consideration of noninvasive ventilation, other aspects of therapy that may eliminate the need for ventilatory assistance should be optimized. A thorough preliminary evaluation is helpful in this regard, identifying the specific defects that may respond to therapy. For example, bronchodilators or a course of corticosteroids may be used to alleviate airway obstruction, with subsequent reversal of hypoventilation. Oxygen therapy is indicated in hypoxemic patients. Enrollment in a pulmonary rehabilitation program may enhance the level of functioning. Sleep evaluation may reveal obstructive sleep apneas that can be treated by CPAP or the addition of PEEP to NPPV. Only after all potentially reversible contributing factors have been adequately treated should initiation of NPPV be considered.

Obstructive Lung Diseases

The lack of controlled studies reporting favorable effects of NPPV in patients with COPD makes selection guidelines highly tentative. However, several relevant observations can be made from the available evidence. First, among NPBV studies showing benefit compared with studies showing no benefit, average initial $PaCO_2$ values were 10 mmHg higher (57 vs. 47 mmHg) (see Tables 2 and 3). Second, patients with little or no carbon dioxide retention, regardless of the severity of airway obstruction, appear to gain little or no benefit from NPPV. Further support for the idea that hypercarbic patients are most likely to benefit derives from the studies showing that hypercarbic patients with diffuse bronchiectasis and cystic fibrosis are stabilized by NPPV. Support also comes from a direct comparison of the two controlled trials of NPPV in patients with severe, stable COPD who used similar 3-month crossover designs. The Meecham-Jones study,[17] the only controlled trial of NPPV in severe stable COPD to obtain favorable results, enrolled patients with more carbon dioxide retention (56 vs. 47 mmHg) but less severe airway obstruction (821 vs. 543 ml FEV_1) than the essentially negative Strumpf study.[22] In addition, patients in the Meecham-Jones study had more severe and frequent episodes of oxyhemoglobin desaturation during sleep than those in the Stumpf study, presumably in relation to more nocturnal hypoventilation. Patients with frequent nocturnal gas exchange disturbances may benefit from NPPV not only because of the amelioration of nocturnal hypoventilation but also because of enhanced sleep quality related to a reduction in the frequency of arousals.

Based on these observations, guidelines for the selection of patients with COPD to receive NPPV have been proposed by consensus groups and include symptom and gas exchange criteria[45] (Table 6). According to these guidelines, patients should undergo a thorough evaluation, and reversible contributing factors should be optimally treated as described above. Patients who have persistent symptoms and gas exchange disturbances

TABLE 6. Guidelines for Selection of Patients with Obstructive Lung Disease to Receive NPPV

1. Evaluation
   - History and physical examination
   - Pulmonary function studies confirming obstructive defect
   - Sleep monitoring
2. Optimization of therapy
   - Reversal of airway obstruction
   - Initiation of supplemental oxygen (if indicated)
   - Consideration of continuous positive airway pressure (in patients with obstructive sleep apnea)
3. Selection factors
   - Motivated patient
   - Symptoms: dyspnea, fatigue, hypersomnolence
   - Gas exchange disturbance: daytime $PaCO_2$ > 55 mmHg *or* daytime $PaCO_2$ > 50 mmHg and nocturnal saturation < 88% on 2 L/min of oxygen

despite optimal therapy and are motivated to undergo a trial are candidates for NPPV. Considering that the average $PaCO_2$ among favorable studies is in the mid-fifties,[16–20] the consensus group suggested that if $PaCO_2$ is between 50 and 54 mmHg, NPPV can be tried if nocturnal oximetry reveals sustained desaturation (< 88%) despite oxygen supplementation. This guideline is consistent with severe hypoventilation at night or sleep-disordered breathing. Patients with $PaCO_2$ less than 50 mmHg should not be considered for a trial with NPPV unless they have symptoms that suggest hypoventilation/sleep-disordered breathing, in which case a sleep study is indicated. The consensus group also recommended that patients found to have predominantly obstructive sleep apneas should undergo a trial of CPAP before consideration of NPPV.

Based on these consensus guidelines, the Durable Medical Equipment Reimbursement Commission (DMERC) of the U.S. Health Care Financing Agency (HCFA), which sets reimbursement policy for Medicare, has promulgated its own guidelines.[46] They differ in that the qualifying baseline $PaCO_2$ is 52 mmHg and all patients must manifest sustained SpO_2 less than 88% for 5 or more minutes of sleep while using their usual oxygen supplementation (Table 7). In addition, all patients must undergo a prerequisite trial of bilevel positive pressure ventilation without a back-up rate (S mode) before a back-up rate (S/T mode) can be considered. These last two requirements serve to minimize use of long-term NPPV in patients with severe COPD. First, oximetry is difficult to obtain in the home. The vendors supplying NPPV equipment are not reimbursed for performing the qualifying oximetry study. Furthermore, constraining the patient to use an S-mode device halves the reimbursement compared with the S/T-mode device, making it difficult for home respiratory vendors to provide adequate follow-up for patients with COPD, who often have difficulty in adapting to NPPV and require frequent adjustments of the interface and ventilator.[33]

No selection guidelines for initiation of NPPV have been formulated for patients with cystic fibrosis or diffuse bronchiectasis. As reviewed earlier, the studies reported thus far have been uncontrolled but suggest that NPPV effects sustained improvements in gas

TABLE 7. Current Health Care Financing Agency Guidelines for NPPV in Severe Stable Chronic Obstructive Pulmonary Disease

1. Diagnosis of severe chronic obstructive pulmonary disease.
2. Daytime $PaCO_2$ > 52 mmHg while patient breathes usual FiO_2, *and*
3. Sleep oximetry showing oxygen saturation < 88% for > 5 consecutive minutes at usual FiO_2, *and*
4. Obstructive sleep apnea has been considered and excluded.

$PaCO_2$ = partial pressure of carbon dioxide in arterial blood, FiO_2 = fractional concentration of oxygen in inspired gas.

exchange and functional capacity in patients with chronic carbon dioxide retention.[29–32,34] Thus, guidelines similar to those for patients with COPD can be applied to patients with other forms of chronic hypercapnic lung disease.

Before completion of this discussion of indications for NPPV in patients with obstructive lung diseases, it must be acknowledged that no controlled studies have yet compared NPPV and CPAP directly. Considering that CPAP can reduce ventilatory work by counterbalancing auto-PEEP and enhance expiratory flows by maintaining airway patency during expiration (similar to pursed-lip breathing), CPAP alone may be effective in patients with severe obstructive lung diseases.[47] Pending trials that compare the modes directly, however, NPPV with PEEP is preferred to CPAP alone because of the greater capacity of NPPV to augment minute volume and the more numerous studies supporting its efficacy.

Restrictive Lung Diseases

Patients with restrictive thoracic diseases respond well to NPPV, and consensus groups have agreed on guidelines for patient selection.[45] On the other hand, no reports of the successful long-term use of NPPV have appeared for patients with restrictive lung diseases. Gas exchange impairment in patients with interstitial lung diseases usually affects oxygenation initially; hypoventilation occurs terminally. Thus, noninvasive ventilation would not be expected to play an important role, and no guidelines are available. NPPV conceivably may ameliorate dyspnea in such patients during acute exacerbations related to respiratory infections or during the terminal stages, but this possibility has not been tested.

In the author's experience, patients with a combination of obstructive and restrictive processes may respond favorably to NPPV. Such patients, particularly those with old tuberculosis, may have a combination of parenchymal scarring and cystic areas, and the scarred areas may contribute to parenchymal restriction. The predominant pathophysiologic defects are usually airway obstruction and restriction related to chest-wall deformity or pleural fibrosis. Although no consensus guidelines have been offered, current HCFA guidelines lump these patients with the COPD group. However, in the author's experience (see above), patients with a combination of obstructive and restrictive processes respond to NPPV more like patients with restrictive thoracic disease. They should be started on NPPV when they develop symptoms and daytime hypercapnia ($PaCO_2 > 45$ mmHg) or nocturnal oxyhemoglobin desaturation and should not have to wait until $PaCO_2$ rises above 52 mmHg.

INITIATION OF NONINVASIVE VENTILATION IN PATIENTS WITH PARENCHYMAL LUNG DISEASE

For many patients, NPPV can be initiated most conveniently in the outpatient setting and at home (see Chapter 7). The following discussion focuses on aspects relevant to patients with parenchymal lung diseases, particularly those with COPD. Most practitioners agree that successful implementation of NPPV is more difficult for these patients than for patients with restrictive thoracic diseases, whose symptoms are easier to alleviate with treatment.[33] This difficulty reinforces the necessity of good compliance. In addition, ventilatory assistance may be more effective when the ventilatory pump is dysfunctional but the lungs are normal (as is the case with restrictive thoracic disorders) than when the lung parenchyma is diseased. Regardless of the reason, successful initiation of NPPV in patients with lung disease requires careful patient selection and perseverance on the part of the practitioner.

Selection of an Interface

Some investigators argue that oronasal facemasks are preferred because patients with dyspneic COPD are mouth breathers. Others favor use of the nasal masks because patients with COPD who use nasal ventilation become accustomed to breathing nasally. In the absence of studies demonstrating the superiority of one interface type over another, practitioner preference and patient comfort are probably the most important selection factors.

Selection of a Ventilator

Although NPBVs were used in earlier studies and certain centers in Spain and Italy still use them for management of acute respiratory failure in patients with COPD, they often are poorly tolerated by patients with severe stable COPD.[12–14] Most practitioners agree that NPPV is the preferred modality. Recent studies have provided NPPV with portable positive-pressure bilevel ventilators set to deliver pressure-support or pressure-assist ventilation (i.e., ventilation is provided spontaneously or spontaneously with a back-up rate).[17,18,22,24,25] Studies in patients with acute exacerbations of COPD demonstrate that, although pressure- and volume-limited modes are equally efficacious, the pressure-support mode is more comfortable.[48] For this reason, despite the lack of studies in the chronic setting, pressure-limited ventilation is preferred for patients with COPD.

Ventilation Settings

During the use of the pressure-limited mode, the inspiratory pressure should be set at a tolerable level but high enough to provide ventilatory assistance. Initial inspiratory pressures of 8–12 cmH_2O are typical, with gradual increases to 12–18 cm H_2O over a period of weeks. The increases are made as tolerated and according to blood gas results. If volume-limited ventilation is used, typical tidal volumes range from 10 to 20 ml/kg, starting at the lower end and increasing gradually as tolerated. Expiratory pressure of 4–5 cmH_2O should be added, particularly for patients with COPD. This strategy is adopted in part to ensure that a continuous airflow is provided during expiration so that carbon dioxide rebreathing is avoided during use of bilevel ventilators and in part to counterbalance auto-PEEP in patients with severe COPD.

Many portable positive-pressure ventilators offer selection of a back-up rate. The need to use a back-up rate has not been established for patients with lung disease. The one controlled trial in patients with severe stable COPD that has shown favorable results used no back-up rate.[17] Indications for a back-up rate include frequent central apneas or sustained nocturnal hypoventilation despite use of a spontaneous mode. If a back-up rate is used, usually it be below the patient's spontaneous rate to permit patient triggering but rapid enough to provide adequate ventilatory assistance in the event of apnea (typically 12–16 per minute).

Oxygen Supplementation

Most patients who meet the proposed guidelines for use of NPPV in COPD also meet Medicare guidelines for oxygen supplementation. The ventilator is used only at night by most patients, whereas oxygen supplementation is provided continuously. For ventilators lacking an oxygen blender, oxygen is easily delivered by attaching an oxygen cannula directly to the mask or to the ventilator tubing via a T-connector. Oxygen flow rate usually must be slightly higher during the use of NPPV than during unassisted breathing, but it can be adjusted according to nocturnal oximetry results.

Adaptation and Monitoring

The first few weeks after initiation of NPPV are critical for successful adaptation, particularly for patients with COPD. Some practitioners use a brief initial hospitalization to optimize settings and promptly address adaptation problems. Others initiate NPPV on an outpatient basis but rely heavily on respiratory home care vendors to reinforce compliance. This approach requires home therapists who are experienced and skilled in the application of NPPV so that mask-fitting and ventilator settings are properly adjusted. For patients with COPD, small upward adjustments in expiratory pressure may enhance patient-ventilator synchrony if auto-PEEP is present. In addition, limiting the inspiratory time to a second or less may enhance ventilator synchrony with the onset of patient expiration in COPD.[49]

Patients also should visit the physician every few weeks initially. In addition to routine monitoring of symptoms and vital signs, the physician should obtain periodic blood gases. The patient should be asked about problems with adaptation to the ventilator, such as mask discomfort and oronasal dryness or congestion. Air leakage through the mouth is a common problem with nasal NPPV, particularly in edentulous patients. Chin straps or alternative interfaces may be helpful.

The physician also should ask about hours of use and consult with the home care vendor, who can check the ventilator usage timer. If the patient is not using the device for at least a few hours nightly within the first month or two, cessation of therapy should be considered. If the patient is using the device at least several hours nightly, monitoring during sleep should be considered to determine effects on nocturnal gas exchange and breathing pattern. Nocturnal oximetry should be considered, but home monitoring with multichannel recorders may be preferable because of the additional information about chest-wall motion and airflow. Full polysomnography probably can be reserved for patients in whom unexplained abnormalities are detected on home monitoring; such patients may benefit from mask or ventilator readjustment in a laboratory setting.

CONCLUSION

Noninvasive ventilation has been used to assist breathing in patients with severe parenchymal lung disease for many decades. Over the past decade, NPBVs have been largely supplanted by NPPV. Recently, increasing numbers of patients with parenchymal lung disease have been treated at home with NPPV despite controversy about its efficacy. Controlled studies have yielded conflicting results; only one study has reported favorable results in patients with COPD.

Based on available evidence, the use of NPPV for treatment of COPD should be reserved for patients with substantial daytime carbon dioxide retention ($PaCO_2 > 50$ mmHg or 52 mmHg [current Medicare guideline]) and corroborating evidence of nocturnal oximetry or blood gas monitoring. When use of NPPV is reserved for patients meeting these guidelines, the likelihood of benefit is increased, although many patients still are unable to tolerate or adapt successfully to the modality. These guidelines also may be used for patients with obstructive lung diseases other than COPD, such as cystic fibrosis or diffuse bronchiectasis, for whom NPPV has been advocated as a bridge to transplantation. Patients with combined restrictive and obstructive ventilatory defects also may benefit from NPPV, but it appears to have little or no role in patients with restrictive lung diseases such as pulmonary fibrosis.

The controversial and conflicting nature of the evidence supporting the use of NPPV by patients with parenchymal lung disease renders any recommendations or proposed guidelines highly tentative. Additional studies are needed, particularly in regard to the types of patients who are apt to benefit and selection guidelines. Future studies should examine not only effects on symptoms, gas exchange, sleep quality, and functional capacity but also utilization of health care resources, survival, and the NPPV techniques most likely to be successful. Controversy is apt to persist for many years to come.

REFERENCES

1. Feinlieb M, Rosenberg HM, Collins JG, et al: Trends in COPD morbidity and mortality in the United States. Am Rev Respir Dis 140:59–68, 1989.
2. Rochester DF, Braun NMT, Arora NS: Respiratory muscle strength in chronic obstructive pulmonary disease. Am Rev Respir Dis 119:151–154, 1979.
3. Ranieri VM, Grasso S, Fiore T, et al: Auto positive end-expiratory pressure and dynamic hyperinflation. Clin Chest Med 17:379–394, 1996.

4. Braun NM, Marino WD: Effect of daily intermittent rest of respiratory muscles in patients with severe chronic airflow limitation (CAL). Chest 85:59S–60S, 1984.
5. Fleetham J, West P, Mezon B, et al: Sleep, arousals and oxygen desaturation in chronic obstructive pulmonary disease. Am Rev Respir Dis 126:429–433, 1982.
6. Catterall JR, Douglas NJ, Calverley PMA, et al: Transient hypoxemia during sleep in chronic obstructive pulmonary disease is not a sleep apnea syndrome. Am Rev Respir Dis 128:24–29, 1983.
7. Bach JR: A historical perspective on the use of noninvasive ventilatory support alternatives. Am Rev Respir Dis 22:161–181, 1996.
8. Gutierrez M, Berolza T, Contreras G, et al: Weekly cuirass ventilation improves blood gases and inspiratory muscle strength in patients with chronic air-flow limitation and hypercarbia. Am Rev Respir Dis 138:617–623, 1988.
9. Cropp A, Dimarco AF: Effects of intermittent negative pressure ventilation on respiratory muscle function in patients with severe chronic obstructive pulmonary disease. Am Rev Respir Dis 135:1056–1061,1987.
10. Scano G, Gigiotti F, Duranti R, et al: Changes in ventilatory muscle function with negative pressure ventilation in patients with severe COPD. Chest 97:322–327, 1990.
11. Ambrosino N, Montagna T, Nava S, et al: Short term effect of intermittent negative pressure ventilation in COPD patients with respiratory failure. Eur Respir J 3:502–508, 1990.
12. Zibrak JD, Hill NS, Federman ED, et al: Evaluation of intermittent long-term negative pressure ventilation in patients with severe chronic obstructive pulmonary disease. Am Rev Respir Dis 138:1515–1518, 1988.
13. Celli B, Lee H, Criner G, et al: Controlled trial of external negative pressure ventilation in patients with severe airflow obstruction. Am Rev Respir Dis 140:1251–1256, 1989.
14. Shapiro SH, Ernst P, Gray-Donald K, et al: Effect of negative pressure ventilation in severe chronic obstructive pulmonary disease. Lancet 340:1425–1429, 1992.
15. Similowski T, Yan S, Gauthier AP, et al: Contractile properties of the human diaphragm during chronic hyperinflation. N Engl J Med 325:917–923, 1991.
16. Elliott MW, Mulvey DA, Moxham J, et al: Domiciliary nocturnal nasal intermittent positive pressure ventilation in COPD: Mechanisms underlying changes in arterial blood gas tensions. Eur Respir J 4:1044–1052, 1991.
17. Meecham-Jones DJ, Paul EA, Jones PW: Nasal pressure support ventilation plus oxygen compared with oxygen therapy along in hypercapnic COPD. Am J Respir Crit Care Med 152:538–544, 1995.
18. Krachman SL, Quaranta AJ, Berger TJ, Criner GJ: Effects of noninvasive positive pressure ventilation on gas exchange and sleep in COPD patients. Chest 112:623–628, 1997.
19. Jones SE, Packham S, Hebden M, Smith AP: Domiciliary nocturnal intermittent positive pressure ventilation patients with respiratory failure due to severe COPD: long term follow up and effect on survival. Thorax 53:495–498, 1998.
20. Sivasothy P, Smith IE, Shneerson JM: Mask intermittent positive pressure ventilation in chronic hypercapnic respiratory failure due to chronic obstructive pulmonary disease. Eur Respir J 11:34–40, 1998.
21. Clini E, Sturani C, Porta R, et al: Outcome of COPD patients performing nocturnal non-invasive mechanical ventilation. Respir Med 92:1215–1222, 1998.
22. Strumpf DA, Millman RP, Carlisle CC, et al: Nocturnal positive-pressure ventilation via nasal mask in patients with severe chronic obstructive pulmonary disease. Am Rev Respir Dis 144:1234–1239, 1991.
23. Gay P, Hubmayr RD, Stroetz RW: Efficacy of nocturnal nasal ventilation in stable, severe chronic obstructive pulmonary disease during a 3-month controlled trial. May Clin Proc 71:533–542, 1996.
24. Lin CC: Comparison between nocturnal nasal positive pressure ventilation combined with oxygen therapy and oxygen monotherapy in patients with severe COPD. Am J Respir Crit Care Med 154:353–358, 1996.
25. Casanova C, Celli BR, Tost L, et al: Long-term controlled trial of nocturnal positive pressure ventilation with severe COPD. Chest 118:1582–1590, 2000.
26. Muir JF, Cuvelier A, Tengang B, et al: Long-term home nasal intermittent positive pressure ventilation (NPPV) + oxygen therapy (LTOT) versus LTOT alone in severe hypercapnic COPD. Preliminary results of a European multicenter trial. Am J Resp Crit Care Med 155:A408, 1997.
27. Clini E, Sturani C: The Italian multicenter study of noninvasive nocturnal pressure support ventilation (NPSV) in COPD patients. Am J Resp Crit Care Med 259:A295, 1999.
28. Granton JT, Kesten S: The acute effects of nasal positive pressure ventilation in patients with advanced cystic fibrosis. Chest 113:1013–1108, 1998.
29. Hodson ME, Madden PB, Steven HM, et al: Non-invasive mechanical ventilation for cystic fibrosis patients: a potential bridge to transplantation. Eur Respir J 4:524–527, 1991.
30. Piper AJ, Parker S, Torzillo PJ, et al: Nocturnal nasal IPPV stabilizes patients with cystic fibrosis and hypercapnic respiratory failure. Chest 102:846–850, 1992.
31. Padman R, Nadkarni VM, Von Nessen S, Goodill J: Noninvasive positive pressure ventilation in end-stage cystic fibrosis: A report of seven cases. Respir Care 39:736–739, 1994.
32. Gozal D: Nocturnal ventilatory support in patients with cystic fibrosis: comparison with supplemental oxygen. Eur Respir J 10:1999–2003, 1997.
33. Criner GJ, Brennan K, Travaline JM, Kreimer D: Efficacy and compliance with noninvasive positive pressure ventilation in patients with chronic respiratory failure. Chest 116:667–675, 1999.

34. Benhamou D, Muir JF, Raspaud C, et al: Long-term efficiency of home nasal mask ventilation in patients with diffuse bronchiectasis and severe chronic respiratory failure A case-control study. Chest 112:1259–1266, 1997.

35. Leger P, Bedicam JM, Cornette A, et al: Nasal intermittent positive pressure: Long-term follow-up in patients with severe chronic respiratory insufficiency. Chest 105:100–105, 1994.

36. Simonds AK, Elliott MW: Outcome of domiciliary nasal intermittent positive pressure ventilation in restrictive and obstructive disorders. Thorax 50:604–609, 1994.

37. Robert D, Gerard M, Leger P, et al: La ventilation mechanique à domicile definitive par tracheostomie de l'insuffisant respiratoire chronique. Rev Fr Mal Resp 11:923–936, 1983.

38. Dolmage TE, Goldstein RS: Proportional assist ventilation and exercise tolerance in subjects with COPD. Chest 111:948–954, 1997.

39. Petrov BJ, Calderini E, Gottfried SB: Effect of CPAP on respiratory effort and dyspnea during exercise in severe COPD. J Appl Physiol 69:179–188, 1990.

40. Keilty SEF, Ponte J, Fleming TA, et al: Effect of inspiratory pressure support on exercise tolerance and breathlessness in patients with severe stable chronic obstructive pulmonary disease. Thorax 49:990–994, 1994.

41. Maltais F, Seissman H, Gottfried SB: Pressure support reduced inspiratory effort and dyspnea during exercise in chronic airflow obstruction. Am J Respir Crit Care Med 151:1027–1033, 1995.

42. Bianchi L, Foglio K, Pagani M, et al: Effects of proportional assist ventilation on exercise tolerance in COPD patients with chronic hypercapnia. Eur Respir J 11:422–427, 1998.

43. Garrod R, Mikelsons C, Paul EA, Wedjicha JA: Randomized controlled trial of domiciliary noninvasive positive pressure ventilation and physical training in severe chronic obstructive pulmonary disease. Am J Respir Crit Care Med 162:1335–1341, 2000.

44. Kirshblum SC, Bach JR: Walker modification for ventilator assisted individuals. Am J Phys Med Rehabil 71:304–306,1992.

45. Consensus Conference: Clinical indications for noninvasive positive pressure ventilation in chronic respiratory failure due to restrictive lung disease, COPD, and nocturnal hypoventilation: A Consensus Conference Report. Chest 116:521–534, 1999.

46. Region B: DMERC supplier manual medical policy. Respir Assist Dev (RAD) Rev 20:199–210, 1999.

47. Petrov BJ, Legere M, Goldberg P, et al: Continuous positive airway pressure reduced work of breathing and dyspnea during weaning from mechanical ventilation in severe chronic obstructive pulmonary disease. Am Rev Resp Dis 141:281–289, 1990.

48. Girault C, Richard J-C, Chevron V, et al: Comparative physiologic effects of noninvasive assist-control and pressure support ventilation in acute hypercapnic respiratory failure. Chest 111:1639–1648, 1997.

49. Calderini E, Confalonieri M, Puccio PG, et al: Patient-ventilator asynchrony during noninvasive ventilation: the role of expiratory trigger. Intens Care Med 25:662–667, 1999.

13 —— Chest Physical Therapy: Mucus-mobilizing Techniques

CEES P. VAN DER SCHANS, P.T., PH.D.
JOHN R. BACH, M.D.
BRUCE K. RUBIN, M.D.

The effective elimination of airway mucus and other debris is the most important factor that permits successful use of noninvasive ventilation for patients with either ventilatory or oxygenation impairment. As noted in Chapter 10, for young patients with primarily ventilatory impairment, 90% of episodes of respiratory failure are a result of inability to clear airway mucus effectively during intercurrent chest colds.[1] Although the use of respiratory muscle aids is the single most important intervention for eliminating airway secretions in patients with inspiratory and expiratory muscle weakness, these aids, like normal coughing, may not adequately expel secretions from the very small peripheral airways more than six divisions from the trachea; the flows they create may not be sufficient to eliminate liquid secretions that line the airways; and effective cough flows may not be generated in severely obstructed or collapsed airways. In these situations, as well as in patients with severe bulbar muscle dysfunction who aspirate upper airway secretions and cannot generate cough flows to eliminate them, it is important to consider other methods that gradually move mucus and airway debris.

NORMAL AIRWAY SECRETION TRANSPORT FROM THE LOWER RESPIRATORY TRACT

In adults, at least 10,000 liters of air per day expose airway membranes to toxic gases, dust, and microorganisms, some of which are deposited in the lower airways. Effective mechanisms are required to clear the airways and maintain lung sterility. One of the most important lung defense mechanisms is the production of airway mucus. Mucus continuously transports debris from the peripheral to the central airways and eventually to the oropharynx. Airway mucus is a heterogeneous fluid that consists of about 95% water and 5% electrolytes, amino acids, sugars, and macromolecules.[2–7]

Airway mucus is produced throughout the bronchial tree by serous cells, goblet or mucus cells, Clara cells, and type II alveolar cells.[3,5,6,8] It consists of a colloidal suspension of water, DNA, proteins, glycoproteins, proteoglycans, and lipids.[4,6] The amount of mucus produced at any level of the bronchial tree depends on the number of mucus-producing cells at that level and the number of these cells in relation to the total airway surface. Airway surface decreases from the peripheral to the central airways. Thus, more mucus is produced in the peripheral than in the central airways. The total amount of mucus that reaches the trachea is normally about 10–100 ml/day.[3,9] The parasympathetic nervous system increases mucus production.

Transport of material is governed by mechanical and inertial forces and friction. Rheology is the study of how energy is stored in materials and how materials deform as a result of applied forces. Usually, the most important frictional forces are determined by the rheologic properties of the fluid. Surface interfacial and adhesive forces between mucus and epithelium are important determinants of mucus transport in the airways.

One of the most important rheologic properties of mucus is viscosity (resistance to flow). Viscosity represents the capacity of a material to absorb energy while it moves. In an "ideal" or Newtonian fluid, viscosity is a constant; mucus, however, is not a Newtonian fluid. Viscosity depends on the shear rate, that is, the velocity at which the shear stress is applied. The shear modulus is a measure of the stress needed to induce alterations in the shape of the material. When the shear modulus is high, at comparable forces, less energy is stored in deformation. Consequently, mucus with a high shear modulus may be more easily transported.[10] Elasticity is the capacity to store the energy used to move or deform material. The ratio between viscosity and elasticity appears to be an important determinant of the transport rate. This ratio is called "tangent d" or the "loss tangent" and is related inversely to mucus recoil.

Bronchial secretions in the airways are in the periciliary sol layer or the overlying periciliary gel layer (Fig. 1). Although the rheology of the sol layer has not been studied, it has a low concentration of glycoproteins and presumably a low viscosity. It is, therefore, always liquid and has no elastic properties. The gel layer consists mainly of mucus. Its concentration of cross-linked glycoproteins is high, making it a non-Newtonian viscoelastic gel. Only the gel layer appears to be transported. The sol layer, however, is also essential for mucus transport[11] because it provides a low resistance medium for ciliary beating to move debris up the airway.

The transporting surface at any level in the bronchial tree is determined by the cross-sectional diameter of the airways as well as by the number of airways at any level of the bronchial tree. From the central to the peripheral airways, airway diameter decreases, but the number of airways increases exponentially.[12] The transporting surface is also somewhat reduced at bifurcations in the peripheral airways.[13] As a result, the transporting surface of the airways decreases from the peripheral to the central airways. Accumulation of mucus in the central airways is normally countered by the higher rate of mucus transport centrally than peripherally[14,15] and possibly by a greater reabsorption of watery constituents centrally.[16,17] In

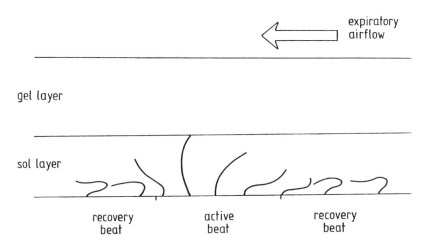

FIGURE 1. Respiratory secretions in the airways are separated into two layers: a sol layer and a gel layer. Respiratory cilia have an effective beat in the direction of the trachea (to the left) and a recovery beat in the direction of the bronchiole (to the right). (Modified from Sleigh MA: The nature and action of respiratory tract cilia. In Brain JD, Proctor DF, Reid LM (eds): Respiratory Defense Mechanisms. New York, Marcel Dekker, 1977, p 247.)

healthy people, mucus transport is decreased during sleep.[18] The reasons for this decrease are as yet unknown. However, it may be explained, at least in part, by diminished tidal volumes, which decrease airway pressure-dependent transport from the peripheral airways, particularly during non-rapid-eye-movement (non-REM) sleep.

The most important mechanism of mucus transport in the bronchial tree is mucociliary transport, which takes place by coordinated activity of cilia that cover the bronchial surface of the airways.[19] Ciliated cells are found in the airways from the trachea to terminal bronchioles. Each cell contains about 200 cilia,[20–22] all of which end in little claws.[23] The cilia beat in the direction of the oropharynx with a frequency of about 8–15 Hz. The claws of the cilia reach the mucus gel layer and push it toward the oropharynx (see Fig. 1). The recovery beat in the direction of the bronchioles takes place only in the periciliary sol layer.[24] The cilia normally move the mucus at 1 mm/min in smaller airways and at up to 2 cm/min in the trachea.[25]

Mucus transport by ciliary beating is influenced by the viscoelastic and surface properties of the mucus.[26] Theoretical models suggest that a decrease in the ratio of viscosity to elasticity can result in an increase in mucociliary transport.[27] According to a recent report, diffuse or focal areas of lung underventilation result in diffuse or focal impairment of mucociliary clearance.[28] Although the decrease in total airway surface and concentration density of ciliated cells in central airways results in less mucus transport by ciliary beat,[23] this deficit is compensated in part by a higher ciliary beat frequency in the central airways.[29]

Relative humidity is the amount of water vapor in a gas relative to the maximal amount that the gas can hold at a particular temperature. Normally the upper airway warms, humidifies, and filters inspired air. Two-thirds of this process is done by the nose; by the time the air reaches the nasopharynx, gas temperature is about 30°C and relative humidity is 95%. At the level of the main bronchi, air is fully saturated with water and at body temperature. Numerous studies have demonstrated that air conditioned to core body temperature and 100% relative humidity promotes optimal mucociliary transport velocity.[30] With decreasing humidity mucus thickens, mucociliary transport velocity slows and ultimately stops, cilia stop, and with severe dehydration cells are damaged and atelectasis occurs.[30] On the other hand, if inspired gas is warmer than 37°C and is 100% saturated, condensation occurs, causing reduced mucus viscosity and increased pericellular fluid depth. As a result, cilia may lose contact with the mucus, which may be too liquid to be properly engaged by the cilial tips, again decreasing mucociliary transport velocity. Excessive heat also may cause cell damage. Exposure time to suboptimal conditions is also a factor. Optimal humidity, by maximizing airway clearance, prevents the formation of pools of mucus, which are an ideal environment for pathogen replication. Other factors that hamper mucociliary function include infection, ciliary-inhibitory factors seen in certain disease states, and medications such as ipratropium.

MUCUS HYPERSECRETION AND IMPAIRMENT OF MUCUS ELIMINATION

Even for patients without airways disease, stasis of secretions in the airways because of a dysfunctional cough or severe glottic dysfunction greatly increases the risk of pneumonia and acute respiratory failure. Sudden accumulation of mucus in airways during chest infections can quickly collapse a lung, even in the absence of long-term lung or airway pathology. For patients with chronic airway disease, mucus stasis can contribute to bronchial obstruction, and chronic expectoration can be a physically and socially disabling problem. Mucus retention also can cause pathologic changes in the lungs[31] and is thought to contribute to the progression of airway disease.[32] It is not surprising, therefore, that in patients with chronic airway disease mucus hypersecretion has been associated with increased mortality[33]; it also is thought to contribute to the development of respiratory tract infections.

In healthy people the amount of mucus in the bronchial tree is small. In pathologic conditions such as bronchitis, however, mucus production increases considerably.[34] Sputum formation arises from a mixture of mucus, inflammatory cells, cellular debris, and sometimes bacteria. Hypersecretion can be caused by inhalation of smoke, antigens, or other airway irritants that trigger inflammation or by mechanical stimulation of the upper airways.[35,36] Irritation of the airways also causes changes in the molecular constituents of bronchial secretions. Initially, the increased volume of mucus results from increased secretion by each secretory cell. With chronic stimulation, hypersecretion is also due to an increased number of secretory cells.[37,38]

Mucus transport is often decreased in patients with pulmonary diseases such as asthma,[39] chronic obstructive pulmonary disease (COPD),[34,40–42] and cystic fibrosis (CF)[43–45] as well as in patients with dysfunctional cough or glottic control. The causes of reduced mucus transport vary, depending on the disease processes.

Asthma

Asthma is characterized by sudden episodes of dyspnea and bronchospasm that usually can be reversed almost completely by medical therapy. The hypersecretion that is usually present during these episodes is a result of mediator release after antigen exposure. Even with resolution of dyspnea and pulmonary dysfunction, airway inflammation and hyperplasia of the mucus glands and cells persist. Bronchodilation probably has no effect on bronchial mucus transport in such patients.[46] A ciliary-inhibiting factor that reduces ciliary activity, disorganizes ciliary beating and, thereby, reduces the efficacy of ciliary activity[47] has been postulated to be present during asthmatic episodes.[48,49] This "factor" may be the result of abnormal physical properties of mucus rather than an intrinsic ciliary inhibitor. Mucus hypersecretion and changes in the flow or surface properties of mucus also may cause a reduction of ciliary activity.[1,50,51] Mucociliary transport, therefore, can be severely reduced in such patients, with a further reduction during sleep.[52] After an exacerbation, when patients are symptom-free, mucus transport may recover[53] and become comparable to that of healthy people, or it may remain reduced[39,54–56] despite favorable changes in mucus viscoelasticity.

Chronic Obstructive Pulmonary Disease

Patients with COPD have day-to-day variability in the extent of airway obstruction. Mucus transport also may be decreased by smoking-induced ciliary paralysis[48,57,58] and by bacterial infections.[59–61] Lower airway collapse with coughing and the inability to generate effective cough flows also result in mucus retention. In contrast to patients with asthma, mucociliary transport does not fully recover and may decrease progressively because of a loss of ciliated epithelium due to recurrent infections and progressively severe airway instability.[61] Hypersecretion, which is usually present in patients with COPD, also may reduce mucociliary transport.

Cystic Fibrosis

Patients with CF initially have normally functioning cilia and an efficient cough.[43] During the course of the disease, however, the bronchial mucus transport rate decreases with the degree of pulmonary function impairment.[62] An inverse correlation between residual volume as a percentage of total lung capacity and bronchial mucus clearance rate has been described.[62] Because the coefficient of correlation was low (– 0.39), however, only about 16% of the variance in pulmonary function can be explained by differences in the mucus clearance rate. Although bronchial mucus is considered to be a bigger problem in CF than in COPD, the rheologic characteristics of CF mucus are comparable to those of mucus from patients with chronic bronchitis.[63] Mucus hydration has been postulated to be decreased, but experimental evidence does not support this contention.[64] It is more likely that poor mucus clearance in CF-affected airways results from abnormal mucus adhesiveness and tenacity.[65] The small peripheral airways can be completely obstructed by mucus. Recurrent respiratory tract infections in combination with hypersecretion and chronic airway obstruction can further reduce mucociliary transport by the mechanisms described above as well as by their tendency to result in dysfunctional coughing.

Neuromuscular Dysfunction of the Coughing Mechanism

Airway mucus elimination can be impaired by factors external to the lungs and airways. Patients with bulbar or expiratory muscle weakness often cannot generate sufficient peak cough flow (PCF) to eliminate airway mucus (see Chapter 2). Severe bulbar dysfunction most commonly occurs in patients with amyotrophic lateral sclerosis, spinal muscle atrophy type 1, and the pseudobulbar palsy of central nervous system origin. Inability to close the glottis and vocal cords results in complete loss of the ability to cough. Patients with central nervous system diseases such as multiple sclerosis can lose volitional cough but retain effective reflex coughs. Cerebellar and basal ganglia diseases often result in ineffective, uncoordinated coughing mechanisms.

PATIENT EVALUATION

The following parameters should be evaluated in each patient:
- Balance between mucus production and mucus transport and expectoration. Mucus expectoration itself is not an indication for intervention. The indication for intervention is retention of mucus in the airways, which can be ascertained by auscultation and percussion and from the fact that it can decrease pulmonary function and SpO_2.
- Ease of expectoration. The patient should be asked if it takes a long time or a lot of effort to expectorate mucus. The patient's methods for mobilizing secretions are evaluated.
- Impact of mucus retention on pulmonary function and gas exchange. Severe mucus retention can cause an acute decrease in vital capacity, forced vital capacity, and flow rates as well as SpO_2. Airway obstruction due to mucus retention also can reduce cough flows and exacerbate difficulties with expectoration.
- Strength and function of respiratory and bulbar muscles. Patients who suffer primarily from oxygenation impairment may have a marked reduction in PCF due to collapsing airways and a decrease in functioning lung but usually not due to respiratory muscle or bulbar muscle dysfunction. However, patients who suffer primarily from ventilatory impairment often have even greater expiratory than inspiratory muscle dysfunction and also may have bulbar muscle dysfunction, resulting in decreased assisted PCF. Maximal insufflation capacity and assisted PCF correlate with the soundness of bulbar muscle function (see Chapters 2 and 7).
- Possible contraindications to specific interventions. Mechanical facilitation of secretion elimination may be hazardous for critically ill patients. Abdominal thrusts should not be applied to a full stomach.

FACILITATION OF MUCUS ELIMINATION

Approaches to preventing retention of airway secretions include the use of medications to reduce mucus hypersecretion or to liquefy secretions and the facilitation of mucus mobilization. Mucus mobilization can be facilitated by the use of special breathing techniques, manual or mechanical chest percussion or vibration, direct oscillation of the air column, and postural drainage, all with or without directed and assisted coughing. The goal is to transport mucus from the peripheral to the central airways, from which it can be more easily eliminated.

Postural Drainage

Gravitational forces can enhance mucus transport when bronchi are vertically positioned. Postural drainage is the facilitation of airway drainage by having the patient assume gravity-assisted positions. It is probably most effective for relatively large quantities of mucus with low adhesiveness. Nine postural positions have been described for draining the large bronchi (Fig. 2).[66] Localization of airway mucus is essential. The goal is vertical positioning of the secretion-encumbered bronchi for a sufficient time, generally about 20 minutes, to allow drainage. The time required probably depends on the quantity of mucus, its viscoelasticity, and its adhesiveness. The patient should sleep in a postural drainage position if it can be tolerated.

Results of Clinical Studies

In an animal model, Chopra et al.[67] found an increase in tracheal mucus transport velocity during postural drainage. Other studies found improved mucus transport in patients with CF,[68,69] but in a study of patients with chronic bronchitis, no improvement was seen.[70] Postural drainage positioning can affect ventilation, perfusion, and SpO_2.[71–75] One study of patients with COPD showed that lung volumes were conserved and that dyspnea and decreases in SpO_2 did not occur in postural drainage positions.[76] Many patients who suffer primarily from ventilatory impairment, however, have less and often no breath volume in various postural drainage positions. Thus, the effect of postural drainage positioning on oxygenation demands close monitoring of alveolar ventilation and SpO_2. Positioning also can place the patient at risk for skin and cardiac complications, cerebral blood flow or intracranial pressure changes, and gastroesophageal reflux. Nevertheless, postural drainage may be useful when forced expirations, assisted coughing, and exercise are impossible or

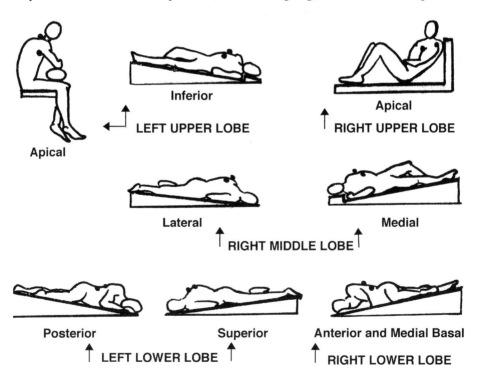

FIGURE 2. The nine positions for drainage of large airways. Percussion and vibration are applied to areas demarcated by the points.

inadequate. Disadvantages are that postural drainage is relatively time-consuming and may necessitate use of a specially modified bed or table.

Manual Chest Percussion and Postural Drainage (Chest Physical Therapy)

Chest percussion is the manual application of rhythmic clapping to the ventral, lateral, and dorsal side of the thorax at a frequency of approximately 3–6 Hz. It is often prescribed and used for 10- to 20-minute treatment sessions in patients with auscultatory or oximetry evidence of airway secretion retention. As for mechanical vibration and oscillation methods (see below), its efficacy may be due to its effect on decreasing mucus viscosity and inducing small coughs or resonance with ciliary action.[77]

Results of Clinical Studies

Animal studies demonstrated that the use of chest percussion combined with postural drainage increases tracheal mucus transport velocity.[67] Likewise, chest percussion[78] and the combination of percussion and postural drainage have been found to improve mucus transport in the airways of patients with COPD.[79] Compared with coughing, however, the results are conflicting. Some authors found an improvement in mucus transport using chest percussion and directed coughing in comparison with coughing alone in patients with COPD.[80,81] In other studies, no difference in mucus transport was found after the addition chest percussion to directed coughing in patients with CF[82] or COPD[78] (Fig. 3). Differences in application and treatment duration as well as differences in disease pathology may account for the different outcomes.

Likewise, improvements in pulmonary function parameters, gas exchange, or both in patients with COPD[83,84] or CF were described with the use of chest percussion and postural drainage.[84–87] Other studies failed to confirm beneficial effects of this treatment in patients with COPD[88–92] or CF.[93,94] In some studies of CF, chest percussion and coughing appeared to have similar effects on pulmonary function.[95,96] In general, improvements in mucus transport and mucus expectoration were not found to be associated with improvements in pulmonary function.

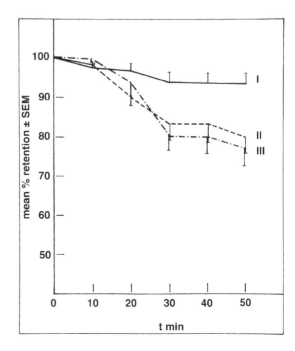

FIGURE 3. Clearance of a radioactive tracer, deposited on airway mucus, from the peripheral lung regions, expressed as percentages of the starting value (mean and standard error of the mean [SEM]) in patients with COPD during three different protocols. During protocol I, chest percussion performed for 20–30 minutes resulted in a small but statistically significant increase in mucus clearance. During protocol II, patients were lying in a 20° head-down position, and percussion, breathing exercises, and coughing were performed for 10–30 minutes. Clearance was significantly greater than with protocol I. Protocol III was the same as protocol II but without percussion. No significant differences were found between protocols II and III. (From van der Schans CP, Pilas DA, Postma DS: Effect of manual percussion on tracheobronchial clearance in patients with chronic airflow obstruction and excessive tracheobronchial secretion. Thorax 41:448–452, 1986, with permission.)

During acute exacerbations of COPD[88] and in patients with acute pulmonary disease,[97] undesirable side effects, such as increased bronchial airway obstruction and oxyhemoglobin desaturation, have been associated with chest percussion. In patients in critical condition with severe hypoxia or bronchial hyperreactivity, care must be taken to avoid hypoxia, cardiac arrhythmias, and lung or chest-wall damage.[98] Because it can cause acute hypoxia, supplemental oxygen is often administered, and SpO_2 monitoring should be considered during treatments. Elderly patients and patients with cardiac disorders appear to have an increased risk of arrhythmias during chest percussion.[97]

Chest percussion does not appear to benefit patients during recovery from acute exacerbations of COPD[92,99] or pneumonia.[100,101] Both conditions are characterized by interstitial pathology that cannot be influenced by physical interventions on the airways. When they are complicated by impaired mucus transport and hypersecretion, however, chest percussion and postural drainage appear to be useful. Inhalation of nebulized saline, water, or terbutaline can further improve the effects of chest percussion and postural drainage on mucus transport in such patients.[102,103] This finding may be due to increased ciliary beat frequency, increased hydration of bronchial mucus, or bronchodilation, which leads to a higher and, thus, more effective airflow. Systemic hydration, however, has been shown to impair mucociliary transport during allergic mucociliary dysfunction.[104]

No evidence indicates that chest physical therapy can decrease hospitalization stays or the likelihood of pulmonary complications for any patient. Likewise, no studies have suggested that chest physical therapy is effective in patients with cough impairment due to expiratory muscle weakness. Although chest percussion is not likely to cause harm and may be beneficial, the main strategy for eliminating airway secretions in patients who suffer primarily from ventilatory impairment is to assist inspiratory and expiratory muscle function to increase cough flows (see Chapter 7).

Mechanical Vibration and High-frequency Oscillation

Vibration can be applied externally to the chest wall or abdomen by rapidly oscillating pressure changes in a vest (e.g., the ThAIRapy Vest, American Biosystems, Inc., St. Paul, MN), by cycling oscillating pressures under a chest shell (e.g., the Hayek oscillator, Breasy Medical Equipment, Inc., Stamford, CT), or by using chest vibrators (Fig. 4). The ThAIRapy Vest provides oscillation at 5–25 Hz. Mechanical vibration is performed at frequencies up to 40 Hz. Vibration is applied during the entire breathing cycle or during expiration only. The adjustable inspiratory-expiratory ratio of the Hayek oscillator permits asymmetric inspiratory and expiratory pressure changes (e.g., + 3 to – 6 cmH_2O), which favor higher exsufflation flow velocities to mobilize secretions. Baseline pressures can be set at negative, atmospheric, or positive values, thus commencing oscillation above, at, or below the functional residual capacity (FRC).

Oscillations to 16 Hz or higher also can be applied at the mouth by high-frequency positive-pressure ventilation or jet ventilation. One such air column oscillator based on high-frequency jet ventilation was developed by the Bird Corporation (Exeter, UK). This hand-held device delivers 30-ml sine wave oscillations through a mouthpiece at 20 Hz. Lower-frequency air-column oscillators are the Intrapulmonary Percussive Ventilator, Percussionator, Impulsator, and Spanker Respirators (Percussionaire Corp., Sandpoint, ID). They can deliver aerosolized medications while providing intrapulmonary percussive ventilation; that is, high-flow mini-bursts of air are delivered to the lungs at a rate of 2–7 Hz (Fig. 5).[105]

It has been reported that high-frequency oscillations break down high-molecular-weight DNA in sputum samples of patients with CF to the same extent as the use of rhDNase treatment.[106] High-frequency oscillations may act like a physical mucolytic, reducing both the spinability and viscoelasticity of mucus and enhancing clearance by coughing.[107] The effect of combining rhDNase with oscillation may be complementary.[108] An in vitro study also suggested that shearing at the air mucus interface may be a factor in

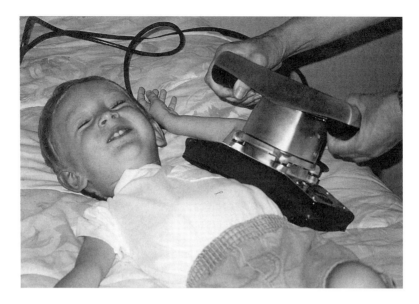

FIGURE 4.   Use of a Jeanie Rub Vibrator M69-315A (Morfam, Inc., Mishawaka, IN) on a 5½-year-old boy with spinal muscular atrophy type 2.

the enhanced tracheal mucus clearance during high-frequency chest-wall oscillation.[109] Hansen et al. suggested that mucus transport is enhanced in three ways: by altering crosslinkage density of mucus glycoproteins, by creating a cough-like expiratory flow bias, and by increasing the strength of ciliary beat through resonance.[77] Whereas huffing can be a much more effective means of expelling airway mucus for patients with collapsible airways, Warwick noted that high-frequency chest compression essentially moves mucus by means of sustained staccato coughs.[110]

Contraindications for high-frequency oscillation are head or neck injuries that have not been stabilized and active hemorrhage with hemodynamic instability. Relative contraindications

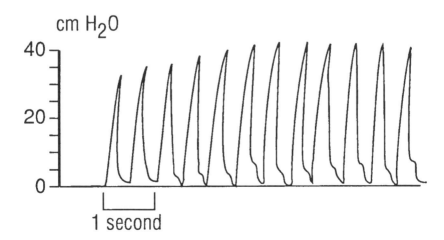

FIGURE 5.   Pressure delivery pattern of the Intrapulmonary Percussive Ventilator (Percussionaire Corp., Sandpoint, ID).

include active or recent gross hemoptysis, pulmonary embolism, subcutaneous emphysema, bronchopleural fistula, esophageal surgery, recent epidural spinal infusion, spinal surgery, spinal anesthesia or acute spinal injury, presence of a transvenous or subcutaneous pacemaker, increased intracranial pressures, uncontrolled hypertension, suspected or confirmed pulmonary tuberculosis, bronchospasm, empyema or large pleural effusion, pulmonary edema due to congestive heart failure, burns, open wounds, infection or recent thoracic skin grafts, osteoporosis, osteomyelitis, coagulopathy, rib fracture, lung contusion, distended abdomen, and chest-wall pain.

Chest vibrators (see Fig. 4) may be the most practical and effective method of chest percussion. They vibrate the chest at optimal frequencies and are inexpensive (about $100 or less), small, light, and easy to use.

Results of Clinical Trials

Mucociliary clearance in anesthetized sheep receiving asymmetric (expiratory-biased) high-frequency oscillation directly to the airway at 15 Hz with peak expiratory flows of 3.8 L/sec and peak inspiratory flows of 1.3 L/sec was greatly affected by posture. Mucus clearance during head-down tilt postural drainage was 3.1 ml/10 min. The rate was 3.5 ml/10 min with use of expiratory-biased high-frequency oscillation in the horizontal position and 11 ml/10 min with expiratory-biased high-frequency oscillation with a head-down tilt. No clearance occurred with inspiratory-biased high-frequency oscillation during head-down tilt. Mucus clearance was less at lower and higher frequencies.[111] In other animal models, frequencies of 13 Hz[109,112,113] and 25–35 Hz[114] were safe and most effective in enhancing mucus transport.[102,115] Differences in the animals used in these models may be responsible for the different results. Nevertheless, only mechanical methods can provide these high frequencies.

High-frequency oscillation to the airways also has been reported to increase mucus transport in healthy humans.[53] For humans, too, its effectiveness seems to be frequency-dependent.[36,112–114] In most studies, frequencies of 10–15 Hz seem to have the greatest effect on mucus transport.[116] Chest vibration at 2 and at 41 Hz was reported to have no effect on mucus transport in patients with COPD.[117] Vibratory-shaking or percussion also had no effect on mucus transport in a mixed group of patients with hypersecretion.[118]

Although some studies of patients with COPD or CF have failed to demonstrate any clear benefit of chest-wall vibration in mucus transport (see Fig. 3),[78,119–121] one study reported improvements in the rate of expectoration of mucus, expressed as grams per minute, when chest vibration was added to manual percussion and postural drainage in patients with chronic bronchitis.[122] In a study of patients with CF, the intrathoracic pressures induced by vibration appeared to be frequency-dependent; the highest pressures were reached at frequencies of about 15 Hz.[123] The experiments of Chang et al.[109] indicate that intervention is more effective for thicker mucus layers. Oscillation and vibration also have been reported to be more effective when expiratory flows are greater than inspiratory flows.[109,111,124,125] In addition, they may be useful in patients with primarily ventilatory impairment during intercurrent chest infections.[126,127]

Intrapulmonary percussive ventilation (Percussionaire, Bird, Inc., Exeter, UK; see Fig. 5) has been reported to be more effective than chest percussion in the treatment of postoperative atelectasis and secretion mobilization in patients with COPD.[128] In one study of 12 inpatients and 8 outpatients, sputum volume and forced vital capacity increased during regular use of intrapulmonary percussive ventilation (IPV). The increase in forced vital capacity, however, was 6% and seen only with inpatients over the 5-day study period. The majority of the patients believed that the treatments were helpful.[129] Several abstracts and a recent publication also favorably compared the use of IPV with chest percussion and postural drainage for patients with COPD or intrinsic lung disease.[130]

In a study of patients with CF recovering from acute pulmonary exacerbations, equivalent improvements in pulmonary function and amount of expectorated mucus were found with conventional chest percussion and postural drainage and with high-frequency chest-wall compression.[131–135] On the other hand, Anbar et al.[136] and Warwick and Hansen[137] found short-term and long-term increases, respectively, in forced vital capacity and forced expiratory volume in one second (FEV_1) in patients with CF who were treated with high-frequency chest-wall compression compared with conventional chest percussion and postural drainage alone. The improved pulmonary function was thought to be related to improved mucus clearance. At least two studies reported that chest-wall vibration effectively mobilized mucus in patients for whom chest percussion and postural drainage were less effective or ineffective.[138,139] It also has been suggested that patient compliance is better with chest-wall vibration (50%) than with flutter (37%) or chest percussion (13%).[140] The addition of positive end-expiratory pressure (PEEP) during high-frequency chest compression has been suggested to augment its effectiveness in clearing mucus.[141] Thus, although evidence of clinical efficacy is controversial, this method, when used with head-down posture, appears to facilitate airway secretion clearance. One study reported that health care costs for patients with CF who use chest-wall vibration were one-half the costs incurred before its use.[142]

Beneficial effects of vibration also may result from mechanisms not related to mucus transport. Piquet et al.[143] found an improvement in gas exchange during high-frequency oscillation, probably due to changes in breathing pattern. Sibuya et al.[144] found that chest-wall vibration decreased dyspnea, and Holody et al.[145] reported an increase in oxygenation in acutely ill patients with atelectasis or pneumonia.

Side effects of percussion and vibration include increased obstruction to airflow in patients with COPD.[88,94] In an animal model, the application of vibration and percussion was associated with the development of atelectasis.[146]

Although patients often report subjective benefits with their use, the expense of most chest-wall vibrators and air-column oscillators and the failure to prove clinically significant benefits make it difficult to justify routine use. Further study is needed to establish both the efficacy and the safety of these methods.

Positive Expiratory Pressure Breathing

Application of positive expiratory pressure (PEP) breathing is based on the hypothesis that mucus in peripheral small airways is mobilized more effectively by coughing or forced expirations if alveolar pressure and volume behind mucus plugs are increased. PEP is usually applied by breathing through a face mask or mouthpiece with an inspiratory tube containing a one-way valve and an expiratory tube containing variable expiratory resistance. It results in positive expiratory pressure throughout expiration. Expiratory pressures of 10–20 cmH_2O are generally used. PEP increases the pressure gradient between open and closed alveoli, thus tending to maintain alveoli patency. It also increases FRC, thus reducing the resistance in collateral and small airways.[147,148]

Results of Clinical Trials

The results of studies of the effect of PEP breathing are conflicting. One study in patients with CF suggests that the addition of PEP increases mucus expectoration more than conventional chest percussion and postural drainage or coughing,[130] but other studies failed to confirm this finding in patients with CF[149–153] or COPD.[154,155] Some authors have reported that the use of PEP along with chest percussion improves pulmonary function in patients with CF[130,156,157] and arterial blood gas values in patients with various disorders.[158] Other studies were unable to confirm these results.[149,151,152,159] PEP breathing is one of the few interventions for which long-term effects have been investigated.[160,161] The results of two studies, however, are conflicting. E. F. Christensen et al.[160] found a decrease in exacerbations of lung disease and use of antibiotics over a 12-month treatment period. H. R. Christensen et al.,[161] however, found no effect of PEP on frequency of exacerbations or antibiotic use over a 6-month treatment period.

A variation of PEP breathing has been developed by Oberwaldner et al.[162] In this high-pressure technique, the patient is asked to expire forcefully through a PEP mask. The purpose of this maneuver is to prevent airway compression during forced expiration. The authors believed that airway compression leads to airway collapse in patients with CF, making mucus transport impossible, and that airway collapse is preventable.

The possible benefit of PEP and high-pressure PEP for mucus transport remains to be proved. However, PEP is useful in patients with indications to increase lung volume at least temporarily.

Flutter Breathing

Flutter breathing is a combination of PEP and air-column oscillation applied at the mouth. It is an inexpensive means of oscillating the air column in conjunction with providing positive expiratory pressure. The patient exhales through a small pipe. The expiratory opening of the pipe is closed by a small stainless steel ball. During expiration the stainless steel ball is pushed upward, producing a positive expiratory pressure, and falls downward again, producing an interruption of the expiratory flow. The mucus-mobilizing effect is thought to be due to both widening of the airways by increased expiratory pressure and airflow oscillations due to the oscillating ball.[163] Flutter breathing is analogous to huffing.

Results of Clinical Trials

The results of clinical trials have been conflicting. Konstan et al.[164] found a significantly greater amount of expectorated sputum in patients with CF during flutter breathing compared with voluntary coughing or chest percussion. However, they found no improvement in pulmonary function or patient well-being. Pryor and colleagues[165] found that the active cycle of breathing technique (see below) resulted in a significantly greater amount of expectorated mucus than flutter breathing in patients with CF, but they, too, failed to demonstrate changes in lung function or oxygenation. In another study, the use of flutter along with expiration with the glottis open in the lateral position resulted in greater sputum expectoration than did chest percussion and postural drainage.[166] Use of the flutter device is demanding; it cannot be easily used by patients with severe lung disease. Carefully controlled studies need to be conducted before this technique can be widely recommended.

Forced Expirations and Coughing

Cough is the primary defense mechanism against foreign bodies in the lower airways. It is also an important compensating mechanism when production and clearance of mucus are out of balance (see Chapter 2). In patients with COPD, the high thoracoabdominal pressures required to cough exacerbate airway collapse, which can render cough ineffective (see Chapter 2).

When a forced expiration technique known as "huffing" is used, forced expiratory flows are created through an open glottis, and the intrapulmonary pressures are much lower than during cough.[167] Coughing and huffing may be performed from different lung volumes. Forced expirations combined with breath control (diaphragmatic breathing) exercises are known as the forced expiration technique (FET). FET combined with thoracic expansion exercises is known as the active cycle of breathing (ACB).[66]

Forced expirations and coughing derive from the fact that airflow through a tube lined with viscous liquid can transport the liquid. This phenomenon is called two-phase gas-liquid flow.[168,169] Mucus transport by two-phase gas-liquid flow can arise in airways that are closed by mucus as well as in open airways thickly lined with mucus. Mucus transport in a closed airway can be achieved only during forced expirations because it requires a high pressure. Mucus transport in an open airway can be achieved by forced expirations and, to some degree, by tidal breathing.[170-172]

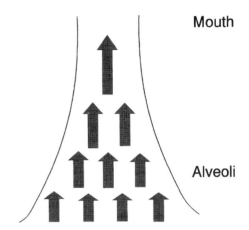

FIGURE 6. Total airway diameter decreases from the peripheral to the central airways. Consequently, air flows increase from the peripheral to the central airways.

   The higher tidal volumes and flows that normally occur during exercise have been reported to increase secretion mobilization up to 41%[173] by increasing parasympathetic activity and fluid secretion and thereby reducing secretion viscosity[174]; by increasing the circulation of endocrines that change the volume and viscosity of secretions[173]; and by increasing airway flows.[173] Mucus is especially well mobilized by flow velocities greater than 2.5 L/sec.[168] High airflow velocities are reached when airflow is high and airway diameter is small. In healthy people, the total airway diameter depends on the airway level and dynamic compression. Because the total airway diameter decreases from the peripheral to the central airways, airflow velocity increases centrally (Fig. 6). Forced expirations and coughing, therefore, are mainly effective in the central airways to about the sixth division.[175]
   During a forced expiration or cough, dynamic compression of the airways occurs. The alveolar pressure, which is the sum of the elastic recoil pressure and the pleural pressure, is the driving pressure to produce expiratory flow. During the coughing maneuver the pressure in the bronchi decreases from the peripheral airways to the mouth because of frictional pressure loss and convective acceleration pressure loss.[176] At a certain point within the airways, the intrabronchial pressure equals the pleural pressure. This point is called the equal pressure point (EPP) (Fig. 7). Upstream, in the direction of the alveoli, bronchial pressure is higher than pleural pressure and no compression takes place. Downstream, in the direction of the mouth, the surrounding pleural pressure is higher than the bronchial pressure and compression of the airways may take place, depending on the stiffness of the airway wall.[177]

FIGURE 7. During a forced expiration, the point in the airways at which bronchial pressure (Pbr) equals pleural pressure (Ppl) is called the equal pressure point (EPP). Downstream from the EPP, compression of the airways can lead to high linear airflow velocities. Palv = alveolar pressure.

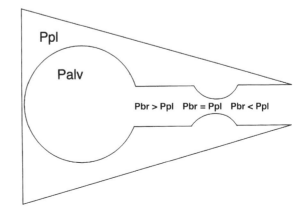

In the event of severe obstruction to airflow, the frictional pressure loss in the bronchi is higher and results in a shift of the EPP in the direction of the alveoli. A lower elastic recoil pressure—as seen in pulmonary emphysema, forced expiration from a lower lung volume, and higher pleural pressures due to higher expiratory forces—leads to an upstream shift of the EPP. Less obstruction to airflow, higher elastic recoil pressure, and lower pleural pressures lead to a shift of the EPP downstream in the direction of the mouth. The degree of compression is related to the compliance of the airway wall. The more compliant the peripheral airways in comparison with the central airways, the greater the degree of compression when the EPP is located more upstream. Dynamic compression contributes to the development of local high airflow velocities in these airways. Experimental animal models have demonstrated that cough-induced mucus transport is much greater when airways are constricted[178,179] (Fig. 8). This finding supports the hypothesis that dynamic compression of the airways can be used to assist mucus clearance during chest percussion and that maneuvers attempting to maintain maximal airway patency may reduce cough effectiveness.

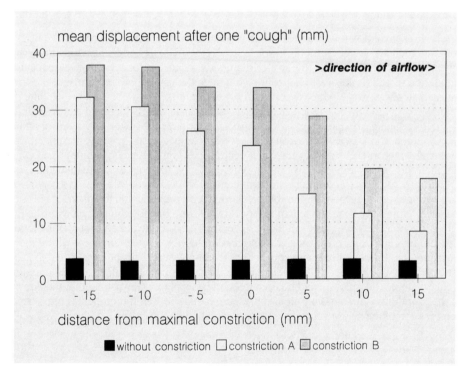

FIGURE 8. Cough-induced transport of a mucus simulant gel (MSG) with viscoelastic properties similar to human sputum was measured in an artificial trachea. A constriction with a length of 73 mm and a maximal diameter of 7.5 mm (constriction A) and a constriction with a length of 87 mm and a maximal diameter of 10 mm (constriction B) were used. MSG samples of 40 μl were spread linearly over the width of the trachea under the point of maximal constriction and 5, 10, and 15 mm both upstream and downstream from the point of maximal constriction. Measurements without the constriction were made at the same positions. Displacement of the MSG was measured after a single simulated cough. The application of the constrictive elements significantly increased mucus displacement (ANOVA p < 0.001). The position of the MSG relative to the point of maximal airway constriction significantly influenced cough displacement with constriction A (ANOVA p < 0.001) and constriction B (ANOVA p < 0.001). The displacement was higher in the upstream positions than in the downstream positions. Without constriction the displacement was unrelated to the position of the MSG (ANOVA p > 0.2). (From van der Schans CP, Ramirez OE, Postma DS, et al: Effect of airway constriction on the cough transportability of mucus. Am J Respir Crit Care Med 149:A1023, 1994, with permission.)

When the force of the expiratory muscles is severely reduced, leading to lower pleural pressures during coughing, the dynamic compression of the airways is less pronounced and cough effectiveness is reduced.[180] When airway compression is too great, airways collapse, as often occurs in patients with severe pulmonary emphysema, and cough-induced mucus transport is reduced.[181] In certain pathologic states, smooth muscle contraction, inflammatory processes and edema, and dynamic compression reduce the diameter of the peripheral airways. Reduced diameter limits peripheral airflow and, thereby, airflow velocity in the more central airways and may result in airway collapse.

In addition, during a forced expiration a high expiratory flow is generated within approximately 0.1 seconds, thereby creating a high shear rate. Mucus viscosity varies inversely with shear rate. This phenomenon is called pseudoplastic flow or shear thinning. Viscosity of mucus in the same sample may vary by a factor of up to 500 depending on the applied shear. This decrease in mucus viscosity can be explained by a temporary realignment of macromolecular glycoproteins[6] as a result of the applied force or "thixotropy." Repeated forced expiratory flows, therefore, may improve mucociliary and cough-induced transport by temporarily reducing mucus viscosity. This hypothesis is supported by the work of Zahm et al.,[182] who found in an experimental model that transport of a mucus gel stimulant in an artificial trachea was higher when the interval between the coughs was reduced. Bennett et al.[183] found that in healthy people both forced expirations and forced inspirations increase mucus transport. The explanation for this surprising phenomenon is not entirely clear, but it may be explained, at least in part, by the reduction in mucus viscosity due to the additional shear effects of the forced inspirations.

Mucus transport by expiratory airflow also depends on the properties of the mucus layer. The critical airflow to transport mucus decreases with increasing thickness of the mucus layer.[170] Thus, patients with more hypersecretion probably need less effort to expectorate mucus by coughing than patients with less pronounced hypersecretion. It may be that with lung and airway disease and the destruction of normal mucociliary function, the teleologic response of the lungs is to thicken the airway mucus so that it can be coughed out more easily. Excessive pharmacologic liquification of airway mucus, therefore, may be hazardous.

Results of Clinical Trials

Forced expirations and coughing are probably the most effective aspects of physical therapy for improving mucus transport.[82,96,184–186] They are effective even in patients who do not expectorate any mucus.[187] Probably for this reason, Lannefors et al.[188] found no difference in mucus transport in a study of patients with CF when they compared forced expirations plus postural drainage, forced expirations plus PEP mask use, and forced expirations plus physical exercise. Forced expirations have been shown to be as effective as coughing for patients with COPD or bronchiectasis, even though patient effort is less when forced expirations are performed.[189] However, a long-term study of patients with CF demonstrated that the annual decrease in the forced expiratory flow of the middle one-half of the expiratory volume ($FEF_{25–75\%}$) was less in the group that received chest percussion, postural drainage, and FET than in the group that applied self-administered FET. No statistically significant differences between the two groups were found in decline in forced vital capacity or FEV_1 or in number of hospitalizations.[190] The reasons for the difference between the groups is not clear, although both treatment efficacy and differences in patient compliance may be responsible.

Zach et al.[191] suggested that in patients with CF the use of bronchodilators may decrease the stability of the airway wall and, thus, reduce the effectiveness of forced expirations and coughing because of airway collapse. This suggestion, however, was not confirmed in a recent study by Desmond et al.[192] Bennett and coworkers[193] showed that mucus clearance by cough in patients with stable COPD was diminished after inhalation of ipratropium bromide. According to the authors, this finding may have resulted from alteration of airway compression characteristics or possibly from changes in the rheologic properties of the mucus. From the present data it can be concluded that bronchodilation does not a priori increase the effectiveness of forced expirations and coughing. The effects of bronchodilators on the effectiveness of forced expirations and coughing need to be investigated to determine which, if any, patients benefit.

Practice

Forced expirations or coughing are considered the first choice of physical therapeutic intervention. Each patient learns to perform the techniques most effective for himself or herself. The first factor to determine is whether to use or decrease dynamic airway compression. In patients with severe airflow obstruction or reduced elastic recoil of lung tissue, compression may collapse the airways, reduce forced expiration and cough effectiveness, and cause a sudden cessation of airflow. Collapse of airways, however, is not homogeneous and may be difficult to assess without pulmonary function testing. In the generation of a maximal expiratory flow volume curve, airway collapse is reflected by a typical sharp bend convex to the volume axis at a volume shortly after the peak expiratory flow (PEF) has been reached (Fig. 9). When signs of airway collapse are present, forced expiration should be started from a lung volume nearer the total lung capacity (TLC) and with submaximal or less expiratory force. In this way, the compression takes place predominantly in the large central airways and collapse may be partly prevented.

In patients with less severe airflow obstruction and normal or increased elastic recoil of lung tissue, forced expiration and coughing can be performed with higher force and initiated at lower lung volumes. Thus, the site of dynamic airway compression is shifted toward the small peripheral airways. The force and lung volume should be chosen so that the patient can hear or feel mucus mobilization. Lung volume and expiration force may be varied more easily by using forced expirations than by coughing. Patients with tracheostoma also can be taught more effective coughing by capping the tracheostomy tube or, preferably, by removal of the tube and placement of a button, if necessary. Thus the obstructing tube is cleared from the airway. Patients then can learn to use forced expirations for effective expectoration of mucus.

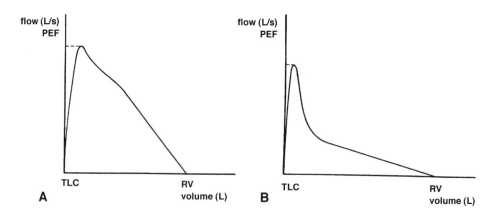

FIGURE 9. *A*, Relationship between expiratory airflow and lung volume during a forced expiration in a healthy person. A maximal forced expiration is performed after a maximal inspiration. Peak expiratory flow (PEF) is reached at high lung volume. Thereafter, the flow decreases. *B*, Relationship between expiratory airflow and lung volume during a forced expiration in a patient with pulmonary emphysema. The PEF is mildly reduced, but after the PEF is reached, the airflow suddenly is curtailed severely because of airway collapse.

If the experimental data of Zahm et al.[182] are clinically relevant, it is important that repetitive forced expirations be performed at short intervals and that high expiratory flows be reached quickly for a high shear rate. This goal can be attained more easily by coughing than by forced expiration with an open glottis.

In cases of severe respiratory muscle weakness, inspiration can be supported by glossopharyngeal breathing,[66] and expiration can be assisted by manual compression of the thorax and abdomen or by mechanical exsufflation.[194–196] In patients with COPD or spinal cord tetraplegia, evidence indicates that the pectoralis muscles have expiratory function and that training of these muscles may contribute to active coughing.[197–201]

Exercise

Many patients with chronic hypersecretion and impaired mucus transport improve expectoration by general physical exercise such as running or bicycling. The increased expiratory flow rates, minute volumes, and sympathetic activity during exercise increase ciliary beat, decrease mucus viscosity, and increase mucus transport.[202] Assuming that the expiratory flows are the most important factor, the exercise must have sufficient intensity and duration to increase ventilatory demand.

Results of Clinical Trials

Exercise may improve bronchial mucus transport in healthy people[202] and in patients with COPD[60] or CF.[203] The addition of exercise to chest physical therapy results in a significant increase in the amount of expectorated mucus.[204] Some authors suggest that exercise may be a substitute for chest physical therapy,[205,206] a supposition not supported by the results of some studies of patients with CF.[207,208] Exercise may improve pulmonary function in patients with CF,[203] possibly by improving mucus transport or by the bronchodilating effect of exercise itself.[201] Exercise reconditioning is considered in Chapter 16.

Autogenic Drainage

Autogenic drainage is based on the hypothesis that a mucus-mobilizing "milking" or squeezing effect occurs in the peripheral airways when the patient breathes with low expiratory flows at lung volumes between the FRC and residual volume. After this so-called "mobilizing phase," a "collection phase" follows, during which mucus is thought to be transported to the larger airways by increasing tidal volumes. The last phase of this technique is the "expectoration phase," during which mucus is expectorated by low-volume forced expirations.[209] There are no studies of the effect of this intervention on mucus transport or mucus expectoration.

Tracheal Suctioning Via the Upper Airway

Nasotracheal suctioning is the last resort when other methods have failed to improve mucus transport. It should be considered only for patients with fixed upper or lower airway obstruction—never for patients with predominantly ventilatory impairment who can effectively use manually and mechanically assisted coughing. A catheter is passed via the upper airway through the vocal cords into the trachea and a mainstem bronchus, and mucus is suctioned. It is easier to enter the right mainstem bronchus than the left mainstem bronchus for anatomic reasons.[210] The procedure may induce coughing, which may mobilize mucus from more peripheral airways. During the procedure saline may be instilled through the suction catheter into the trachea to liquefy the mucus. The instillations usually reach only as far as the trachea because of the cough reflex and probably have no liquefying or diluting effect on mucus in the mainstem bronchi.[211] The practice of introducing saline into an endotracheal tube and driving it into the airway by positive pressure "bagging" is to be condemned; this technique may cause mucus to be loosened and driven deeper into the airway, occluding airways beyond the reach of suction catheters. The direct bronchoscopic aspiration of secretions may be preferable to endotracheal or nasotracheal suctioning because the bronchoscope permits visual inspection of the airway and direction of the suction pressure. Manually and mechanically assisted coughing should eliminate the need for deep airway suctioning in patients with assisted PCF over 160 L/min.

Results of Clinical Trials

Nasotracheal suctioning can lead to damage of the bronchial epithelium[212–214] and to hypersecretion of mucus.[35] The procedure also can cause respiratory distress and severe oxyhemoglobin desaturation,[215,216] severe hemodynamic complications,[217–220] bronchospasm, and bacteremia[221] as well as tracheal puncture, suction catheter granuloma formation with airway obstruction, and inadvertent esophageal intubation with blind introduction of the catheter. Autopsies of patients with long-term indwelling tracheostomy tubes who have undergone frequent transtracheal suctioning have demonstrated widespread denuding of the epithelium and widespread airway scarring.

Practice

Nasotracheal suctioning is extremely unpleasant, hazardous, and poorly tolerated. It should be used only when it is absolutely necessary; that is, when there is a risk of acute respiratory insufficiency due to accumulation of mucus in the airways and the patient cannot expectorate the mucus sufficiently even with manual and mechanical assistance. Hypoxic patients should receive supplemental oxygen before starting the procedure. A sterile disposable catheter is brought into the trachea through the nose or mouth. Suctioning is done in intervals of a few seconds with negative pressures between 8 and 20 kPa, depending on the viscoelasticity of the mucus.[66] In case of large airway instability, the negative pressure may lead to tracheobronchial collapse; thus, suction pressures are decreased. A few milliliters of saline can be instilled through the catheter into the trachea. The patient is monitored closely for complications. After removal of the catheter, ventilation is checked in both lungs by auscultation.

Mechanical Insufflation-Exsufflation

Mechanical insufflation-exsufflation involves the use of an airflow generator to provide about 10 L/sec of expiratory flow directly to the airways. It can be applied via an oronasal interface or mouthpiece or directly via an endotracheal or tracheostomy tube. Its application for patients with obstructive and restrictive pulmonary syndromes is discussed in Chapters 7–10 and 15.

Thoracic Mobilization

Manually assisted coughing techniques (see Chapter 7) are examples of thoracic mobilization. In addition to the standard hand placements for applying thrusts to the chest and abdomen to increase cough flows, other placements can be used to apply thrusts to specific lung regions. Likewise, thrusts can be applied to stretch specific areas of the anterior and posterior chest walls. Guidebooks have been published that demonstrate the hand placements and thrusting techniques.[222] Although thoracic mobilization can be used in conjunction with chest percussion and postural drainage, no specific outcome studies are available.

PATIENT COMPLIANCE

In a 10-year study of patients with CF, Patterson and coworkers[223] found that good compliance with daily therapy was associated with a slower rate of loss of FEV_1. The compliance of patients who suffer primarily from respiratory impairment with mucus-mobilizing interventions is generally poor, however.[105,224,225] Independence in administering therapy improves compliance. Methods to facilitate independence and other strategies need to be developed to improve compliance with treatment.

Patients who suffer primarily from ventilatory impairment, on the other hand, tend to embrace enthusiastically the use of assisted coughing methods,[226] especially in conjunction with oximetry as feedback,[227,228] to maintain airway patency and avoid respiratory morbidity. As a result, assisted coughing methods can be highly effective in avoiding hospitalization and the need to resort to tracheostomy.

La primera reacción no está en manos de los hombres. (The first reaction is not in the hands of men.)

Miguel de Cervantes, *Don Quijote de La Mancha*

REFERENCES

1. Adler KB, Wooten M, Dulfano MJ: Mammalian respiratory mucociliary clearance. Arch Environ Health 27:364–369, 1973.
2. Barton AD, Lourenço RV: Bronchial secretions and mucociliary clearance: Biochemical characteristics. Arch Intern Med 131:140–144, 1973.
3. Jeffery PK: The origins of secretions in the lower respiratory tract. Eur J Respir Dis 71(Suppl 153):34–42, 1987.
4. Kaliner M, Marom Z, Patow C, Shelhamer J: Human respiratory mucus. J Allergy Clin Immunol 73:318–323, 1984.
5. Lopez-Vidriero MT, Das I: Airway secretion: Source, biochemical and rheological properties. In Brain JD, Proctor DF, Reid LM (eds): Respiratory Defense Mechanisms. New York, Marcel Dekker, 1977, pp 288–301.
6. Lopez-Vidriero MT: Airway mucus production and composition. Chest 80:799–804, 1981.
7. Richardson PS: The physical and chemical properties of airway mucus and their relation to airway function. Eur J Respir Dis 61(Suppl 111):13–15, 1980.
8. Jeffery PK: The respiratory mucous membrane. In Brain JD, Proctor DF, Reid LM (eds): Respiratory Defense Mechanisms. New York, Marcel Dekker, 1977, p 193.
9. Toremalm NG: The daily amount of tracheobronchial secretions in man. Acta Oto-Laryngol (Suppl 185):43–53, 1960.
10. King M, Macklem PT: Rheological properties of microliter quantities of normal mucus. J Appl Physiol 42:797–802, 1977.
11. Litt M: Mucus rheology relevance to mucociliary clearance. Arch Intern Med 126:417–423, 1970.
12. Weibel ER: Morphometry of the Human Lung. Berlin, Springer-Verlag, 1963.
13. Hilding AC: Ciliary streaming in the lower respiratory tract. Am J Physiol 191:404–410, 1957.
14. Asmundsson T, Kilburn KH: Mucociliary clearance rates at various levels in dogs lungs. Am Rev Respir Dis 102:388–397, 1970.
15. Lee PS, Gerrity TR, Hass FJ, Lourenço RV: A model for tracheobronchial clearance of inhaled particles in man and comparison with data. IEEE Transactions on Biomedical Engineering 26:624–630, 1979.
16. Kilburn KH: A hypothesis for pulmonary clearance and its implications. Am Rev Respir Dis 98:449–463, 1968.
17. Van As A: Pulmonary airway clearance mechanisms: A reappraisal. Am Rev Respir Dis 115:721–726, 1977.
18. Pavia D, Agnew JE, Clarke SW: Physiological, pathological and drug-related alterations in tracheobronchial mucociliary clearance. In Isles AF, von Wichert P (eds): Sustained-release Theophylline and Noctural Asthma. Amsterdam, Exerpta Medica, 2000, p 44.
19. van As A: Pulmonary airway defense mechanisms: An appreciation of integrated mucociliary activity. Eur J Respir Dis 61(Suppl 111):21–24, 1980.
20. Newhouse M, Sanchis J, Bienenstock J: Lung defense mechanisms. N Engl J Med 195:990–998, 1976.
21. Sleigh MA: The nature and action of respiratory tract cilia. In Brain JD, Proctor DF, Reid LM (eds): Respiratory Defense Mechanisms. New York, Marcel Dekker, 1977, p 247.
22. Wanner A: Clinical aspects of mucociliary transport. Am Rev Respir Dis 115:73–125, 1977.
23. Jeffery PK, Reid L: New observations of rat airway epithelium: A quantitative and electron microscopic study. J Anat 120:295–320, 1975.

24. Hilding AC: Phagocytosis, mucous flow, and ciliary action. Arch Environ Health 6:67–79, 1963.
25. Hoffman LA: Ineffective airway clearance related to neuromuscular dysfunction. Nurs Clin North Am 22:151–166, 1987.
26. Rubin BK, Ramirez O, King M: Mucus-depleted frog palate as a model for the study of mucociliary clearance. J Appl Physiol 69:424–429, 1990.
27. Rubin BK, King M: Rheology of airway mucus: Relationship with clearance function. In Takishima T, Shimura S (eds): Airway Secretion: Physiological Bases for the Control of Mucus Hypersecretion. Marcel Dekker, New York, 1994, pp 283–297.
28. Giugliano MA, Russo R, Palladino A, et al: Mucociliary activity evaluation by ventilatory lung scintigraphy in Duchenne patients. Eighth Journées Internationales de Ventilation à Domicile, abstract 155, March 7, 2001, Hôpital de la Croix-Rousse, Lyon, France.
29. Rutland J, Griffin WM, Cole PJ: Human ciliary beat frequency in epithelium from intrathoracic and extrathoracic airways. Am Rev Respir Dis 125:100–105, 1982.
30. Williams R, Rankin N, Smith T, et al: Relationship between the humidity and temperature of inspired gas and the function of the airway mucosa. Crit Care Med 24:1920–1929, 1996.
31. Mullen JBM, Wright JL, Wiggs BR, et al: Structure of central airways in current smokers and ex-smokers with and without mucus hypersecretion: Relation to lung function. Thorax 42:843–848, 1987.
32. Mossberg B, Camner P, Afzelius BA: The immotile-cilia syndrome compared to other obstructive lung diseases: A clue to their pathogenesis. Eur J Respir Dis 64(Suppl 127):129–136, 1983.
33. Lange P, Nyboe J, Appleyard M, et al: Relation of ventilatory impairment and of chronic mucus hypersecretion to mortality from obstructive lung disease and from all causes. Thorax 45:579–585, 1990.
34. Iravani J, van As A: Mucus transport in the tracheobronchial tree of normal and bronchitic rats. J Pathol 116:81–93, 1972.
35. Phipps RJ, Richardson PS: The effects of irritation at various levels of the airway upon tracheal mucus secretion in the cat. J Physiol 261:561–581, 1976.
36. Richardson PS, Peatfield AC: The control of airway secretion. Eur J Respir Dis 71(Suppl 153):43–51, 1987.
37. Reid LM, O'Sullivan DD, Bhaskar KR: Pathophysiology of bronchial hypersecretion. Eur J Respir Dis 71(Suppl 153):19–25, 1987.
38. Rubin BK, Ramirez O, Zayas JG, et al: Respiratory mucus from asymptomatic smokers is better hydrated and more easily cleared by mucociliary action. Am Rev Respir Dis 145:545–547, 1992.
39. Bateman JRM, Pavia D, Sheahan NF, et al: Impaired tracheobronchial clearance in patients with mild asthma. Thorax 38:463–467, 1983.
40. Camner P, Mossberg B, Philipson K: Tracheobronchial clearance and chronic obstructive lung disease. Scand J Resp Dis 54:272–281, 1973.
41. Goodman RM, Yergin BM, Landa JF, et al: Relationship of smoking history and pulmonary function tests to tracheal mucous velocity in nonsmokers, young smokers, ex-smokers, and patients with chronic bronchitis. Am Rev Respir Dis 117:205–214, 1978.
42. Santa Cruz R, Landa J, Hirsch J, Sackner MA: Tracheal mucous velocity in normal man and patients with obstructive lung disease: Effects of terbutaline. Am Rev Respir Dis 109:458–463, 1974.
43. Kollberg H, Mossberg B, Afzelius BA, eet al: Cystic fibrosis compared with the immotile-cilia syndrome: A study of mucociliary clearance, ciliary ultrastructure, clinical picture and ventilatory function. Scand J Respir Dis 59:297–306, 1978.
44. Wood P, Wanner A, Hirsch J, Farrel P: Tracheal mucociliary transport in patients with cystic fibrosis and its stimulation by terbutaline. Am Rev Respir Dis 111:733–738, 1975.
45. Yeates D, Sturgess J, Kahn S, et al: Mucociliary transport in the trachea of patients with cystic fibrosis. Arch Dis Child 51:28–33, 1976.
46. Isawa T, Teshima T, Hirano T, et al: Effect of bronchodilation on the deposition and clearance of radioaerosol in bronchial asthma in remission. J Nucl Med 28:1901–1906, 1987.
47. Wilson R, Roberts D, Cole P: Effect of bacterial products on human ciliary function in vitro. Thorax 40:125–131, 1985.
48. Dulfano MJ, Luk CK: Sputum and ciliary inhibition in asthma. Thorax 37:646–651, 1982.
49. Wanner A: The role of mucociliary dysfunction in bronchial asthma. Am J Med 67:477–485, 1979.
50. Pucchelle E, Polu JM, Zahm JM, Sadoul P: Role of the rheological properties of bronchial secretion in the mucociliary transport at the bronchial surface. Eur J Respir Dis 61(Suppl 111):29–34, 1980.
51. Rubin BK: Immotile cilia syndrome (primary ciliary dyskinesia) and airways inflammation. Clin Chest Med 9:657–668, 1988.
52. Pavia D, Lopez-Vidriero MT, Clarke SW: Mediators and mucociliary clearance in asthma. Bull Eur Physiopathol Respir 23(Suppl 10):89s–94s, 1987.
53. George RJD, Johnson MA, Pavia D, et al: Increase in mucociliary clearance in normal man induced by oral high frequency oscillation. Thorax 40:433–437, 1985.
54. Messina MS, O'Riordian TG, Smaldone GC: Changes in mucociliary clearance during acute exacerbations of asthma. Am Rev Respir Dis 143:993–997, 1991.

55. Pavia D, Lopez-Vidriero MT, Clarke SW: Mediators and mucociliary clearance in asthma. Bull Eur Physiopathol Respir 23(Suppl 10):90s–94s, 1987.
56. Pavia D, Bateman JRM, Sheahan NF, et al: Tracheobronchial mucociliary clearance in asthma: Impairment during remission. Thorax 40:171–175, 1985.
57. Iravani J, Melville GN: Long-term effect of cigarette smoke on mucociliary function in animals. Respiration 31:358–366, 1974.
58. Rubin BK, King M: The physiologic effects of smoking in COPD. Eur J Respir Dis 4:S19, 1993.
59. Dormehl I, Ras G, Taylor G, Hugo N: Effect of Pseudomonas aeruginosa-derived pyocyanin and 1-hydrox-yphenazine on pulmonary mucociliary clearance monitored scintigraphically in the baboon model. Nucl Med Biol 18:455–459, 1991.
60. Wilson R, Sykes DA, Currie D, Cole PJ: Beat frequency of cilia from sites of purulent infection. Thorax 41:453–458, 1986.
61. Wilson R: Secondary ciliary dysfunction. Clin Sci 75:113–120, 1988.
62. Regnis JA, Robinson M, Bailey DL, et al: Mucociliary clearance in patients with cystic fibrosis and in normal subjects. Am J Respir Crit Care Med 150:66–71, 1994.
63. King M: Is cystic fibrosis mucus abnormal? Pediatr Res 15:120–122, 1981.
64. Tomkiewicz RP, App EM, Boucher RC, et al: Amiloride inhalation therapy in cystic fibrosis: Its influence on ion content, hydration and rheology of sputum. Am Rev Respir Dis 148:1002–1007, 1993.
65. Rubin BK: A superficial view of mucus and the cystic fibrosis defect. Pediatr Pulmonol 13:4–5, 1993.
66. Webber BA, Pryor JA: Physiotherapy skills: Techniques and adjuncts. In Webber BA, Pryor JA (eds): Physiotherapy for Respiratory and Cardiac Problems. London, Churchill Livingstone, 1993, p 113.
67. Chopra SK, Taplin GV, Simmons DH, et al: Effects of hydration and physical therapy on tracheal transport velocity. Am Rev Respir Dis 115:1009–1014, 1977.
68. Verboon JML, Bakker W, Sterk PJ: The value of the forced expiration technique with and without postural drainage in adults with cystic fibrosis. Eur J Respir Dis 69:169–174, 1986.
69. Wong JW, Keens TG, Wannamaker EM, et al: Effects of gravity on tracheal mucus transport rates in normal subjects and in patients with cystic fibrosis. Paediatrics 60:146–152, 1977.
70. Oldenburg FA, Dolovich MB, Montgomery JM, Newhouse MT: Effects of postural drainage, exercise and cough on mucus clearance in chronic bronchitis. Am Rev Respir Dis 120:730–745, 1979.
71. Chang SC, Chang HI, Shiao GM, Perng RP: Effect of body position on gas exchange in patients with uni-lateral central airway lesions: Down with the good lung. Chest 103:787–791, 1993.
72. Dhainaut JF, Bons J, Bricard C, Monsallier JF: Improved oxygenation in patients with extensive unilateral pneumonia using the lateral decubitus position. Thorax 35:792–793, 1980.
73. Gillespie DJ, Rehder K: Body position and ventilation-perfusion relationships in unilateral pulmonary dis-ease. Chest 92:75–79, 1987.
74. Mahler DA, Snyder PE, Virgulto JA, Loke J: Positional dyspnea and oxygen desaturation related to carci-noma of the lung: Up with the good lung. Chest 83:826–827, 1983.
75. Ross J, Dean E, Abboud RT: The effect of postural drainage positioning on ventilation homogeneity in healthy subjects. Phys Ther 72:794–799, 1992.
76. Marini JJ, Tyler ML, Hudson LD, et al: Influence of head-dependent positions on lung volume and oxygen saturation in chronic air-flow obstruction. Am Rev Respir Dis 129:101–105, 1984.
77. Hansen LG, Warwick WJ, Hansen KL: Mucus transport mechanisms in relation to the effect of high fre-quency chest compression (HFCC) on mucus clearance. Pediatr Pulmonol 17:113–118, 1994.
78. van der Schans CP, Piers DA, Postma DS: Effect of manual percussion on tracheobronchial clearance in patients with chronic airflow obstruction and excessive tracheobronchial secretion. Thorax 41:448–452, 1986.
79. Bateman JRM, Newman SP, Daunt KM, et al: Regional lung clearance of excessive bronchial secretions during chest physiotherapy in patients with stable chronic airways obstruction. Lancet 1:294–297, 1979.
80. Bateman JRM, Newman SP, Daunt KM, et al: Is cough as effective as chest physiotherapy in the removal of excessive tracheobronchial secretions? Thorax 36:683–687, 1981.
81. Sutton PP, Parker RA, Webber BA, et al: Assessment of the forced expiration technique, postural drainage and directed coughing in chest physiotherapy. Eur J Respir Dis 64:62–68, 1983.
82. Rossman CM, Waldes R, Sampson D, Newhouse MT: Effect of chest physiotherapy on the removal of mucus in patients with cystic fibrosis. Am Rev Respir Dis 126:131–135, 1982.
83. Cochrane GM, Webber BA, Clarke SW: Effects of sputum on pulmonary function, Br Med J 2:1181–1183, 1977.
84. Feldman J, Traver GA, Taussig LM: Maximal expiratory flows after postural drainage. Am Rev Respir Dis 119:239–245, 1979.
85. Desmond KJ, Schwenk WF, Thomas E, et al: Immediate and long-term effects of chest physiotherapy in patients with cystic fibrosis. J Pediatr 103:538–542, 1983.
86. Tecklin JS, Holsclaw DS: Evaluation of bronchial drainage in patients with cystic fibrosis. Phys Ther 55:1081–1084,1975.

87. Weller PH, Bush E, Preece MA, Matthew DJ: Short-term effects of chest physiotherapy on pulmonary function in children with cystic fibrosis. Respiration 40:53–56, 1980.

88. Campbell AH, O'Connell JM, Wilson F: The effect of chest physiotherapy upon the FEV I in chronic bronchitis. Med J Aust 1:33–35, 1975.

89. March H: Appraisal of postural drainage for chronic obstructive pulmonary disease. Arch Phys Med Rehabil 52:528–530, 1971.

90. Mazzocco MC, Owens GR, Kirilloff LH, Rogers RM: Chest percussion and postural drainage in patients with bronchiectasis. Chest 88:360–363, 1985.

91. Mohsenifar Z, Rosenberg N, Goldberg HS, Koerner SK: Mechanical vibration and conventional chest physiotherapy in outpatients with stable chronic obstructive lung disease. Chest 87:483–485, 1985.

92. Newton DAG, Stephenson A: Effect of physiotherapy on pulmonary function. Lancet 228–230, 1978.

93. Kerrebijn KF, Veentjer R, Bonzet-van de Water E: The immediate effect of physiotherapy and aerosol treatment on pulmonary function in children with cystic fibrosis. Eur J Respir Dis 63:35–42, 1982.

94. Zapletal A, Stefanova J, Horak J, et al: Chest physiotherapy and airway obstruction in patients with cystic fibrosis: A negative report. Eur J Respir Dis 64:426–433, 1983.

95. Bain J, Bishop J, Olinsky A: Evaluation of directed coughing in cystic fibrosis. Br J Dis Chest 82:138–148, 1988.

96. de Boeck C, Zinman R: Cough versus chest physiotherapy: A comparison of the acute effects on pulmonary function in patients with cystic fibrosis. Am Rev Respir Dis 129:182–184, 1984.

97. Hammon WE, Connors AF, McCaffree DR: Cardiac arrhythmias during postural drainage and chest percussion of critically ill patients. Chest 102:1836–1841, 1992.

98. Tyler ML: Complications of positioning and chest physiotherapy. Respir Care 27:458–466, 1982.

99. Anthonisen P, Riis P, Søgaard-Andersen T: The value of lung physiotherapy in the treatment of acute exacerbations in chronic bronchitis. Acta Med Scand 175:715–719, 1964.

100. Britton S, Bejstedt M, Vedin L: Chest physiotherapy in primary pneumonia. Brit Med J 290:1703–1704, 1985.

101. Graham WGB, Bradley DA: Efficacy of chest physiotherapy and intermittent positive pressure breathing in the resolution of pneumonia. N Engl J Med 199:624–627, 1978.

102. Conway JH, Fleming JS, Perring S, Holgate SD: Humidification as an adjunct to chest physiotherapy in aiding tracheo-bronchial clearance in patients with bronchiectasis. Respir Med 86:110–116, 1992.

103. Sutton PP, Gemell HG, Innes N, et al: Use of nebulized saline and nebulized terbutaline as an adjunct to chest physiotherapy. Thorax 43:57–60, 1988.

104. Marchette LC, Marchette BE, Abraham WM, Wanner A: The effect of systemic hydration on normal and impaired mucociliary function. Pediatr Pulmon 1:107–111, 1985.

105. Currie DC, Munro C, Gaskell D, Cole PJ: Practice, problems and compliance with postural drainage: A survey of chronic sputum producers. Br J Dis Chest 80:249–253, 1986.

106. App EM, Lohse P, Matthys H, King M: Physiotherapy and mechanical breakdown of the excessive DNA load in CF sputum: An anti-inflammatory therapeutic strategy. Pediatr Pulmonol 17(Suppl):349, 1998.

107. Tomkiewicz RP, Biviji AA, King M: Effects of oscillating air flow on the rheological properties and clearability of mucous gel stimulants. Biorheology 31:511–520, 1994.

108. Dasgupta B, Tomkiewicz RP, Boyd WP, et al: Effects of combined treatment with rhDNAase and airflow oscillations on spinability of cystic fibrosis sputum in vitro. Pediatr Pulmonol 20:78–82, 1995.

109. Chang HK, Weber ME, King M: Mucus transport by high frequency nonsymetrical airflow. J Appl Physiol 65:1203–1209, 1988.

110. Warwick W: High-frequency chest wall compression moves mucus by means of sustained staccato coughs. Pediatr Pulmonol 6(Suppl):283, 1991.

111. Freitag L, Long WM, Kim CS, Wanner A: Removal of excessive bronchial secretions by asymmetric high-frequency oscillations. J Appl Physiol 67:614–619, 1989.

112. King M, Phillips DM, Gross D, et al: Enhanced tracheal mucus clearance with high frequency chest wall compression. Am Rev Respir Dis 128:511–515, 1983.

113. Rubin EM, Scantlen GE, Chapman GA, et al: Effect of chest wall oscillation on mucus clearance: comparison of two vibrators. Pediatr Pulmonol 6:123–127, 1989.

114. Radford R, Barutt J, Billingsley JG, et al: A rational basis for percussion augmented mucociliary clearance. Respir Care 27:556–563, 1982.

115. Gross D, Zidulka A, O'Brien C, et al: Peripheral mucociliary clearance with high frequency chest-wall compression. J Appl Physiol 58:1157–1163, 1985.

116. Jones RL, Lester RT, Brown NE: Effects of high-frequency chest compression on respiratory system mechanics in normal subjects and cystic fibrosis patients. Can Respir J 2:40–46, 1995.

117. Pavia D, Thomson ML, Phillipakos D: A preliminary study of the effect of a vibrating pad on bronchial clearance. Am Rev Respir Dis 113:92–96, 1976.

118. Sutton PP, Lopez-Vidriero MT, Pavia D, et al: Assessment of percussion, vibratory-shaking and breathing exercises in chest physiotherapy. Eur J Respir Dis 66:147–152, 1985.

119. Pryor JA, Parker RA, Webber BA: A comparison of mechanical and manual percussion as adjuncts to postural drainage in the treatment of cystic fibrosis in adolescents and adults. Physiotherapy 6:140–141, 1981.

120. Sutton PP, Parker RA, Webber BA, et al: Assessment of the forced expiration technique, postural drainage and directed coughing in chest physiotherapy. Eur J Respir Dis 64:62–68, 1983.
121. van Hengstum M, Festen J, Beurskens C, et al: No effect of oral high frequency oscillation combined with forced expiration maneuvers on tracheobronchial clearance in chronic bronchitis. Eur Respir J 3:14–18, 1990.
122. Gallon A: Evaluation of chest percussion in the treatment of patients with copious sputum production. Respir Med 85:45–51, 1991.
123. Flower KA, Eden RI, Lomax L, et al: New mechanical aid to physiotherapy in cystic fibrosis. Br Med J 2:630–631, 1979.
124. King M, Phillips DM, Zidulka A, Chang HK: Tracheal mucus clearance in high-frequency oscillation. Am Rev Respir Dis 130:703–706, 1984.
125. King M, Zidulka A, Phillips DM, et al: Tracheal mucus clearance in high-frequency oscillation: Effect of peak flow rate bias. Eur Respir J 3:6–13, 1990.
126. Castagnino M, Vojtova J, Kaminski S, Fink R: Safety of high-frequency chest wall oscillation in patients with respiratory muscle weakness. Chest 110:S65, 1996.
127. Chiappetta A, Beckerman R: High-frequency chest-wall oscillation in spinal muscular atrophy. J Respir Care Pract 8:112–114, 1995.
128. Toussaint M, De Win H, Steens M, Soudon P. A new technique in secretion clearance by the percussionaire for patients with neuromuscular disease. [abstract]. In Programme des Journées Internationales de Ventilation à Domicile, Hôpital de la Croix Rousse, Lyon, France, 1993, p 27.
129. McInturff SL, Shaw LI, Hodgkin JE, et al: Intrapulmonary percussive ventilation in the treatment of COPD. Respir Care 30:885, 1985.
130. Falk M, Kelstrup M, Andersen JB, et al: Improving the ketchup bottle method with positive expiratory pressure (PEP): A controlled study in patients with cystic fibrosis. Eur J Respir Dis 65:57–66, 1984.
131. Arens R, Gozal D, Omlin KJ, et al: Comparison of high frequency chest compression and conventional chest physiotherapy in hospitalized patients with cystic fibrosis. Am J Respir Crit Care Med 150:1154–1157, 1994.
132. Braggion C, Cappelletti LM, Cornacchia M, et al: Short-term effects of three chest physiotherapy regimens in patients hospitalized for pulmonary exacerbations of cystic fibrosis: A cross-over randomized study. Pediatr Pulmonol 19:16–22, 1995.
133. Burnett M, Takis C, Hoffmeyer B, et al: Comparative efficacy of manual chest physiotherapy and a high-frequency heat compression vest in inpatient treatment of cystic fibrosis. Am Rev Respir Dis 147(Suppl):A30, 1993.
134. Scherer TA, Barandun J, Martinez E, et al: Effect of high-frequency oral airway and chest wall oscillation and conventional chest physical therapy on expectoration in patients with stable cystic fibrosis. Chest 113:1019–1027, 1998.
135. Whitman J, Van Beusekom R, Olson S, et al: Preliminary evaluation of high-frequency chest compression for secretion clearance in mechanically ventilated patients. Respir Care 38:1081–1087, 1993.
136. Anbar RD, Powelkl KN, Iannuzzi DM: Short-term effect of ThAIRapy Vest on pulmonary function of cystic fibrosis patients. Am J Respir Crit Care Med 157:A130, 1998.
137. Warwick WJ, Hansen LG: The long-term effect of high-frequency chest compression therapy on pulmonary complications of cystic fibrosis. Pediatr Pulmonol 11:265–271, 1991.
138. Hull KK, Warren RH: ThAIRapy Vest vs. conventional chest physical therapy: Case report. Respir Care 36:1266–1267, 1991.
139. Kluft J, beker L, Castagnino M, et al: A comparison of bronchial drainage treatments in cystic fibrosis. Pediatr Pulmonol 22:271–274, 1996.
140. Oermann CM, Accurso F, Castile R, Sockrider MM: Evaluation of the safety, efficacy and impact on quality of life of the ThAIRapy Vest and flutter compared to conventional chest physical therapy in patients with cystic fibrosis. Am J Respir Crit Care Med 155(Suppl 4):A638, 1997.
141. Perry RJ, Man GCW, Jones RL: Effects of positive end-expiratory pressure on oscillated flow rate during high-frequency chest compression. Chest 113:1028–1033, 1998.
142. Klous DR, Boyle M, Hazelwood A, McComb RC: Chest vest and CF: Better care for patients. Adv Mgrs Respir Care 2:45–50, 1993.
143. Piquet J, Brochard L, Isabey D, et al: High frequency chest wall oscillation in patients with chronic air-flow obstruction. Am Rev Respir Dis 136:1355–1359, 1987.
144. Sibuya M, Yamada M, Kanamaru A, et al: Effect of chest wall vibration on dyspnea in patients with chronic respiratory disease. Am J Respir Crit Care Med 149:1235–1240, 1994.
145. Holody B, Goldberg HS: The effect of mechanical vibration physiotherapy on arterial oxygenation in acutely ill patients with atelectasis or pneumonia. Am Rev Respir Dis 124:372–375, 1981.
146. Zidulka A, Chrome JF, Wight DW, et al: Clapping or percussion causes atelectasis in dogs and influences gas exchange. J Appl Physiol 66:2833–2838, 1989.
147. Menkes HA, Traystman RJ: Collateral ventilation. Am Rev Respir Dis 116:287–309, 1977.
148. Peters RM: Pulmonary physiologic studies of the perioperative period. Chest 76:576–584, 1979.

149. Hofmeyer JL, Webber BA, Hodson ME: Evaluation of positive expiratory pressure as an adjunct to chest physiotherapy in the treatment of cystic fibrosis. Thorax 41;951–954, 1986.
150. Mortensen J, Falk M, Groth S, Jensen C: The effects of postural drainage and positive expiratory pressure physiotherapy on tracheobronchial clearance in cystic fibrosis. Chest 100:1350–1357, 1991.
151. Tyrrell JC, Hiller EJ, Martin J: Short reports: Face mask physiotherapy in cystic fibrosis. Arch Dis Child 61:598–611, 1986.
152. van Asperen PP, Jackson L, Hennessy P, Brown J: Comparison of positive expiratory pressure (PEP) mask with postural drainage in patients with cystic fibrosis. Aust Paediatr J 23:283–284, 1987.
153. van der Schans CP, van der Mark ThW, de Vries G, et al: Effect of positive expiratory pressure breathing in patients with cystic fibrosis. Thorax 46:252–256, 1991.
154. Olséni L, Midgren B, Hörnblad Y, Wollmer P: Chest physiotherapy in chronic obstructive pulmonary disease: forced expiratory technique combined with either postural drainage or positive expiratory pressure breathing. Respir Med 88:435–440, 1994.
155. van Hengstum M, Festen J, Beurskens C, et al: The effect of positive expiratory pressure versus forced expiration technique on tracheobronchial clearance in chronic bronchitis. Scand J Gastrenterol 23(Suppl 143):114–118, 1988.
156. Groth S, Stafanger G, Dirksen H, et al: Positive expiratory pressure (PEP mask) physiotherapy improves ventilation and reduces volume of trapped gas in cystic fibrosis. Bull Eur Physiopathol Respir 21:339–343, 1985.
157. Tonnesen P, Stovring S: Positive expiratory pressure (PEP) as lung physiotherapy in cystic fibrosis: A pilot study. Eur J Respir Dis 65:419–422, 1984.
158. Herala M, Gislason T: Chest physiotherapy. Evaluation by transcutaneous blood gas monitoring. Chest 93:800–802, 1988.
159. Kaminska TM, Pearson SB: A comparison of postural drainage and positive expiratory pressure in the domiciliary management of patients with chronic bronchial sepsis. Physiotherapy 74:251–254, 1988.
160. Christensen EF, Nedergaard T, Dahl R: Long-term treatment of chronic bronchitis with positive expiratory pressure mask and chest physiotherapy. Chest 97:645–650, 1990.
161. Christensen HR, Simonsen K, Lange P, et al: PEEP-mask in patients with severe obstructive pulmonary disease: A negative report. Eur J Respir Dis 3:267–272, 1990.
162. Oberwaldner B, Evans JC, Zach MS: Forced expirations against a variable resistance: A new chest physiotherapy method in cystic fibrosis. Pediatr Pulmonol 2:358–367, 1986.
163. Schibler A, Casaulta C, Kraemer R: Rationale of oscillatory breathing in patients with cystic fibrosis. Paediatr Pulmonol 8:301S, 1992.
164. Konstan MW, Stern RC, Doershuk CF: Efficacy of the flutter device for airway mucus clearance in patients with cystic fibrosis. J Pediatr 124:689–693, 1994.
165. Pryor JA, Webber BA, Hodson ME, Warner JO: The Flutter VRP1 as an adjunct to chest physiotherapy in cystic fibrosis. Respir Med 88:677–681, 1994.
166. Bellone A, Lascioli R, Raschi S, Guzzi L, Adone R: Chest physical therapy in patients with acute exacerbation of chronic bronchitis: Effectiveness of three methods. Arch Phys Med Rehabil 81:558–560, 2000.
167. Langlands J: The dynamics of cough in health and in chronic bronchitis. Thorax 22:88–96, 1967.
168. Clarke SW, Jones JG, Oliver DR: Resistance to two-phase gas-liquid flow in airways. J Appl Physiol 9:359–372, 1970.
169. Leith DE: Cough. Phys Ther 48:439–447, 1968.
170. Kim CS, Rodriguez CR, Eldridge MA, Sackner MA: Criteria for mucus transport in the airways by two-phase gas-liquid flow mechanism. J Appl Physiol 60:901–907, 1986.
171. Sackner MA, Kim CS: Phasic flow mechanisms of mucus clearance. Eur J Respir Dis 71(Suppl 153):159–164, 1987.
172. Warwick WJ: Mechanisms of mucous transport. Eur J Respir Dis 64(Suppl 127):162–167, 1983.
173. Wolff RK, Dolovich MB, Obminski G, Newhouse MT: Effects of exercise and eucapnic hyperventilation on bronchial chearance in man. J Appl Physiol 43:46–50, 1977.
174. Clarke SW: Rationale of airway clearance Eur Respir J 7(Suppl):599s–603s, 1989.
175. Scherer PW: Mucus transport by cough. Chest 80:830–833, 1981.
176. Pedersen OF, Nielsen TM: The critical transmural pressure of the airway. Acta Physiol Scand 97:426–446, 1976.
177. Mead J, Turner JM, Macklem PT, Little JB: Significance of the relationship between lung recoil and maximum expiratory flow. J Appl Physiol 22:95–108, 1967.
178. Agarwal M, King M, Rubin BK, Shukla JB: Mucus transport in a miniaturized simulated cough machine: effect of constriction and serous layer simulant. Biorheology 26:977–988, 1989.
179. van der Schans CP, Ramirez OE, Postma DS, et al: Effect of airway constriction on the cough transportability of mucus. Am J Respir Crit Care Med 149:A1023, 1994.
180. Arora NS, Gal TJ: Cough dynamics during progressive expiratory muscle weakness in healthy curarized subjects. J Appl Physiol 51:494–498, 1981.
181. van der Schans CP, Piers DA, Beekhuis H, et al: Effect of forced expirations on mucus clearance in patients with chronic airflow obstruction: Effect of lung recoil pressure. Thorax 45:623–627, 1990.

182. Zahm JM, King M, Duvivier C, et al: Role of simulated repetitive coughing in mucus clearance. Eur Respir J 4:311–315, 1991.

183. Bennett WD, Foster WM, Chapman WF: Cough-enhanced mucus clearance in the normal lung. J Appl Physiol 69:1670–1675, 1990.

184. Pryor JA, Webber BA, Hodson ME, Batten JC: Evaluation of the forced expiration technique as an adjunct to postural drainage in treatment of cystic fibrosis. Br Med J 2:417–418, 1979.

185. van Hengstum M, Festen J, Beurskens C, et al: Conventional physiotherapy and forced expiration maneuvers have similar effects on tracheobronchial clearance. Eur J Respir Dis 1:758–761,1988.

186. Webber BA, Hofmeyer JL, Morgan MD, Hodson ME: Effects of postural drainage: Incorporating forced expiration technique on pulmonary function in cystic fibrosis. Br J Dis Chest 80:353–359, 1986.

187. Hasani A, Pavia D, Agnew JE, Clarke SW: The effect of unproductive coughing/FET on regional mucus movement in the human lungs. Respir Med 85:23–26, 1991.

188. Lannefors L, Wollmer R: Mucus clearance with three chest physiotherapy regimens in cystic fibrosis: A comparison between postural drainage, PEP and physical exercise. Eur Respir J 5:748–753, 1992.

189. Hasani A, Pavia D, Agnew JE, Clarke SW: Regional lung clearance during cough and forced expiration technique (FET): Effects of flow and viscoelasticity. Thorax 49:557–561, 1994.

190. Reisman JJ, Rivington-Law B, Corey M, et al: Role of conventional physiotherapy in cystic fibrosis. J Pediatr 113:632–636, 1988.

191. Zach MS, Oberwaldner B, Forche G, Polgar G: Bronchodilators increase airway stability in cystic fibrosis. Am Rev Respir Dis 131:537–543, 1985.

192. Desmond KJ, Demizio DL, Allen PD, et al: Effect of salbutamol on gas compression in cystic fibrosis and asthma. Am J Respir Crit Care Med 149:673–677, 1994.

193. Bennett WD, Chapman WF, Mascarella JM: The acute effect of ipratropium bromide bronchodilator therapy on cough clearance in COPD. Chest 103:488–495, 1993.

194. Bach JR: Mechanical insufflation-exsufflation: Comparison of peak expiratory flows with manually assisted and unassisted coughing techniques. Chest 104:1553–1562, 1993.

195. Bach JR, Smith WH, Michaels J, et al: Airway secretion clearance by mechanical exsufflation for post-poliomyelitis ventilator assisted individuals. Arch Phys Med Rehabil 74:170–177, 1993.

196. Barach AL, Beck GJ: Exsufflation with negative pressure. Arch Intern Med 93:825–841, 1954.

197. Estenne M, van Muylem A, Gorini M, et al: Evidence of dynamic airway compression during cough in tetraplegic patients. Am J Respir Crit Care Med 150:1081–1085, 1994.

198. Estenne M, Knoop C, Vanvaerenbergh J, et al: The effect of pectoralis muscle training in tetraplegic subjects. Am Rev Respir Dis 139:1218–1222, 1989.

199. Estenne M, De Troyer A: Cough in tetraplegic subjects: An active process. Ann Intern Med 112:22–28, 1990.

200. Estenne M, Van Muylem A, Gorini M, et al: Evidence of dynamic airway compression during cough in tetraplegic patients. Am J Respir Crit Care Med 150(4):1081–1085, 1994.

201. van der Schans CP, Piers DA, Mulder GA: Efficacy of coughing in tetraplegic patients. Spine 25:2200–2203, 2000.

202. Wolff RK, Dolovich MB, Obminski G, Newhouse MT: Effects of exercise and eucapnic hyperventilation on bronchial clearance in man. J Appl Physiol 43:46–50, 1977.

203. Zach MS, Purrer B, Oberwaldner B: Effect of swimming on forced expiration and sputum clearance in cystic fibrosis. Lancet 2:1201–1203, 1982.

204. Baldwin DR, Hill AL, Peckham DG, Knox AJ: Effect of addition of exercise to chest physiotherapy on sputum expectoration and lung function in adults with cystic fibrosis. Respir Med 88:49–53, 1994.

205. Cerny F: Relative effects of bronchial drainage and exercise for in-hospital care of patients with cystic fibrosis. Phys Ther 69:633–639, 1989.

206. Zach MS, Oberwaldner B, Häusler F: Cystic fibrosis: Physical exercise versus chest physiotherapy. Arch Dis Child 57:587–589, 1982.

207. Bilton D, Dodd M, Abbot JV, Webb AK: The benefits of exercise combined with physiotherapy in the treatment of adults with cystic fibrosis. Respir Med 86:507–511, 1992.

208. Salh W, Bilton D, Dodd M, Webb AK: Effect of exercise and physiotherapy in aiding sputum expectoration in adults with cystic fibrosis. Thorax 44:1006–1008, 1989.

209. Schöni MH: Autogenic drainage: A modern approach to physiotherapy in cystic fibrosis, J Royal Soc Med 82(Suppl 16):32–37, 1989.

210. Haberman PB, Green JP, Archibald C, et al: Determinants of successful selective tracheobronchial suctioning. N Engl J Med 289:1060–1063, 1973.

211. Hanley MV, Rudd T, Butler J: What happens to intratracheal saline instillations. Am Rev Respir Dis 117(Suppl):124, 1978.

212. Hilding AC: Experimental bronchoscopy in calves: Injury and repair of tracheobronchial epithelium after passage of bronchoscope. Am Rev Respir Dis 98:646–652, 1968.

213. Jung RC, Gottlieb LS: Comparison of tracheobronchial suction catheters in humans. Visualization by fiberoptic bronchoscopy. Chest 69:179–181, 1976.

214. Sackner MA, Landa JF, Greeneltch N, Robinson MJ: Pathogenesis and prevention of tracheobronchial damage with suction procedures. Chest 64:284–290, 1973.
215. Petersen GM, Pierson DJ, Hunter PM: Arterial oxygen saturation during nasotracheal suctioning. Chest 76:283–287, 1979.
216. Rindfleisch SH, Tyler ML: Duration of suctioning: An important variable. Respir Care 28:457–459, 1983.
217. Boutros AR: Arterial blood oxygenation during and after endotracheal suctioning in the apneic patient. Anaesthesiology 32:114–118, 1970.
218. Gunderson LP, Stone KS, Hamlin RL: Endotracheal suctioning-induced heart rate alterations. Nurs Res 40:139–143, 1991.
219. Shim C, Fine Fernandez R, Williams MH: Cardiac arrhythmias resulting from tracheal suctioning. Ann Intern Med 71:1149–1153, 1969.
220. Stone KS, Preuser BA, Groch KF, et al: The effect of lung hyperinflation and endotracheal suctioning on cardiopulmonary hemodynamics. Nurs Res 40:76–80, 1991.
221. LeFrock JL, Klainer AS, Wu WH, Turndor FH: Transient bacteremia associated with nasotracheal suctioning. JAMA 236:1610–1611, 1976.
222. Hubert J: Kinesitherapie Respiratoire. Les Editions Medicales et Paramedicales de Charleroi, Montignies-sur-Sambre, Belgium, 1989.
223. Patterson JM, Budd J, Goetz D, Warwick WJ: Family correlates of a 10-year pulmonary health trend in cystic fibrosis. Pediatrics 91:383–389, 1993.
224. Fong SL, Dales RE, Tierney MG: Compliance among adults with cystic fibrosis. Drug Intell Clin Pharm 24:689–692, 1990.
225. Passero MA, Remor B, Salamon J: Patient-reported compliance with cystic fibrosis. Clin Pediatr 20:264–268, 1981.
226. Garstang SV, Kirshblum SC, Wood KE: Patient preference for in-exsufflation for secretion management with spinal cord injury. J Spinal Cord Med 23:80–85, 2000.
227. Tzeng AC, Bach JR: Prevention of pulmonary morbidity for patients with neuromuscular disease. Chest 118:1390–1396, 2000.
228. Bach JR, Ishikawa Y, Kim H: Prevention of pulmonary morbidity for patients with Duchenne muscular dystrophy. Chest 112:1024–1028, 1997.

14 —— Nutrition

IRVING I. HABER, D.O.
JOHN R. BACH, M.D.
JILL GAYDOS, M.S.

Severe catabolism and loss of lean body mass are well-recognized complications of chronic obstructive pulmonary disease (COPD). Loss of lean body mass also occurs in patients with neuromuscular disease (NMD). In fact, malnutrition and weight loss are independent and significant determinants of morbidity and mortality for people with pulmonary impairment, whether due to intrinsic lung disease or respiratory muscle dysfunction.[1]

In addition to loss of lean muscle in patients with NMD, weight loss can be caused by imbalance between caloric intake and energy expenditure. Some NMDs also are associated with inborn errors of metabolism. Significant weight loss has been reported in 10–26% of outpatients and up to 47% of hospitalized patients with COPD. Likewise, weight loss to a mean total body weight of 70 lb has been reported in patients with Duchenne muscular dystrophy (DMD) at the point when ventilator use is required.[2]

NUTRITIONAL REQUIREMENTS

Recommended daily allowances (RDAs) are used to estimate nutrient needs. They are designed to provide a margin of safety. Even in the general population, however, RDAs may not be adequate. Elderly people often have inadequate gastrointestinal absorption of specific nutrients. Younger patients can develop malabsorption abnormalities, especially with the presence of gastrointestinal or certain other medical conditions. In addition, many people eating overly processed foods and few vegetables and fruit simply may not receive enough of many nutrients. It also has been estimated that up to 70% of all children do not receive adequate calcium from their daily diets.

Nutrient requirements of the normal infant and child are complicated by rate of growth, physical activity, and increased basal energy expenditure. The RDAs for children were estimated using intakes of normally growing infants and the nutrient content of human milk. The needs for children with NMD or generalized medical conditions can be quite different.

The best way to measure adequacy of nutrient intake is to monitor growth. Infancy is a period of rapid growth. Calorie needs per unit of body size are greater than those for adults. Normally, infants aged 0–5 months require 108 kcal/kg, 2.2 gm/kg of protein, and 100 ml/kg of fluid per day. Six- to 12-month-old infants normally require 98 kcal/kg, 1.6 gm/kg of protein, and 100 ml/kg of fluid. Older children require 1000 ml plus 50 ml/kg if they weigh more than 10 kg. As the rate of growth slows, calorie needs per unit of body weight decline. Protein needs per unit of body weight are also greater for an infant than for an adult. The increased requirement allows tissue replacement and growth. Protein intake recommendations are based on the composition of human milk. Fluid needs are determined by the amount of water lost through the skin, lungs, urine, and feces as well as the amount needed for growth. The renal concentrating capacity of the infant is less than that of an older child, placing infants at greater risk for water imbalance.

Although breast milk is usually ideal, infant formulas provide the appropriate distribution of essential nutrients under normal conditions when breast-feeding is contraindicated. As in human milk, it is recommended that infants receive at least 30–50% of total calories from fat. Fat is an important source of calories for the young infant and helps to spare protein for tissue synthesis. Infant formulas are grouped into standard, soy, protein hydrolysate, and elemental formulas. When noninfant formulas are used for infants, they must be supplemented to ensure that the RDA is achieved for all essential nutrients.

PATHOPHYSIOLOGIC EFFECTS OF WEIGHT LOSS OR GAIN

As little as 10% weight loss from ideal levels is associated with loss of physiologic adaptability and high morbidity.[3] The greater the weight loss, the poorer the prognosis for any degree of lung disease (Fig. 1). Short-term starvation decreases lung connective

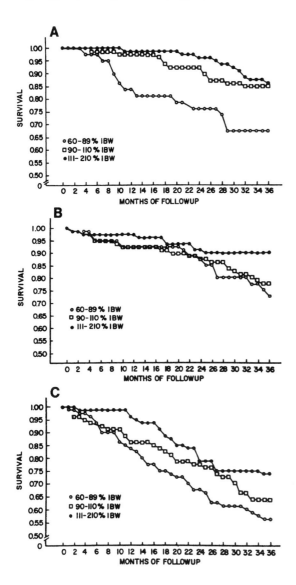

FIGURE 1. Survival curves for patients with mild *(A)*, moderate *(B)*, and severe *(C)* airflow obstruction. (From Wilson DO, Rogers RM, Wright EC, Anthonisen NR: Body weight in chronic obstructive pulmonary disease: The National Institutes of Health intermittent positive pressure breathing trial. Am Rev Respir Dis 139:1435–1438, 1989, with permission.)

tissue, protein synthesis, and surfactant.[4-6] Three weeks of semistarvation in rats led to increases in lung compliance, surface forces, and alveolar volume.[6-8] Forty-percent weight loss was associated with reduction of elastic recoil pressures, enlargement of terminal air spaces, and smaller alveolar surface areas.[9] In addition, the resulting reduction in lung RNA and RNA-to-DNA ratios implies a diminished response to illness or injury.[10] This result is particularly detrimental for patients with respiratory or ventilatory impairment, who have a high risk of lung injury when intercurrent respiratory infections result in pulmonary infiltrates and scarring because of impaired pulmonary defense mechanisms. In addition, rats restricted to one-third of normal caloric intake for 6 weeks developed emphysema-like lung changes,[11] which resembled the lesions found in victims of starvation from the Warsaw ghetto.[12] Such changes may result from lung damage due to protease-induced protein catabolism caused by the alpha$_1$-antitrypsin deficiency associated with malnutrition.[13]

Prolonged food or nutritional deprivation impairs respiratory muscle function by reducing available energy substrates. In chronic starvation, branched-chain amino acids, a component of muscle tissues, become an important energy substrate for diaphragm activity. The rate of the degradation of branched-chain amino acids by the diaphragms of semi-starved rats is 10–20 times greater than normal (Fig. 2).[14] In certain NMDs associated with impaired fatty acid oxidation, even a few hours of fasting can result in degradation of muscle protein.

Malnutrition impairs cell-mediated and humoral immunity,[15,16] and alveolar macrophage phagocytic activity decreases.[17,18] Bacterial adherence to the lower airways increases in undernourished patients with indwelling tracheostomy tubes.[19] In addition, deficiencies in specific nutrients can have repercussions for respiratory function. Hypophosphatemia, which may be due to malnutrition or rapid glucose loading, can trigger acute respiratory insufficiency or difficulty in weaning from assisted ventilation.[20] Similarly, excessive carbohydrate intake increases carbon dioxide production. The additional load can pose a problem for patients with intrinsic lung disease and scoliotic patients, whose hypercapnia cannot be easily corrected by the use of inspiratory muscle aids. Drug pharmacokinetics, intestinal absorption, metabolism, and volume of distribution also can be altered, leading to a decrease in response to medication.[21]

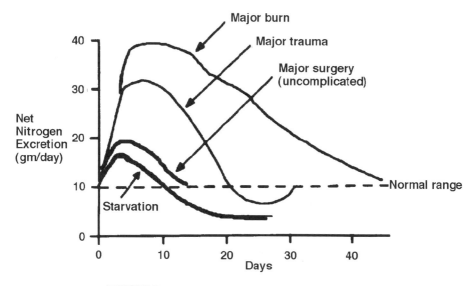

FIGURE 2.   Nitrogen loss associated with undernutrition.

Nutritional deficiencies lead to muscle wasting and impairment of physiologic functioning of the diaphragm and other respiratory and skeletal muscles. Maximal diaphragm isometric strength,[22,23] endurance, maximal static inspiratory and expiratory pressures,[23,24] and maximal voluntary ventilation decrease during fasting.[24] In addition, semistarvation blunts hypoxic[25,26] and hypercapnic[27] ventilatory drive. It is not surprising that ventilatory failure can result from starvation alone.

Obesity is also a frequently encountered problem, especially early in the course of NMD. Obesity can compromise ventilatory dynamics and central regulation of both spontaneous and assisted ventilation and also impairs mobility and leads to skin pressure problems.

Thus, a combination of the direct biochemical effects of undernutrition and the indirect effects of under- or overnutrition can predispose patients to respiratory tract infections, atelectasis, chronic alveolar hypoventilation, and impaired pulmonary defense and repair mechanisms.

CAUSES OF MALNUTRITION AND WASTING

The underlying mechanisms for wasting include decreased oral intake of nutrients, malabsorption of nutrients, and altered metabolism of nutrients, all of which increase resting energy expenditure (REE) or favor the preservation of adipose tissue over lean body mass. In addition, many patients with lung disease or NMD are treated with glucocorticoids. Glucocorticoids can further potentiate loss of type II muscle fiber mass and decrease lean body mass. Type I oxidation fibers, because they are in continuous use, may have an advantage in maintaining relative mass. Recent data in rat studies show a significant decrease in diaphragmatic muscle strength even with minimal dosing of methylprednisolone over a relatively short time.[28] A cortisol-related decrease in androgenic hormones also can result in loss of lean body mass.

Several studies indicate that the hypermetabolism due to the high work of breathing[29] rather than reduced caloric intake is the primary cause of malnutrition in patients with COPD[29] (Fig. 3). However, despite the hypercatabolic state, patients with COPD also may

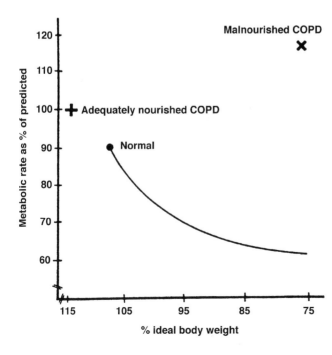

FIGURE 3. Metabolic rate as a function of body weight in normal volunteers subjected to semistarvation and well-nourished and undernourished patients with chronic obstructive pulmonary disease. (From Wilson DO, Donahoe M, Rogers RM, Pennock BE: Metabolic rate and weight loss in chronic obstructive lung disease. J Parent Ent Nutr 14:7–11, 1990, with permission.)

decrease food intake because of dyspnea, gastrointestinal side effects of medications, anorexia, and difficulty with meal preparation due to related energy expenditure. Folate and vitamin B_{12} deficiencies, as well as other forms of avitaminoses, are common in patients with COPD. Lowered antioxidant levels also can potentiate emphysematous changes in lung parenchyma.

Decreased nutrient intake also may be related to eating difficulties resulting from cognitive impairments, central nervous system infections, neurologic or psychiatric abnormalities (e.g., dysphagia, depression, dementia), pharyngeal or esophageal disease, or loss of appetite that in patients with COPD and occasionally in patients with NMD may be associated with medications, bloating, and shortness of breath. Decreased nutrient intake also can result from vomiting or diarrhea.[21] Chronic undernutrition is also quite common in patients with NMD because skeletal muscle weakness, upper extremity musculotendinous contractures, and hand deformities impair the ability to feed oneself.[30,31] Bulbar muscle weakness or the presence of an indwelling tracheostomy tube also may impair swallowing.

In addition to the many reasons for malnutrition, patients with NMD, especially children, may have little tolerance for fasting. They have low muscle buffering capacity with little muscle carbohydrate, protein, and mineral stores. Normally, liver glycogen is metabolized to glucose to sustain blood glucose levels for 6–8 hours after a meal. With continued fasting, muscle degrades protein to amino acids, which enter the blood and are converted to glucose by the liver. Within 3 hours of a normal meal, blood glucose and amino acid levels of infants with spinal muscle atrophy (SMA) decrease to levels that would not be reached until after at least 8 hours of fasting in unaffected children.[32] Patients with SMA, therefore, tend to have low blood glucose levels. When blood glucose and amino acid levels are low, muscle protein is catabolized; when blood glucose and amino acid levels are high, muscle protein is synthesized. Furthermore, infants with SMA type 1 do not efficiently metabolize fatty acids, another major source of energy during fasting. As discussed below, these children may have high levels of fatty acid byproducts in urine and blood after overnight fasting. For the average unaffected child or adult, the amount of muscle protein that is degraded in one day of fasting may be only 1% of total muscle mass, whereas for a child with NMD who may have less than 10% of normal mass, a much greater proportion is sacrificed. Thus, even the small net loss of protein during normal overnight fasting may be significant for a child with SMA.

Likewise, more than the RDA intake of vitamins, minerals, and protein may be necessary.[33] Vitamin D functions in the absorption of calcium and phosphorous. Deficiencies of vitamin D, calcium, and magnesium lead to reduced bone mineral content. Even though intake of vitamin D and calcium may be adequate, decreased intestinal absorption of calcium and vitamin D, along with drug interactions and lack of physical activity, can decrease bone calcium adsorption and greatly increase the risk of fracture with minor trauma. For this reason, bone density evaluations is important.[34] Decreased exposure to sunlight also impairs the conversion of skin 7-dehydrocholesterol to 1,25-dehydroxycholecalciferol (vitamin D).

Although vitamin supplements can be critical for children on modified elemental amino acid diets, the fat-soluble vitamins A, D, and K should be administered with caution. Excessive storage of these vitamins in the liver and adipose tissues can reach toxic levels.[35]

Because of inadequate bone buffering, serum potassium and phosphate quickly decrease to hazardous and potentially lethal levels during respiratory tract infections or episodes of fever and diarrhea or vomiting (see Chapter 2).[36] Thus, it is particularly important to monitor and replace electrolytes and metabolites during intercurrent illnesses.

ABNORMALITIES IN FATTY ACID OXIDATION AND SPINAL MUSCLE ATROPHY

In addition to decreased muscle nutrient stores, metabolic aspects of immobility, systemic illness, and muscle denervation and atrophy, children with SMA also have abnormalities in muscle mitochondrial fatty acid oxidation and carnitine metabolism and impaired insulin regulation, all of which point to the potential for muscle loss and progressive weakening.[32] Any process that increases cytoplasmic free fatty acid levels, such as fasting or defects in fatty acid transport or beta-oxidation, can increase hepatic and renal production and excretion of possibly toxic dicarboxylic acids. Fasting ketosis reflects normal ketogenesis by the liver's utilization of free fatty acids. However, children with SMA can be catabolic without developing ketosis because of enhanced gluconeogenesis at the expense of muscle mass and a downregulated insulin response.

Dicarboxylic acid levels are elevated in the urine of infants with SMA and in the blood and urine after fasting overnight. The extent of dicarboxylic aciduria is a function of SMA severity. Patients with SMA type 1 tolerate only the briefest fasting without ketosis and dicarboxylic aciduria, whereas patients with SMA type 3 patients express these abnormalities only during prolonged fasting, illness, and physiologic stress. The quantity of fatty acid metabolites generated in SMA type 3 may be considerably lower, reflecting a lower percentage of atrophic muscle fibers, than in SMA types 1 and 2. These metabolites may be taken up by the liver and metabolized, whereas in the more severe types of SMA the absolute levels of the metabolites are higher or the capacity of the liver is saturated. As a result, the excess is detected in serum and urine.[37] Metabolic analyses, including the appearance of relatively early ketosis, selective renal loss of carnitine,[37] and fatty vacuolization of the liver, suggest that the abnormalities are caused by changes in cellular physiology related to the molecular defects of the SMA-pathogenic survival motor neuron gene or neighboring genes. Abnormal fatty acid metabolism also appears to resolve with age independently of disease severity.[38]

Improved motor function and developmental milestones can develop without treatment in infants with SMA.[39] Likewise, from ages 10 to 19 years, muscle strength, when measured dynametrically, can remain constant and SMA can be considered a nonprogressive disease.[40] However, very often before 10 years of age or during periods of physiologic stress (e.g., intercurrent respiratory tract infections), patients with SMA suddenly lose muscle strength at a high rate.[40] During these episodes loss of strength tends to become progressive and is most severe in infants. Infants with SMA also weaken rapidly when nutrition is compromised by swallowing impairment. The sudden exacerbations of muscle weakness may be due to relative fasting; if so, the weakening can be abated or averted with proper nutrition.

METABOLIC RESPONSE TO STRESS AND UNDERNUTRITION

Energy balance equals energy intake minus energy expenditure. Quantitative comparison of starvation with the stress response helps to demonstrate the marked difference in the rates of protein loss, mostly from muscle, and fat loss.[1,41] The metabolic response to starvation aims to preserve lean body mass. This response is characterized by decreased energy expenditure, initial use of alternative fuel sources (e.g., stored glycogen and glucose synthesized from amino acids and fatty acids), and ultimately the use of ketones and glycerol to reduce protein wasting.[41–43] Because 85–90% of calories come from fat and 1 gram of fat produces 9–10 calories, one-half of a pound of fat can provide the needed calories for one day. Normally only 200 calories per day come from protein, but this amount corresponds to one-half of a pound of muscle (4 calories/gm protein). However, the starving body burns fat and protein in a 1:1 ratio. One-half of a pound of both protein and fat is lost each day.

Stress in otherwise normal people produces hypermetabolism and increased need for calories. The fuel source is mixed,[41–43] with 20% normally coming from protein, 30% from carbohydrates, and 50% from fats. With stress and fasting the ratio of fat-to-muscle loss is 1:4. In hypermetabolism with administered nutrition, on the other hand, the fat-to-muscle-loss ratio is 4:1. For patients with pulmonary dysfunction who use 3,000 calories per day,

TABLE 1. Comparison of Starvation and Hypermetabolism

State	Catabolized Protein/Fat Gram Ratio	Catabolized Muscle/Fat Gram Ratio	Calories Expended	Estimated Muscle Mass Lost Per Day
Starvation	1:1	4:1	2000	>220 gm
Hypermetabolism	4:1	16:1	3000	>450 gm
Extreme hyper-metabolism	8:1	32:1	4500	?

From Demling RH, DeSanti L: Use of anticatabolic agents for burns. Curr Opin Crit Care 2:482–491, 1996, with permission.

600 (20%) of these calories normally come from protein and 1,500 from fat. However, the patient can lose a pound of muscle, but only one-third of a pound of fat, for each day of fasting. Therefore, weight loss is not an accurate reflection of loss of lean mass. Loss of lean mass is even worse without provision of carbohydrates. In a starved-stress state, eight times more muscle than fat can be lost[44] (Table 1).

Increased caloric expenditure and protein catabolism are quite common in the stress states of patients with COPD. Fuel substrate is mobilized at rates of 2–3 times normal.[45] Much of the fuel substrate and oxygen requirement of patients with COPD is due to the energy cost of breathing associated with respiratory muscle dysfunction. The effect is exacerbated in patients with less than ideal body weight (Fig. 4). Protein consumption due to increased catabolism can exceed 200 gm/day, a significant sum considering that the average man has only about 4,500 grams of skeletal muscle protein and 8,500 grams of other protein.[45] Hypermetabolism in COPD is marked by 30% fuel oxidation from amino acids, 40% from glucose, and 30% from fat.[42] The increased use of protein for fuel may be seen as a maladaptive response to injury.[46] Although glucose oxidation increases, the fraction of calories coming from glucose is lower compared with starvation.[42]

In the hypermetabolic state, muscle loss occurs especially quickly over a period of about 3–4 weeks. The average lean tissue loss can be 10 kilograms. Unfortunately, the time required to regain the lost muscle is 5–10 times longer than the time required to lose

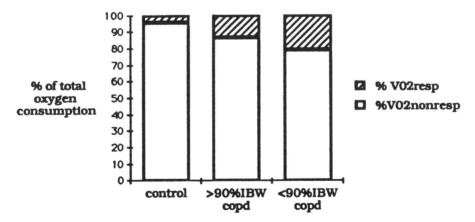

% of total oxygen consumption

■ % VO2resp
□ %VO2nonresp

control   >90%IBW copd   <90%IBW copd

FIGURE 4. Bar graphs comparing respiratory muscle and nonrespiratory muscle oxygen consumption (VO$_2$ resp and VO$_2$ nonresp) during dead space-induced ventilation in control subjects and well (> 90% ideal body weight) and undernourished (< 90% ideal body weight) patients with chronic obstructive pulmonary disease. The measurements are expressed as a percentage of the total VO$_2$. (From Donahoe M, Roger RM, Wilson DO, Pennock B: Oxygen consumption of the respiratory muscles in normal and malnourished patients with chronic obstructive pulmonary disease. Am Rev Respir Dis 140:385–391, 1989, with permission.)

it, Net positive muscle gain does not occur until the recovery phase when the hypermeta-bolic state dissipates and endogenous anabolism exceeds catabolism. At that point, with exercise and optimal nutrition, maximal muscle gain is about 100 gm/day (approximately 1–1.5 pounds per week).[47]

COPD also causes metabolic disturbances, including an increase in glucose produc-tion.[42,48] Because the gluconeogenesis is in excess of the required amount, much of the glucose is recycled to lactate and then back to glucose—a highly ineffective form of energy production. The gluconeogenesis is driven by the high levels of cortisol and cate-chols. Relative insulin resistance often results in hyperglycemia.[42] The substrates for glu-coneogenesis come from the tissue amino acid pool; therefore, proteolysis is markedly amplified to produce the substrate.[49]

Low serum testosterone is a common endocrine abnormality in men with COPD.[21] Significantly lower testosterone levels were found in patients with COPD and wasting than in a similar group without wasting (p < 0.001).[43] Reduced testosterone has been cor-related with weight loss and decreased survival.[50] Possible causes of low testosterone in-clude testicular failure or resistance to gonadotropins, breakdown of the blood-testis barrier, and medications. Reduced testosterone also may be a response to chronic infec-tion, stress, and malnutrition.[41] The use of corticosteroids in the treatment of COPD and NMDs also induces gonadal suppression. Sequelae of male hypogonadism contribute to a worsened quality of life and include sexual dysfunction, fatigue, mental depression, osteo-porosis, decreased muscle mass and strength, and loss of facial and body hair.[49]

EVALUATION AND MONITORING

History and Physical Examination

Questions about appetite and nutrient intake should be routine for prompt detection of nu-tritional deficits. Assessments are performed every three months in asymptomatic respiratory patients, at every visit in symptomatic patients, and every three days in hospitalized patients.[51]

The history and physical examination are performed with special attention to nutrient balance. Questions are asked about previous nutritional status, history of opportunistic in-fections, current medications, and any past or present substance abuse.[51] Baseline weight is obtained. Early recognition of weight changes is a good way to detect nutritional imbal-ance. Conditions must be the same each time that weight is measured. It is important to use the same scale and to ensure that the scale is properly calibrated. Braces, casts, catheter bags and tubing, clothing, wheelchair weight, seat cushions, pillows, blankets, and time since the patient has eaten or been fed must be considered. Weight also can be af-fected by hydration and edema.

Height is important for understanding the effects of nutrition on growth and for com-parison with predicted normal values of many physiologic parameters. When height is dif-ficult to assess in patients with NMD because of scoliosis or other musculoskeletal abnormalities, knee height measurements from beneath the foot to the top of the femoral condyle can be used to estimate height using the following formulas[52]:

Boys' height = 64.19 – [0.04 × age] + [0.02 × knee height in cm]
Girls' height = 84.88 [0.24 × age] + [1.83 × knee height in cm]

Alternate techniques for assessing body size have been suggested, such as arm span and single arm length.[53] Although the measurement of arm span permits prediction of height for scoliotic children,[54] it does not seem to be applicable to patients with DMD. In addi-tion, arm articulations may be contracted, rendering measurements more difficult.[55]

The appearance of the hair, eyes, skin, and teeth is noted. Changes in skin or hair color and texture and tongue and gingival lesions may signal specific nutritional deficiencies.

Swallowing ability, taste, and smell are evaluated. Bowel routines are reviewed and difficulties addressed. Xerosis indicates dehydration or suboptimal levels of vitamin C or zinc.[51] Dehydration due to compromised fluid intake can be exacerbated by excessive fluid losses (e.g., from vomiting and drooling). In one study, salivary losses of an 8-year-old girl were measured at 320 ml/day, or 25% of the girl's maintenance fluid requirement.[34] Urine specific gravity is assessed to determine hydration status. A 24- to 72-hour food and fluid intake diary is kept and assessed.

Calorie and nutrient ingestion is quantitated and compared with ideal quantities for age-, gender-, and stature-matched peers. Caloric and nutrient assessments are expressed as a percentage of the RDA over a 3-day period.[56] The ideal calorie intake levels of patients with hypermetabolic COPD or inactive patients with NMD often vary considerably from those of the general population.

A number of indices have been developed to assess nutritional status and quantitate body fat and lean mass. Examples include determination of skinfold thickness, midarm circumference, bioelectric resistive impedance, creatine-height index, body mass index (weight divided by height squared), and weight for zero muscle mass (ZMM; see below).

Tape and caliper anthropometry is commonly available, cost-effective, and accurate within ± 3%. Suprailiac and subscapular skinfolds are often easier to obtain and can be more reliable than the triceps fold measurement because of the often present contractures of the upper arm. If obtainable, mid-arm muscle circumference (mid-arm circumference minus 3.14 × triceps skinfold) can be used as an indicator of muscle mass. Standards for anthropometric measurements are available.[52] The 50th percentile for fat stores is considered ideal for children with NMD.[34] Weight, height, and anthropometric measurements are complementary.

Clinical anthropometry is complicated for patients with NMD because the largest body compartment, the muscle mass, is affected by the primary pathologic processes. Although subcutaneous body fat theoretically may be represented by the adipose layer measured at the usual sites, such measures may not take into account perimuscular and intramuscular lipid infiltration. Therefore, generally accepted anthropometric equations for determining body fat mass[57,58] are not reliable in patients with NMD.[59,60]

A recent study demonstrated that in patients with DMD or ALS, ZMM more effectively takes into account muscle fat composition and more successfully indicates overweight status (excessive body fat composition) than BMI.[61] ZMM is determined by using a creatine-free diet for 6 days and then measuring total urinary creatinine excretion for the next 3 days. This protocol permits the estimation of the contribution of muscle to body weight by dividing the patient's body weight for zero muscle mass by the theoretical body weight for zero muscle mass. Of a total of 7 patients with ALS and 34 with DMD, BMI was normal (20–25 kg/m²) for all 7 patients with ALS and for 29 patients with DMD, whereas 5 patients with ALS and 30 patients with DMD were classified as overweight by ZMM.

Assessment for pediatric patients with NMD also is complicated by altered growth dynamics and metabolism as well as by atrophied muscle mass and limb contractures and weakness. Children require more frequent assessment of physical examination parameters, caloric and nutrient intake, anthropometric measurements, and biochemical analyses related to deficiency in the muscle mass "buffer" for carbohydrates, protein, and minerals. Concomitant abnormalities of fatty acid metabolism and insulin regulation also complicate the clinical picture for patients with SMA and certain other pediatric conditions.

Laboratory Evaluation

Undernutrition reduces hepatic protein synthesis. Serum levels of albumin and iron transport protein (transferrin) reflect protein availability to the liver for protein synthesis. Both protein and transferrin have half-lives just under 2 weeks. Therefore, serum levels reflect long-term but not short-term changes in protein status. Prealbumin and retinol-binding protein are more useful for assessing short-term nutritional interventions because of their shorter half-lives of 2 days and 12 hours, respectively.[62] Levels of urinary nitrogen, a measurement of nitrogen metabolism, are assessed by a 24-hour urine collection.[63] Other tests that assess nutritional status include total iron-binding capacity, cholesterol, and serum vitamin levels, especially of vitamins A, C, and E. Serum vitamin levels are especially important because patients with COPD and NMD have a high incidence of vitamin deficiencies. Delayed cutaneous hypersensitivity is a function of cell-mediated immunity and is the immune response most sensitive to nutritional deprivation. The normal induration and erythematous response to an injected antigen occurs in 24–48 hours. A decreased or absent response is associated with malnutrition, infection, primary immune disease, systemic pathology, or glucocorticoid therapy.

Chlebowski and associates examined the value of using serum albumin levels to predict clinical outcomes in wasting syndromes.[64] They found a median survival of more than 960 days in patients with a baseline serum albumin level equal to or greater than 3.5 gm/dl; survival of 103 days with a baseline of 2.5–3.5 gm/dl; and survival of only 17 days with an albumin level less than 2.5 gm/dl.[64] Ninety-eight percent of their patients were underweight. Sixty-eight percent had experienced a 10% loss of usual body weight. The authors also found that survival in patients with less than 10% loss of usual body weight at admission was 520 days; with 10–20% weight loss, survival was 101 days; and with 20% or more weight loss, survival was only 48 days.[64] A loss of lean body mass greater than 40% was usually fatal.

NUTRITIONAL INTERVENTIONS

Successful nutritional management of pulmonary patients limits wasting, lean body mass depletion, and loss of muscle strength; it also enhances well-being and preserves energy reserves to help resist respiratory complications. By delaying or diminishing wasting, patients are often able to function better and remain independent for a longer time.

Chronic Obstructive Pulmonary Disease

For patients with COPD, protein requirements are between 1.5 and 2 gm/kg/day, or about 2–3 times the normal RDA.[44,47] Glutamine supplementation of approximately 0.5 gm/kg/day or 10 times the RDA[65] has been shown to counter glucocorticoid-induced muscle atrophy.[66] Increased vitamins and minerals, between 5 and 10 times the normal RDA, are also required.[44,47]

Prolonged restriction to 5% dextrose can initiate starvation early in acutely hospitalized patients and can aggravate hypermetabolic decompensatory catabolic cascades. It may lead to or prolong the need for ventilatory support. Restriction to intravenous dextrose, therefore, should be avoided.

Muscle resistance exercise produces a local anabolic effect in muscles that is important for muscle regeneration.[67] In a study of older men, researchers found that vigorous strength training led to muscle hypertrophy at the same rate as in younger men.[67] One study focused on 5 patients with COPD who received nutritional supplementation in combination with resistive breathing.[68] After an initial evaluation that included spirometry, nutritional assessment, anthropometric measurements, and creatinine-height index, the patients received an individually adapted, enriched diet for 2 months. The patients were reevaluated, and then resistive breathing was added for another 2 months, followed by a final evaluation. Although the patients were initially mildly to moderately malnourished, as indicated by skinfold measurements, body weight, and creatinine-height index, after the first 2 months of only nutritional supplementation, significant improvement was noted in respiratory muscle strength and endurance. Forced vital capacity increased from 58.6% to 63.6% of predicted (p < 0.05), and maximal voluntary ventilation, an index of ventilatory endurance, increased from 36.8% to 44.6% of predicted (p < 0.01). The combined treatment that included resistive breathing training further increased forced vital capacity to 69.4% of predicted (p < 0.02)—similar to the improvement after the first two months of nutritional interventions. However, maximal voluntary ventilation (MVV) increased to 57.8% of predicted normal (p < 0.005) after the combined treatment. This increase was significantly greater than the increase after the first two months of nutrition-only supplementation. The authors concluded that nutritional supplementation can improve ventilatory capacity and endurance, but the effects are significantly greater when nutritional supplementation is combined with resistive breathing.[68]

A further increase in anabolic activity can be provided by combining anabolic agents with optimal nutrition and increased muscle activity.[66,69] Anabolic agents increase nitrogen retention, decrease protein catabolism, and increase protein synthesis. Human growth hormone (HGH) can increase anabolic activity and decrease lean tissue loss, but high cost and complications such as hyperglycemia and insulin resistance have prevented its widespread use in pulmonary patients.[41,65,69,70] Because hyperglycemia is often a sign of sepsis, it can be difficult to identify the true clinical status of HGH-treated patients. Infrequently, transient peripheral edema occurs.[71] Asymptomatic hypercalcemia is also seen in critically ill surgical patients who receive HGH therapy.[72] In addition, HGH must be given parenterally,[69,72] and optimal protein intake (1.5–2.0 gm/kg/day) is essential.[65,72] Exogenous HGH is approved for treatment of growth disorders in children and also is used for its anabolic activity, especially in the treatment of burns.[72] Thus far, HGH has been studied in patients with severe catabolism due to illness or injury,[47,65] malnourished patients with catabolic illness,[45] patients with an acute loss of more than 15% of lean body mass, and patients with burns or wounds that heal poorly.[47]

Oxandrolone is an anabolic agent approved for restoration of muscle mass after trauma or severe injury.[47] It also can increase significantly the body weight and muscle function of hypermetabolic patients. Oxandrolone is a testosterone analog. Testosterone, the principal androgen secreted by the testis, possesses two distinct biologic properties: (1) virilizing activity known as androgenic activity and (2) protein-building (anabolic) activity. Shortly after the isolation and synthesis of testosterone, efforts were initiated to modify the parent compound to separate the androgenic from the anabolic properties and to establish therapeutically active androgenic compounds suitable for replacement therapy in patients with low testosterone levels.[73]

In one study, oxandrolone was used in combination with high-calorie and high-protein intake that included a protein hydrolysate with its bioactive peptides to achieve a protein intake of 2 gm/kg/day.[47] This protein intake was unattainable with standard supplements such as Ensure-HN or Sustacal, but it was attained with MET-Rx. The lower carbohydrate and fat content of this supplement also allowed ideal matching of nonprotein calories. A standard resistance and endurance exercise program was used to augment restoration of muscle function.[47] Patients in the study had no active infections, demonstrated stable cardiopulmonary status, were not significantly hypermetabolic, and had no need for life support. Their basal temperatures were less than 99.5°F with a resting metabolic rate of 130% of normal. They received oral diets with supplements or tube feeding. Active participation in physical therapy was required.[47] The study was prospective, and patients were randomized into two groups with an additional group studied retrospectively. Group one received a high-calorie, high-protein, ad-lib oral diet plus a high-protein supplement (MET-Rx) for a total protein intake of 2 gm/kg/day. Group two received the same diet plus a 10-mg oral dose of oxandrolone twice daily. Group three, the retrospective group, had previously received a high-calorie, high-protein, ad-lib oral diet with a high protein supplement (Ensure-HN or Sustacal) for a total protein intake of 1.3–1.5 gm/kg/day. All groups received additional vitamin and mineral supplementation at levels of 10 times the RDA.

The study protocol lasted three weeks, followed by two weeks of patient evaluation.[47] Group 1 patients (high-calorie, high-protein intake) gained an average of 2.5–2.6 pounds per week for a total of approximately 7.5 pounds by the end of the 3-week study. Group 2 patients (high-calorie, high-protein intake plus oxandrolone) gained on average twice as much weight as those in group one— that is, a total of 12.9 pounds by the end of the study period. Group 3 patients gained less weight than patients in either group 1 or group 2. The addition of 20 mg/day of oxandrolone to the protein-rich diet resulted in a marked increase in weight, nearly four times that of controls. The rate of restoration of function also was significantly better in the oxandrolone group compared with the group receiving only MET-Rx. In addition, strength increased and discharge time decreased.[47]

Nutritional supplements high in fat and low in carbohydrate for patients with hypercapnic lung disease who need to limit carbohydrate intake include Respalor (Mead-Johnson, Princeton, NJ), with 20%, 41%, and 39% of calories from protein, fat, and carbohydrate, respectively; NutriVent (Nestle, U.S.A., Inc., Glendale, CA), with 18%, 55%, and 27% of calories from protein, fat, and carbohydrate, respectively; and Pulmocare (Ross, Inc., Columbus, OH), with 16.7%, 55.1%, and 28.2% of calories from protein, fat, and carbohydrate, respectively. All three have about 1.5 kcal/ml.

TREATMENT OF CHILDREN WITH SPECIFIC NEUROMUSCULAR DISORDERS

Spinal Muscular Atrophy

Although caloric requirements vary significantly for both normal children and children with NMD,[34] overall caloric needs for infants with NMD are 80–100 cal/kg. Older children with NMD also require less-than-normal calorie intake. In addition, sufficient fluid intake is required to prevent constipation and urinary system calculi as well as dehydration. Fluid intake is often insufficient because of decreased thirst, difficulty in obtaining or swallowing fluids, or communication impairment.

Three specific dietary goals have been identified: (1) an increase in dietary complex carbohydrates, (2) provision of at least 2 gm/kg/day of protein, and (3) a feeding schedule that limits overnight fasting to 4 hours for a young infant and 8 hours for older children. The child must receive adequate calories with a minimum of 5% of calories from essential fatty acids. Infants with SMA have been reported to regain or retain strength by taking elemental or semi-elemental formulas, such as Tolerex and Pediatric Vivonex (Novartis, Minneapolis, MN), that provide high carbohydrate and elemental amino acids and small-chained polypeptides.[37] They are easier to digest and may allow better utilization of nutrients and spare muscle protein. A late evening supplement of complex carbohydrates, such as uncooked corn starch (1 gm/kg), can sustain blood glucose levels and reduce the effects of overnight fasting.[32] In addition, considering that denervation can cause a decrease in muscle carnitine concentrations and in the abnormalities in fatty acid metabolism associated with infantile SMA, supplements of riboflavin, coenzyme Q10, and L-carnitine have been suggested, along with 200 mg/kg of glutamine and 250 mg/kg of arginine.[37] The elemental formulas, glutamine, and arginine provide extra essential amino acids to shift the ketoacid-amino acid equilibrium in favor of muscle protein retention and synthesis. Glutamine may simultaneously remove ketoacids from degradative pathways. Glutamine supplementation is well established for patients with inborn errors of amino acid and organic acid metabolism, burn patients, and postsurgical care.

Both Tolerex and Pediatric Vivonex have the essential fatty acids, but Tolerex has only 1 gm of fat per 300-calorie packet as opposed to 5 gm per 200-calorie packet for Pediatric Vivonex. Tolerex also has twice as many complex carbohydrates per pack as Pediatric Vivonex. For children, both Tolerex and Pediatric Vivonex are low in calcium, iron, iodine, potassium, vitamin C, B complex and fat-soluble vitamins, and folic acid. Supplements are warranted.

Recent evidence from animal models indicates that such children also may benefit from a greater amount of folic acid and vitamin B_{12} than the RDA. Folic acid should be provided daily: 65 µg for children from 0 to 6 months of age, 80 µg from 7 to 12 months of age, 150 µg from 1 to 3 years of age, 200 µg from 4 to 8 years of age, 300 µg from 9 to 13 years of age, and 400 µg for older people. At the same ages vitamin B_{12} is provided at 0.5 µg, 1.5 µg, 2 µg, and 2.5 µg, respectively; 3 µg is provided from 9 to 13 years of age and after.

In addition to corn starch, minerals, and vitamins, the low fatty content of these elemental formulas is supplemented by adding several grams of primrose or safflower oil with water or white grape juice. Jars of baby fruit and vegetables round out the diet, along with sufficient fluids for good hydration to prevent thickening of airway secretions.

Diets high in carbohydrate, amino acids, and polypeptides and low in fat provide muscle with utilizable energy substrates, thereby reducing dependence on fatty acid oxidation and decreasing dicarboxylic acids.[37] This diet maintains more nearly normal blood glucose levels during fasting, delays fasting-associated ketoacidosis, and has been noted to normalize liver function enzyme levels. Provision of amino acids and short-chain peptides instead of complex dairy proteins facilitates glucogenesis. Most tube-fed children using this dietary strategy do not receive whole protein foods such as eggs, meats, soy, or grains because they exacerbate thickness and possibly quantity of secretions, sweating, and constipation and may cause facial flushing. Harpey et al. believed that strength and function improved significantly in 13 patients treated in this manner.[74]

Caution is recommended in making empiric changes to a diet that may lead to unintended and potentially adverse consequences.[38] Because of limited muscle stores and rapid changes in blood levels, there is a narrow window of optimal blood protein levels. Excessive levels leading to high blood nitrogen content may be hazardous. In addition, the use of protein-hydrolysate formulas containing modified cornstarch results in high levels of oxtenylsuccinic aciduria,[75] the pharmacokinetics, drug interactions, and long-term effects of which are unknown. It also is possible that avoidance of fasting rather than nutrient manipulation per se has played the largest role in preventing ongoing muscle weakening. Nevertheless, 80% of conventionally managed infants with SMA type 1 are dead by 12 months of age; rare patients survive to age 2 years.[76] But of the over 30 infants with uncomplicated SMA type 1 who received these dietary modifications and for whom death and tracheostomy were avoided with the use of respiratory muscle aids (see Chapter 10), 15 are already older than 3 years, 7 are older than 6 years, and only 1 has died. No children are known to have died or suffered from receiving these formulas. Parents report increasing motor function or stabilization of previously deteriorating motor function. Clearly, these children either have fewer life-threatening respiratory tract infections or are able to handle them much better. Thus, it is hard to imagine what can be lost by at least a brief trial of this dietary strategy. Children with SMA type 2 who have not been intubated drink the formula slowly throughout the day, although cooperation can be a problem.

Based on recent studies of mice with SMA, it may be prudent to provide supplemental creatine monohydrate at 0.1 gm/kg/day divided into 2 doses, despite the lack of confirmatory evidence in humans. Creatine, a 3-amino acid peptide, is similar in nature to the elemental amino acid preparations that seem to be beneficial.

Because patients with SMA are often hypoglycemic, it can be tempting to treat them with glucose administration. However, hyperglycemia can be severe because of inadequate insulin release. This scenario indicates the need for insulin therapy (0.05 U/kg/hr) to increase glucose utilization, block protein catabolism, and enhance protein synthesis. The cyclic vomiting that some children with SMA develop responds quickly to glucose plus insulin administration, whereas it may take hours or days of intravenous glucose administration to achieve the same effect.

Because the avoidance of fasting is crucial to the maintenance of muscle strength, fasting and undernutrition must be avoided when children with SMA are acutely ill. Virtually all children with SMA type 1 and many children with type 2 require gastrostomy tubes before 2 years of age. Prophylactic provision of gastrostomy tubes before acute illness or dysphagia-associated weight loss causes deterioration may be an important strategy. Patients who require surgery and have periods of receiving no food by mouth should receive nutrition parenterally.

Many tube-fed infants with SMA 1 receive enough packets of elemental formula for 80–90 cal/kg over 24 hours, initially at 60–90 ml per hour. Eventually small boluses are provided during the day along with a slow drip overnight. Two- to 3-year old children receive 60–70 cal/kg/day and larger boluses. The preparation with supplements is made in a blender every morning and individualized for each child, taking into account patient tolerance as well as effects on strength and function, secretions, and respiratory status.

Duchenne Muscular Dystrophy

Studies suggest that, early on, DMD is a hypercatabolic disease. Compared with controls, patients with DMD have a higher basal metabolic rate, higher maintenance protein requirements, and a higher daily excretion of urinary 3-methylhistidine per unit muscle mass.[77] The reason for hypermetabolism is unknown, but it may be related to functional defects of skeletal muscle mitochondria.[78] Therefore, it is important to take this phenomenon into account when supplementing the diets and calculating caloric needs.

Tilton, Miller, and Khoshoo have found that 54% of 7- to 13-year-old patients with NMD are obese.[34] The most obvious explanation for obesity is that more calories are taken in than expended, but this explanation is still debated. Progression of NMD is associated with loss of lean muscle tissue, which reduces the resting energy expenditure. Hankard et al. have reported reduction of muscle mass up to 71% in patients with DMD.[79] Resting energy expenditure is reduced by 13%, and postabsorptive fat utilization is also reduced in DMD.[79] Furthermore, obesity does not indicate adequate protein stores or adequate vitamin and mineral status. In fact, obesity can mask deficiency states, making the food intake record and biochemical evaluation a vital component of assessment for obese as well as undernourished patients.

The caloric needs of relatively inactive people with NMDs have been estimated from an equation developed to guide the recommended caloric intake of children with DMD:

$$\text{Daily energy intake in kcal} = 2000 - \text{age (years)} \times 50$$

For advanced patients who require ventilatory support, caloric needs may not exceed normal resting energy expenditure, which is estimated at 110% of basal metabolic rate. The reason may be that the oxygen cost of breathing and the energy substrates needed for respiratory function are greatly reduced in many patients for whom ventilators substitute for inspiratory muscle function.

Caloric needs must be modified for obese or undernourished people as well as during respiratory tract infections and after surgical interventions. In the case of obese patients, many physicians hesitate to recommend an overly restrictive diet for fear of aggravating muscle atrophy by relative fasting. However, surveillance of the body composition of two patients with severe caloric restrictions did not demonstrate any deleterious effects on either body composition or muscular function.[80] Accordingly, it seems reasonable to advise a 20% reduction in caloric intake and a monthly weight reduction of 2 kg for obese patients with DMD and perhaps for obese patients with other NMDs. Moderate rather than severe dietary restriction is more likely to favor lean muscle sparing over fat sparing. Cookbooks that contain recipes for appetizing and attractive texture-adapted meals are available.[81,82]

PSYCHOSOCIAL ISSUES

Most children and adolescents with NMD attend school. Adolescents want to eat the same foods and in the same manner as their peers. Inability to do so and weight extremes can decrease self-esteem and cause depression. Depression also can decrease appetite or lead to overeating. Adolescents and children may use eating as a control tactic. Unfortunately, schools are often not equipped or staffed to deal with the special needs of feeding such children, and this problem can contribute to malnutrition. Time constraints and schedules can also adversely affect feeding and eating in the school setting.

CONCLUSION

Malnutrition is common and often contributes to morbidity and mortality in patients with COPD and generalized NMDs. Pediatric patients pose a unique challenge and must be assessed and treated accordingly. Recognition of the problem and appropriate intervention can reverse malnutrition-associated morbidity and enhance quality of life.

ACKNOWLEDGMENT

The work reported in this chapter was performed at University Hospital, Newark, N.J.

REFERENCES

1. Roubenoff R, Kehaylas JJ: The meaning and measurement of lean body mass. Nutr Rev 49:163–175, 1991.
2. Bach JR, Tippett DC, McCrary MM: Bulbar dysfunction and associated cardiopulmonary considerations in polio and neuromuscular disease. J NeuroRehabil 6:121–128, 1992.
3. Blackburn GL, Bistrian BR, Maini BS, et al: Nutritional and metabolic assessment of the hospitalized patient. J Parent Ent Nutr 1:11, 1977.
4. Gacad G, Dickie K, Marraro D: Protein synthesis in the lung: Influence of starvation on amino acid incorporation in protein. J Appl Physiol 33:381–385, 1972.
5. Weiss HS, Jurus E: Effects of starvation on compliance and surfactant of the rat lung. Respir Physiol 12:123–129, 1971.
6. Sahebjami H, MacGee J: Changes in connective tissue composition of the lung in starvation and refeeding. Am Rev Respir Dis 128:644–647, 1983.
7. Sahebjami H, Vassallo CL: Effects of starvation and refeeding on lung mechanics and morphometry. Am Rev Respir Dis 119:443–451, 1979.
8. Sahebjami H, Vassallo CL, Wirman JA: Lung mechanics and ultrastructure in prolonged starvation. Am Rev Respir Dis 117:77–83, 1979.
9. Sahebjami H, Wirman JA: Emphysema-like changes in the lungs of starved rats. Am Rev Respir Dis 124:619–624, 1981.
10. Sahebjami H, MacGee J: Effects of starvation and refeeding on lung biochemistry in rats. Am Rev Respir Dis 126:483–487, 1982.
11. Kerr JS, Riley DJ, Lanza-Jacoby S, et al: Nutritional emphysema in the rat: Influence of protein depletion and impaired lung growth. Am Rev Respir Dis 131:644–660, 1985.
12. Stein J, Fenigstein H: Anatomie pathologique de la maladie de la famine. In Apfelbaum E (ed): Maladie de la famine. Recherches cliniques sur la famine executées dans le ghetto de Varsovie en 1942. Warsaw, 1946, pp 21–27. Published in Laaban JR: Nutrition artificielle chez l'insuffisant respiratoire chronique opéré. Ann Fran Anesthes Reanim 14(Suppl 2):112–120, 1995.
13. Wilson DO, Rogers M, Openbrier D: Nutritional aspects of chronic obstructive pulmonary disease. Clin Chest Med 7:643–656, 1986.
14. Goldberg AL, Odessy R: Oxidation of amino acids by diaphragms from fed and fasted rats. Am J Physiol 233:1384–1396, 1972.
15. McMurray DN, Loomis SA, Casazza LJ, et al: Development of impaired cell mediated immunity in mild and moderate malnutrition. Am J Clin Nutr 34:68–77, 1981.
16. Good RA: Nutrition and immunity. J Clin Immunol 1:3–11, 1981.
17. Moriguchi S, Sonc S, Kishino Y: Changes of alveolar macrophages in protein deficient rats. J Nutr 113:40–46, 1983.
18. Martin TR, Altman LC, Alvares OF: The effects of severe protein-calorie malnutrition on antibacterial defense mechanisms in the rat lung. Am Rev Respir Dis 128:1013–1019, 1983.
19. Niederman MS, Merrill WW, Ferranti RD, et al: Nutritional status and bacterial binding in the lower respiratory tract in patients with chronic tracheostomies. Ann intern Med 100:795–800, 1984.

20. Aubier M, Murciano D, Lecocguie Y, et al: Effect of hypophosphatemia on diaphragmatic contractility in patients with acute respiratory failure. N Engl J Med 313:420–424, 1985.
21. Harris RL, Frenkel RA, Cottam GL, Baxter CR: Lipid perioxidation and metabolism after thermal trauma. J Trauma 22:194–198, 1982.
22. Kelsen SG, Ference M, Kaoor S: Effects of prolonged undernutrition on structure and function of the diaphragm. J Appl Physiol 58:1354–1359, 1985.
23. Rochester DF, Arora NS, Braun NMT: Maximum contractile force of human diaphragm muscle determined in vivo. Trans Am Clin Climatol Assoc 83:200–208, 1981.
24. Arora NS, Rochester DF: Respiratory muscle strength and maximal voluntary ventilation in undernourished patients. Am Rev Respir Dis 126:5–8, 1982.
25. Baier H, Somani P: Ventilatory drive in normal man during semi-starvation. Chest 85:222–225, 1984.
26. Doekel RC Jr, Zwillich CW, Scoggin CH, et al: Clinical semistarvation: Depression of hypoxic ventilatory response. N Engl J Med 295:358–361, 1976.
27. Askanazi J, Rosembaum SH, Hyman AI, et al: Effects of parenteral nutrition on ventilatory drive [abstract]. Anesthesiology 53(Suppl):185, 1980.
28. Balkom R, Dekhuijzen PN, Folgering H, et al: Effects of long-term low-dose methylprednisolone on rat diaphragm function and structure. Muscle Nerve 20:983, 1997.
29. Fitting JW: Energy expenditure in chronic lung disease. In Ferranti RD, Rampulla C, Fracchia C, Ambrosino N (eds): Nutrition and Ventilatory Function. New York, Springer-Verlag, 1992, pp 45–52.
30. Wagner MB, Vignos PJ, Carlozzi C: Duchenne muscular dystrophy: A study of wrist and hand function. Muscle Nerve 12:236–244, 1989.
31. Bach JR, Zeelenberg A, Winter C: Wheelchair mounted robot manipulators: Long term use by patients with Duchenne muscular dystrophy. Am J Phys Med Rehabil 69:59–69, 1990.
32. Kelley R: Nutrition: A new understanding of muscle metabolism in spinal muscular atrophy and other muscle disorders. Direction 7:7, 1993.
33. Fried M, Pencharz P: Energy and nutrient intakes of children with spastic quadriplegia. J Pediatr 119:947–951, 1991.
34. Tilton AH, Miller MD, Khoshoo V: Nutrition and swallowing in pediatric neuromuscular patients. Semin Pediatr Neurol 5:106–115, 1998.
35. Morrison G, Hark L: Medical Nutrition and Disease. Cambridge, MA, Blackwell Science, 1996, pp 48–59.
36. McDonald B, Rosenthal SA: Hypokalemia complicating Duchenne muscular dystrophy. Yale J Biol Med 60:405–408, 1987.
37. Tein I, Sloane AE, Donner EJ, et al: Fatty acid oxidation abnormalities in childhood-onset spinal muscular atrophy: Primary or secondary defects? Pediatr Neurol 12:21–30, 1995.
38. Crawford TO, Sladky JT, Hurko O, et al: Abnormal fatty acid metabolism in childhood spinal muscular atrophy. Ann Neurol 45:337–343, 1999.
39. Iannaccone ST, Browne RH, Samaha FJ, Buncher CR: Prospective study of spinal muscular atrophy before age 6 years. Pediatr Neurol 9:187–193, 1993.
40. Iannaccone ST, Russman BS, Browne RH, et al: Prospective analysis of strength in spinal muscular atrophy. J Child Neurol 15:97–101, 2000.
41. Barton RG: Nutrition support in critical illness. Nutr Clin Pract 9:127–139, 1994.
42. Cerra FB: Hypermetabolism, organ failure, and metabolic support. Surgery 101:1–14, 1987.
43. Wilmore DW, Aulick LH: Metabolic changes in burned patients. Surg Clin North Am 58:1173–1187, 1978.
44. DeBiasse M, Wilmore D: What is optimal nutrition support? New Horizons 2:122–130, 1994.
45. Pasulka PS, Wachtel TL: Nutritional considerations for the burned patient. Surg Clin North Am 67:109–131, 1987.
46. Wilmore DW, Black PR, Muhlbacher F: Injured man: Trauma and sepsis. In Winters RW, Greene HL (eds): Nutritional Support of the Seriously Ill Patient. New York, Academic Press, Bristol-Meyers Nutrition Symposia, 1983, pp 34–52.
47. Demling RH, DeSanti L: Use of anticatabolic agents for burns. Curr Opin Crit Care 2:482–491, 1996.
48. Wilmore DW, Aulick LH, Mason AD, Pruitt BA: Influence of the burn wound on local systemic responses to injury. Ann Surg 186:444–458, 1977.
49. Wilmore DW, Long JM, Mason AD, et al: Catecholamines: Mediator of the hypermetabolic response to thermal injury. Ann Surg 180:653–669, 1974.
50. Tredget EE, Yu YM: The metabolic effects of thermal injury. World J Surg 16:68–79, 1992.
51. Jin L, Lalone C, Demling R: Lung dysfunction after thermal injury in relation to prostanoid and oxygen radical release. J Appl Physiol 61:103–112, 1986.
52. Frisancho AR: Anthropometric Standards for the Assessment of Growth and Nutritional Status. Ann Arbor, MI, University of Michigan Press, 1993.
53. Spender QW, Cronk CE, Charney EB, Stallings VA: Assessment of linear growth of children with cerebral palsy: Use of alternative measures to height or length. Dev Med Child Neurol 31:206–214, 1989.
54. Engstrom FM, Roche AF, Mukherjoe D: Differences between arm span and stature in white children. J Adolesc Health Care 2:19–22, 1981.

55. Miller F, Koreska J: Height measurement of patients with neuromuscular disease and contractures. Dev Med Child Neurol 34:55–60, 1992.
56. National Academy of Sciences: Recommended Dietary Allowances, 10th ed. Washington, DC, National Academy Press, 1989.
57. Slaughter MH, Lohman TG, Boileau RA, et al: Skinfold equations for estimation of body fatness in children and youth. Hum Biol 60:709–723, 1988.
58. Brook CGD: Determination of body composition of children from skinfold measurement. Arch Dis Child 46:182–184, 1971.
59. Tanner JH, Whitehouse RH, Takaishi M: Standards from birth to maturity for height, weight, height velocity, and weight velocity: British Children, Part II, 1965. Arch Dis Child 41:613–635, 1966.
60. Willig TN, Carlier L, Legrand M, et al: Nutritional assessment in Duchenne muscular dystrophy. Dev Med Child Neurol 35:1074–1082, 1993.
61. Pessolano FA, Suarez A, Dubrovsky A, et al: Assessment of the nutritional status in patients with neuromuscular disease. Am J Phys Med Rehabil [in press].
62. Axen KV: Nutrition in chronic obstructive pulmonary disease. In Haas F, Axen K (eds): Pulmonary Therapy and Rehabilitation Principles and Practice, 2nd ed. Baltimore, Williams & Wilkins, 1991, pp 95–105.
63. Kagan RJ: Restoring nitrogen balance after burn injury. Compr Ther 17:60–67, 1991.
64. Coodley GO, Loveless MO, Merrill TM: The HIV wasting syndrome: A review. J Acq Immun Defic Syndr 7:681–694, 1994.
65. Hammarqvist F, Wernerman J, Ali R, et al: Addition of glutamine to total parenteral nutrition after elective abdominal surgery spares free glutamine in muscle, counteracts the fall in muscle protein synthesis, and improves nitrogen balance. Ann Surg 209:455–456, 1989.
66. Ziegler T: Growth hormone administration during nutrition support: What is to be gained? New Horizons 2:244–256, 1994.
67. Frontera WR, Meredith CN, O Reilly KP, et al: Strength conditioning in older men: Skeletal hypertrophy and improved function. J Appl Physiol 64:1038–1044, 1988.
68. Gross E, Meyron E, Shindler D: The effect of resistive breathing training combined with nutritional supplementation in malnourished chronic obstructive pulmonary disease. In Ferranti RD, Rampulla C, Fracchia C, Ambrosino N (eds): Nutrition and Ventilatory Function New York, Springer-Verlag, 1992, pp 197–205.
69. Gatzen C, Scheltinga MR, Kimbrough TD, et al: Growth hormone attenuates the abnormal distribution of body water in critically ill surgical patients. Surgery 12:181–187, 1993.
70. Clayton PE, Shalet SM, Price DA, Addison GM: Growth and growth hormone responses to oxandrolone in boys with constitutional delay of growth and puberty (CDPG). Clin Endocrinol 29:123–130, 1998.
71. Physician's Desk Reference. Montvale, NJ, Medical Economics, 1997, pp 1051–1053.
72. Know JB, Demling RH, Wilmore DW, et al: Increased survival after major thermal injury: the effect of growth therapy in adults. J Trauma Inj Infect Crit Care 39:526–532, 1995.
73. Schwartz FL, Miller RJ: Androgens and anabolic steroids. In Craig CR, Stitzel RE (eds): Modern Pharmacology. Boston, Little, Brown, 1982, pp 905–924.
74. Harpey JP, Charpentier C, Paturneau-Jonas M, et al: Secondary metabolic defects in spinal muscular atrophy type II. Lancet 336:629–630, 1990.
75. Kelley RI. Octenylsuccinic aciduria in children fed protein-hydrolysate formulas containing modified cornstarch. Pediatr Res 30:564–569, 1991.
76. Dubowitz V: Very severe spinal muscular atrophy (SMA type 0): An expanding clinical phenotype. Eur J Paediatr Neurol 3:49–51, 1999.
77. Okada K, Sachinobu M, Sadaichi S, et al: Protein and energy metabolism in patients with progressive muscular dystrophy. J Nutr Sci Vitaminol 38:147–154, 1992.
78. Lin CH, Hudson AJ, Strickland KP: Palmitic acid-1-14C oxidation by skeletal muscle mitochondria of dystrophic mice. Can J Biochem 48:566–572, 1969.
79. Hankard R, Gottrand F, Turek D, et al: Resting energy expenditure and energy and energy substrate utilization in children with Duchenne's muscular dystrophy. Pediatr Res 40:29–33, 1996.
80. Edwards RHT, Round JM, Jackson MJ, et al: Weight reduction in boys with muscular dystrophy. Dev Med Child Neurol 26:384–390, 1984.
81. Appel V, Calvin S, Smith G, Woehr D. Meals for easy swallowing. Muscular Dystrophy Association, Tucson, 1986.
82. Willig TN. Tous à table: Cuisine adaptée aux difficultés d'alimentation. Paris, Association Contre les Myopathies et l'Association des Paralysés de France, 1993.

15 —— Illustrative Case Studies of Respiratory Management

JOHN R. BACH, M.D.

Il n'y a qu'un seul moyen d'enseigner, c'est de donner l'exemple.
(There is only way to teach—that is, to provide the example.)

Gustav Mahler

Most patients with ventilatory impairment are evaluated inappropriately and treated as if they had respiratory impairment or lung disease. The following are the most common errors in the evaluation and management of patients with respiratory muscle dysfunction:

1. Misinterpretation of symptoms
2. Failure to perform spirometry with the patient in various positions and circumstances and failure to evaluate for maximal insufflation capacity (MIC)
3. Failure to evaluate peak cough flow (PCF)
4. Use of arterial blood gas analyses rather than noninvasive monitoring of SpO_2 and carbon dioxide tensions
5. Unnecessary resort to bronchoscopy, endotracheal intubation, and tracheostomy
6. Failure to deflate or eliminate tracheostomy tube cuffs
7. Use of tracheal and airway suctioning rather than mechanically assisted coughing (MAC) with insufflation-exsufflation at optimal spans
8. Administration of oxygen, bronchodilators, and chest physical therapy instead of aiding respiratory muscles
9. Use of body ventilators instead of noninvasive intermittent positive-pressure ventilation (IPPV)
10. Use of continuous airway pressure (CPAP) or pressure-assist ventilation with positive end-expiratory pressure (PIP + PEEP) at suboptimal spans
11. Use of pressure- rather than volume-limited ventilators for patients capable of air-stacking
12. Failure to vary IPPV interfaces for fit, comfort, and efficacy
13. Failure to use mouthpiece IPPV or to extend use of noninvasive IPPV into daytime hours
14. Unnecessary ventilator use or inappropriate weaning
15. Failure to train patients in glossopharyngeal breathing (GPB)
16. Inappropriate resort to electrophrenic pacing (EPR)

Case 1: Misinterpretation of Symptoms/
Lack of Utility of Arterial Blood Gases

In February of 1986, a 36-year-old woman with a 19-year history of multiple sclerosis and a baseline vital capacity of 1500 ml developed rapidly progressive tetraplegia. She was hospitalized and became increasingly anxious and tachypneic. On the morning of the fourth hospital day an arterial blood sample demonstrated pH of 7.38, PaO_2 of 86 mmHg, and $PaCO_2$ of 46 mmHg. During consultation that evening she complained of extreme fatigue and three days of sleeplessness associated with anxiety and inability to breathe when lying down. She had a vital capacity of 180 ml when supine and 250 ml when sitting (6% of predicted normal). She was placed on nasal IPPV for impending ventilatory failure using the synchronized intermittent mechanical ventilation (SIMV) mode at 900 ml and at a rate of 14/min. Expiratory volumes measured at the expiratory valve were 750 ml when she was awake or asleep and with the mouth open or closed. The $PaCO_2$ became 29 mmHg while she used nasal IPPV, and she feel asleep almost immediately. On direct observation during sleep, the delivered air moved her soft palate against the posterior aspect of the tongue, thereby preventing significant insufflation leakage. At no time overnight did end-tidal carbon dioxide exceed 36 mmHg. The next morning vital capacity had decreased to 100 ml, and she was dependent on nasal IPPV with no breathing tolerance. This scenario continued for the next 72 hours, at which point vital capacity began to increase as she responded to treatment with adrenocorticotrophic hormone. After 5 days she no longer required ventilatory support.

This case was the first reported use of nasal IPPV for 24-hour ventilatory support in a patient with no breathing tolerance and negligible vital capacity. Fatigue, anxiety, and sleeplessness typically signal impending ventilatory failure in wheelchair users with decompensating ventilatory impairment. Other symptoms—such as headaches, frequent arousals from sleep, and nightmares—also are commonly ascribed incorrectly to conditions other than ventilatory insufficiency. The mild pretreatment hypercapnia seen in the arterial blood gas sampling did not alert the clinicians to intervene. End-tidal carbon dioxide and oximetry monitoring are generally more useful.

Case 2: Misinterpretation of Symptoms/Inappropriate Ventilator Weaning

In November of 1989 a 53-year-old man with primary congenital lymphedema was hospitalized for shortness of breath, fatigue, and headaches. He reported extreme daytime drowsiness for 10 years. He also had a history of "asthma" with daily wheezing since adolescence and had been taking bronchodilators for 12 years without objective or subjective relief. His vital capacity was 1.15 L (20% of predicted normal); forced expiratory volume in one second (FEV_1), 0.94 L (23% of predicted normal); and FEV_1-to-forced vital capacity (FVC) ratio, 103%. He was intubated and required ventilatory support and hospitalization for 3 weeks. He was subsequently rehospitalized, intubated, and mechanically ventilated; chest tubes were placed for pleural effusions three times during the next two years.

Early during the last of these admissions, an arterial blood gas sample demonstrated pH of 7.43, $PaCO_2$ of 50 mmHg, PaO_2 of 61 mmHg, and bicarbonate level of 33.7 mEq. He developed progressive respiratory failure and was nasotracheally intubated two weeks after admission. Chest tubes were placed bilaterally, and a thoracocentesis biopsy showed pulmonary fibrosis. Because of failure to wean, a tracheostomy tube was placed on the 52nd hospital day, and the nasotracheal tube was removed. He lost all breathing tolerance while using tracheostomy IPPV. Four days after tracheotomy he became septic. He subsequently developed infection with *Klebsiella pneumoniae* in the right lower lobe, from which an abscess was drained. Atelectasis, lobar collapse, and bronchial mucus plugging became persistent problems. Episodes of respiratory arrest during weaning attempts and septic shock necessitated pressor support. Although the effusion and infiltrate eventually cleared and the chest tubes were removed, weaning attempts continued to fail over a period of 3 additional months, with $PaCO_2$ levels quickly exceeding 60 mmHg. Weaning was attempted in the conventional manner of gradually decreasing SIMV rates and volumes while providing pressure support ventilation, PEEP, and supplemental oxygen. These attempts continued despite the following facts: his maximal effort vital capacity was 570 ml; he had no breathing tolerance; and he had extremely hypersecretory airways. He also continued to require full alimentation via a nasogastric tube.

We were consulted during the sixth month of hospitalization. A fenestrated tracheostomy tube was placed and capped to permit him to practice receiving mouthpiece IPPV. After several days, he was able to tolerate mouthpiece IPPV during most of the day and nasal IPPV overnight. Oxygen therapy was discontinued. As he breathed room air, SpO_2 was 90–95% during daytime hours, and he had a mean nocturnal SpO_2 of 93% with typical "sawtooth" desaturations.[1] The tracheostomy tube was then removed and the site buttoned for 5 days before being allowed to close (Fig. 1). Thus, he was converted directly from continuous tracheostomy IPPV to daytime mouthpiece and nocturnal nasal IPPV. PaO_2 was maintained above 60 mmHg by providing adequate ventilatory support and assisting coughing by air-stacking. Because his abdominal muscles were functional, abdominal thrusts were not useful. However, PCF increased from 1.3 L/sec, unassisted, to 4.4 L/sec with maximal air-stacking via a mouthpiece. Transition to continuous noninvasive IPPV and tracheostomy site closure required 2 weeks. Breathing tolerance remained under 5 minutes despite an increase in vital capacity to 640 ml and the alleviation of airway hypersecretion by tracheostomy site closure.

During the six months before this hospitalization the patient was unable to walk 200 feet without assistance and had not been able to go up more than five steps because of dyspnea. At the initiation of his rehabilitation program, he was able to ambulate only a few feet with a walker while using mouthpiece IPPV and was dependent in all activities of daily living (ADLs).

His rehabilitation included training in GPB as well as general strengthening, mobility, and endurance exercises. His ability to walk increased, but vital capacity remained less than 700 ml and he still had no breathing tolerance. Because of inadequate strength to propel himself in a standard wheelchair equipped with a ventilator and unwillingness to use a motorized wheelchair, he used a rolling walker with a tray.[2]

When, after 60 days of rehabilitation, the patient was discharged home, he was independent in ADLs, transfers, and automobile use and could ambulate more than 400 feet

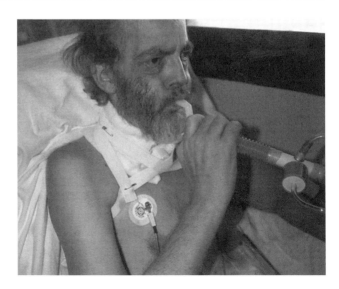

FIGURE 1. Switching a patient with severe restrictive pulmonary impairment and no breathing tolerance from tracheostomy to noninvasive IPPV. As seen, the tracheostomy button was removed and the site is closing under a pressure dressing as the patient ventilates his lungs with mouthpiece IPPV.

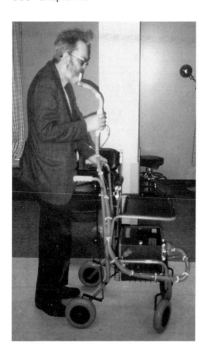

FIGURE 2. A 53-year-old man with congenital lymphedema and chronic alveolar hypoventilation. Symptoms began at 15 years of age. He was decannulated to full-time noninvasive IPPV, which he has required for 15 years. Because his skeletal musculature is generally intact, he walks using a rolling walker to permit continued mouthpiece IPPV.

using mouthpiece IPPV with the rolling walker (Fig. 2). He returned to full-time employment as an accountant despite continuous use of noninvasive IPPV and no breathing tolerance. He has been working and living at home for the past 15 years. He has had no further hospitalizations for respiratory difficulties, pleural effusions, or "asthmatic" episodes and has discontinued all asthma medications. Vital capacity had increased to 1050 ml and he had weaned himself from the ventilator for up to 4 hours of breathing tolerance, but his current vital capacity is 580 ml and he no longer has any breathing tolerance.

This patient demonstrates the following principles:

1. Noninvasive IPPV can be used for long-term full-time ventilatory support.

2. Except in the presence of premorbid chronic bronchitis, chronic aspiration, or other causes of chronic airway hypersecretion, the hypersecretory state of the airways associated with tracheal intubation is reversed by extubation/decannulation and site closure.

3. Decannulation and noninvasive IPPV with oximetry feedback can be used as an alternative to conventional ventilator weaning strategies. The patient simply takes fewer and fewer assisted breaths, as needed, rather than follows a constraining and arbitrary schedule.

4. The conversion to noninvasive IPPV can be made with a nasogastric tube in place. However, such a tube interferes with nasal interface placement, increases air leakage during mouthpiece or nasal IPPV, and tends to gastric insufflation and abdominal distention by opening the gastroesophageal sphincter. In general, nasogastric tubes are removed before transition to noninvasive IPPV.

5. PCF can be greatly increased by air-stacking alone.

6. A rolling walker with a tray can be used by ventilator users who can walk.

7. Under certain circumstances, wheezing that is mistaken for asthma may be due to peribronchial edema or airway mucus. It may be reversible by increasing thoracic pressures with IPPV or by MAC.

8. Despite the presence of symptomatic hypercapnia for over 10 years, he was inappropriately weaned from ventilator use at the cost of hypercapnia on three previous occasions. Hypoventilation was permitted and even exacerbated by oxygen therapy, because

his clinicians were unfamiliar with noninvasive alternatives to tracheostomy, an option that the patient repeatedly refused.

9. Breathing tolerance can decrease rapidly with tracheostomy IPPV but may recover once the patient is decannulated and ventilated noninvasively.

10. Gradual improvements in pulmonary volumes and breathing tolerance can result from effective use of noninvasive muscle aids. Noninvasive IPPV reversed chronic hypercapnia, which in itself has been shown to exacerbate respiratory muscle weakness.[3]

Case 3: Failure to Perform Spirometry with the Patient Supine/Inappropriate Oxygen Therapy/Failure to Offer Various IPPV Interfaces

A man born in 1951 with an undifferentiated myopathy had severe scoliosis and had complained of increasing dyspnea, headaches, orthopnea, leg edema, and decreased ability to concentrate since 1975, from which time he slept in a sitting position and had no breathing tolerance in the supine position. By 1984 he had severe continuous headaches, sleep and arousal dysfunction, violent nightmares, obtundation, and massive pretibial edema despite taking 120 mg of furosemide daily for 2 years. In his own words, "I felt like I was dreaming when I was awake, and I did things without being aware of what I was doing." Falling asleep at 5- to 15-minute intervals, he burned his arm twice on the stove while cooking.

He developed pneumonia in May of 1984 and was intubated for 5 weeks. From August 19, 1984 to May 6, 1985, $PaCO_2$ ranged from 40 to 51 mmHg and SpO_2 from 85% to 92% during the day, and end-tidal carbon dioxide was between 60 and 80 mmHg with a maximum of 90 mmHg during four sleep studies.

In December of 1985 he had jugular vein distention at 45°, massive pretibial edema with severe chronic stasis dermatitis, anasarca, cardiomegaly, a tender and enlarged liver with elevated liver function enzymes, pulmonary congestion, and polycythemia (hematocrit = 52.6). Vital capacity in the sitting position was 1410 ml (31% of normal), and the FEV_1/FVC ratio was 90%. SpO_2 was 87%, whereas $PaCO_2$ was 57 mmHg and increased to 63 mmHg when he received 0.5 L/min of supplemental oxygen by nasal cannula. However, obtundation and cor pulmonale worsened, and he developed pneumonia for which he was hospitalized, intubated, and mechanically ventilated on two further occasions through June 1986.

In June of 1986 polysomnography and capnography (Grass Model 78 D polysomnograph, Grass Instruments, Quincy, MA) were performed in the semisupine position. He had 118 hypopneas per hour, a mean SpO_2 of 55.2%, and end-tidal carbon dioxide levels as high as 91 mmHg. He had neither rapid-eye-movement nor slow-wave sleep.

In August of 1986 he was rehospitalized for dyspnea and obtundation and further elevations of plasma liver enzymes. Furosemide was increased to 160 mg/day, and he was placed on nocturnal nasal IPPV, which he used in the supine position. Two weeks later, polysomnography was repeated while he used nasal IPPV and breathed room air. Total sleep, sleep efficiency, sleep latency, sleep onset, and REM sleep were nearly normal. He had 13 apneas/hypopneas per hour. SpO_2 was 48–63% during the first hour (12–1 AM) and 70–96% for the rest of the night. He was discharged home using nasal IPPV and slept in the supine position. His furosemide dosage was gradually lowered to 60 mg/week. All hypoventilation symptoms had resolved.

In January of 1987, after 5 months of nocturnal nasal IPPV, he had only minimal residual dependent lower extremity edema. Liver size and enzymes were normal, and hematocrit was 40. Vital capacity was 1300 ml in the sitting position and 600 ml in the supine position. Breathing tolerance in the supine position continued to be negligible, but he did not require ventilator use when sitting. Although the baseline end-tidal carbon dioxide level was 45–50 mmHg and SpO_2 was 88–92%, $PaCO_2$ decreased to 33–38 mmHg and SpO_2 was greater than 95% within 2 minutes of using nasal IPPV, in the sitting or supine position, on assist/control mode with a delivered volume of 1150 ml (airway pressure: 30 cmH_2O).

Because during sleep he used nasal IPPV, insufflation leakage caused a decrease in air delivery pressure to a minimum of 26 cmH$_2$O. At this pressure SpO$_2$ dropped to a low of 88%, and end-tidal carbon dioxide rose to a maximum of 49 mmHg. The airway pressure varied from 26 to 28 mmHg during most of the night but was adequate to maintain a mean SpO$_2$ of 95%. His major complaint was that as soon as he discontinued nasal IPPV in the morning he became dyspneic for the rest of the day. Nonetheless, he resisted daytime use of mouthpiece IPPV.

He did well until he was hit by a truck and incurred fractures of the left tibia and fibula in January of 1991. Although he had been unable to walk for 8 years, his fractures were set under general anesthesia. However, because he was left supine and could not be weaned from the ventilator, he remained intubated, developed adult respiratory distress syndrome, self-extubated, and died while he was being reintubated.

This patient demonstrates the following principles:

1. Unessential surgery and general anesthesia should be avoided for patients with minimal ventilatory reserve.

2. Because of failure to assess pulmonary function and ventilatory capacity in the recumbent position and failure to use inspiratory muscle aids in a timely manner, the patient had ventilatory insufficiency for over 10 years, severe cor pulmonale, and ultimately fatal complications.

3. Exacerbation of hypoventilation by oxygen therapy can result in increased respiratory morbidity and hospitalizations.

4. A variety of IPPV interfaces, oral and nasal, should be tried, and the patient should be allowed to choose.

Case 4: Failure to Evaluate or Use PCF as a Criterion for Decannulation

Three tracheostomized patients with spinal cord injury who were breathing room air comfortably and autonomously via the upper airway maintained normal SpO$_2$ and had vital capacities of 1.3, 1.7, and 2.1 L, respectively. In each case the tracheostomy tube was removed and a tracheostomy button was placed. All three developed dyspnea, oxyhemoglobin desaturation, and diminution in vital capacity in less than 24 hours; two also developed fever. The tracheostomy tubes were replaced, and the patients received aggressive mechanical insufflation-exsufflation (MI-E) through the tubes. SpO$_2$ and vital capacity returned to baseline as the airways were cleared of secretions over a period of hours. Further examination revealed that one patient had tracheal stenosis and two had vocal cord adhesions preventing full abduction.

These three patients demonstrate that airway patency can be adequate for ventilation but not for effective coughing. Laryngoscopic evaluation of the upper airway has been advocated in all patients before removal of tracheostomy tubes.[4] However, the ability to generate PCF above 160 L/min generally ensures sufficient airway patency for safe elimination of indwelling tubes, regardless of the extent of respiratory muscle paralysis.[5]

Case 5: Inappropriate Administration of Oxygen, Bronchodilators, and Chest Physical Therapy/Body Ventilator-Associated Sleep Apneas

A patient with complete C4–C5 tetraplegia due to a fall in 1957 at age 14 years developed ventilatory insufficiency in 1969. He complained of hypersomnolence from 1969 to 1974 and was treated by continuous home oxygen therapy. As a result, PaCO$_2$ climbed to 70–80 mmHg, and hypersomnolence worsened. He was first hospitalized for respiratory failure triggered by a chest infection in 1974. He was intubated, temporarily tracheostomized, and received IPPV for 3 weeks. Over the next 9 years he was hospitalized on eight occasions and intubated three times for respiratory failure. In 1983, he developed cor pulmonale and had three episodes of respiratory arrest, resulting in loss of consciousness, during attempts to wean him from IPPV via a nasotracheal tube after urologic surgery. Chest-shell ventilator use permitted extubation. He continued to use it nightly for 4 years, then switched to a negative-pressure wrap-style ventilator nightly until 1989. From 1983 to 1989 he was hospitalized on nine occasions and intubated eight times. He underwent bronchoscopic mucus removal on 13 occasions and had two grand mal seizure episodes associated with theophylline therapy.

In 1989, with a vital capacity of 450 ml in the sitting position and 580 ml in the supine position, arterial blood gases and continuous noninvasive blood gas monitoring were performed to evaluate the effectiveness of nocturnal negative-pressure wrap ventilator use. His awake unaided $PaCO_2$ ranged from 55 to 95 mmHg during periods of fatigue late in the day. PaO_2 values were as low as 40 mmHg. Severe oxyhemoglobin desaturation occurred during sleep as well as throughout daytime hours. He was switched to nocturnal mouthpiece IPPV but refused to use a lipseal (Mallincrodt, Pleasanton, CA) because of inability to remove the retention straps independently for use of a sip-and-puff telephone during the night. His blood gases were not optimal using nocturnal mouthpiece IPPV without a lipseal. Since he retained antigravity strength in his right biceps, a pulley system was set up that allowed him to remove lipseal straps independently (Fig. 3).

Theophylline, oxygen, and ongoing routine chest physical therapy were discontinued. Mouthpiece IPPV with lipseal retention normalized nocturnal SpO_2 and end-tidal carbon dioxide. He also discovered that, by adding oximetry and occasionally capnography, he could normalize SpO_2 and alveolar ventilation with daytime use of mouthpiece IPPV and

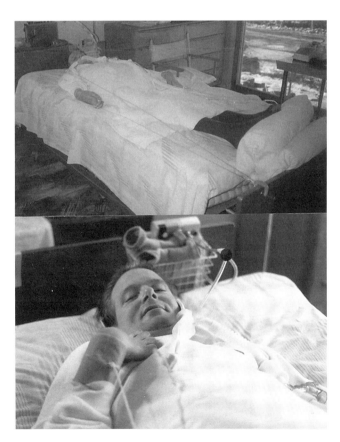

FIGURE 3. Patient with spinal cord injury and late-onset chronic ventilatory failure. He uses a pulley system to remove independently the lipseal retention system used for nocturnal mouthpiece IPPV.

thus relieve fatigue and dyspnea. His vital capacity increased to 720 ml in the sitting position and 760 ml in the supine position 4 months after initiation of noninvasive IPPV in December of 1989, and mandatory ventilator use decreased from 24 hours to 14 hours per day. He had neither respiratory complications nor hospitalizations over the next 10 years while using mouthpiece IPPV and MI-E to clear airway secretions during chest infections. He had no further seizure activity. His maximal unassisted PCF of 0.9 L/sec increased to 1.2 L/sec after maximal insufflation to 1100 ml; with the use of MI-E, it was higher.[6]

This patient demonstrates that noninvasive IPPV and airway secretion management can be effective and prevent respiratory complications and hospitalizations even when assisted PCF is less than 2.7 L/sec—provided that baseline SpO_2 is normal. Both oxygen therapy and theophylline were useless and harmful; ongoing chest physical therapy was a waste of time. As for 40 previously described patients, body ventilator use was or became inadequate, and this patient, too, needed to be switched to noninvasive IPPV with trials of various noninvasive IPPV interfaces.[7]

Case 6: Inappropriate Resort to Electrophrenic Pacing

The longest case of tracheostomy tube decannulation despite full-time ventilator dependence for a patient with high-level spinal cord injury is a man who in March of 1967, at 17 years of age, fell from a horse in a school gymnasium. He sustained a fracture dislocation of C1 on C2 and complete C2 tetraplegia. He was immediately apneic and became permanently ventilator-dependent without breathing tolerance. Phrenic pacemakers were placed bilaterally but proved ineffective. He remained in intensive care for 10 months because of pulmonary infections. He was transferred for rehabilitation in February of 1968 with an indwelling tracheostomy tube and a cuff inflated with 12 ml of air. He developed severe trachiectasis with a cuff-to-trachea diameter ratio of 3:1. He continued to have frequent bronchial mucus plugging, which led to one episode of respiratory arrest that resulted in partial cortical blindness and two episodes of near-arrest. He was highly motivated for tracheostomy site closure.

He began using daytime mouthpiece IPPV with a portable pressure-limited ventilator at a rate of 18 breaths per minute and a pressure of 20 cmH_2O in April of 1968. The tracheostomy tube was plugged. He began nocturnal iron lung use in July of 1968. Both methods provided normal alveolar ventilation and blood gases. Even with the tube plugged, however, tracheal site leakage prevented the patient from attaining more than 5 minutes of breathing tolerance by combining GPB and accessory muscle use. In April of 1969, the tracheostomy site was allowed to close after another two episodes of pneumonia, and the pacemaker was removed. Breathing tolerance increased to greater than 3 hours by GPB, and he developed a GPB maximal single-breath capacity[8] of 1700 ml. The vital capacity (without GPB) increased to 420 ml with accessory muscle use in the sitting position. He was converted from nocturnal iron lung to wrap ventilator use. He continued to use mouthpiece IPPV during the daytime and the Pulmowrap (Respironics, Inc., Murrysville, PA) ventilator overnight until he committed suicide by discontinuing ventilator use and taking morphine in August of 1999. He had suffered three episodes of pneumonia due to chest infections and had resided in a chronic care facility for the past 30 years.

Another patient developed complete C4 spinal cord injury on November 25, 1989, as the result of a tank accident while he was serving in the Greek army. He was dyspneic but breathing spontaneously at the accident site. Once he arrived at a local hospital, however, he had cardiopulmonary arrest and required defibrillation and intubation for ventilatory support. He underwent tracheotomy on the third day after injury. He developed chest infections on and off for 1.5 years and remained hospitalized until he was transferred to the United States to undergo evaluation for EPR on May 7, 1992. At that time he had as much as 4 hours of breathing tolerance by using accessory inspiratory muscles. Since phrenic nerve conduction was absent bilaterally, he underwent intercostal nerve grafts into the

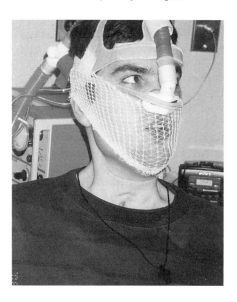

FIGURE 4.   Patient with C4 complete traumatic tetraplegia. He has been continuously ventilator-dependent since his injury in 1989. He was decannulated in 1992 and has been using mouthpiece IPPV during daytime hours and nasal IPPV for sleep. He notes improved sleep with less oral insufflation leakage with the use of a fish-net chin strap to help keep the mouth closed during sleep.

phrenic nerves. He continued using tracheostomy IPPV during the day. After the grafts, EPR increased tidal volumes by 200 ml, and he began to use it overnight but complained that he could not sleep because of shortness of breath. He was transferred to Kessler Institute for Rehabilitation on June 17, 1992 for adjustment to EPR.

On October 29, 1992 we placed him on nocturnal nasal IPPV (Fig. 4) and introduced him to mouthpiece IPPV for use in his wheelchair. He tried to use EPR during daytime hours, but it failed to relieve his dyspnea. When he discovered how easy and comfortable it was to use simple mouthpiece IPPV with the mouthpiece fixed adjacent to his lips while he was in the wheelchair, he refused further attempts at EPR. He used mouthpiece IPPV during the day with 1–2 hours of breathing tolerance in the supine position and up to 4 hours of breathing tolerance in the sitting position. His tracheostomy was sutured closed.

He continues using full-time noninvasive IPPV in Pella, Greece. Vital capacity at the time of site closure was 650 ml in the sitting position and 600 ml in the supine position. In 1998, after closure, it became 780 ml and 740 ml, respectively. However, MIC was 3260 ml. Although unassisted PCF was only 2 L/sec, PCF was 6.8 L/sec from the MIC and became 9.5 L/sec with the addition of an abdominal thrust. He also was able to use GPB up to the MIC. With regular lung expansion and such excellent air-stacking and assisted coughing ability, he has managed to cough effectively during all subsequent chest infections, has not required MI-E, and has had no respiratory morbidity since leaving the U.S., despite lack of improvement in vital capacity or breathing tolerance.

Although pacemakers were placed in both patients—34 and 9 years ago, respectively— more recent results fail to justify this expensive, invasive, and unphysiologic approach[9] except in patients who cannot rotate the neck to grab a mouthpiece for noninvasive IPPV (see Chapter 8). All four traumatic tetraplegic ventilator users with pacemakers and tracheostomy tubes whom we have decannulated converted to noninvasive IPPV and discontinued pacemaker use.

Case 7: Inappropriate Ventilator Use

A 24-year-old man, who had had a spinal cord injury on November 30, 1979, was intubated, then tracheostomized, and used IPPV for 6 months with no breathing tolerance. He was transferred for rehabilitation. Vital capacity increased to 340 ml, and maximal breathing tolerance gradually increased so that he could wean to nocturnal-only IPPV in August of 1980, He was discharged home and instructed to "never stop using nocturnal ventilatory support." He suffered two episodes of lung collapse and pneumonia in 1983 but had no further difficulties and underwent no further pulmonary function testing until January of 1988, when he presented with vital capacity of 2920 ml in the sitting position and 3170 ml in the supine position. At that point he had been using nocturnal tracheostomy IPPV for 9 years. Nocturnal IPPV was discontinued, and nocturnal mean SpO_2 was 96% with a low of 91%. The tracheostomy site was allowed to close. In October of 1992, vital capacity was 4200 ml in the sitting position and 3600 ml in the supine position. He has had no subsequent respiratory difficulties.

Case 8: Inappropriate Ventilator Weaning and Failure to Use Mechanical Insufflation-Exsufflation in a Timely Manner

A 67-year-old man with a 58 pack-year history of cigarette smoking became a complete C4 ventilator-dependent traumatic tetraplegic in July of 1992. He was weaned from ventilator use 2 months after injury and transferred for rehabilitation with an indwelling capped tracheostomy tube and profuse airway secretions. He was receiving supplemental oxygen. Three days after admission to rehabilitation, he developed pneumonia, was rehospitalized, became ventilator-dependent for 3 weeks, then once again was weaned to oxygen supplementation and transferred for rehabilitation. At this time the tracheostomy site was allowed to close, but secretions remained profuse and purulent. He continued antibiotics and supplemental oxygen therapy. Over the next 2 months, two episodes of hypercapnic coma necessitated two further hospitalizations, intubations, and bronchoscopic removal of mucus. He then was referred to a rehabilitation ventilator unit.

A review of earlier hospital and rehabilitation records revealed that vital capacity had ranged from 750 to 1000 ml. On admission to the ventilator unit, vital capacity was 900 ml, oxygen therapy was discontinued, and baseline SpO_2 varied from 80% to 93% with end-tidal carbon dioxide greater than 50 mmHg. He was placed on mouthpiece IPPV with oximetry feedback, nocturnal nasal IPPV to normalize ventilation, and frequent air-stacking for assisted coughing. His maximal unassisted PCF was 1.2 L/sec. He had frequent and sudden episodes of oxyhemoglobin desaturation below 80% that were corrected with the elimination of large volumes of mucus by MAC. As an immediate result of MAC, vital capacity rose to 1200 ml. He required MAC every 15 minutes during daytime hours for 2 days, at which point the airways became virtually free of sputum; SpO_2 remained over 94%; vital capacity increased to 1600 ml or by 77% in 2 days; and he discontinued nocturnal nasal IPPV. He was able to complete his rehabilitation program without further incident and returned home without ventilatory support, largely because of MAC.

This patient had been intubated to resuscitate him from hypercapnic coma. However, we have used lipseal IPPV rather than intubation to resuscitate two patients with "do not resuscitate" orders from hypercapnic coma (see Case 19). Nasal ventilation also was recently reported to be effective in relieving another comatose patient in hypercapnic respiratory failure for whom reintubation was ruled out for ethical reasons.[10]

Case 9: Overreliance on Tracheostomy/Failure to Deflate Cuff/Failure to Evaluate for Home Care

A patient with DMD who had lost the ability to walk at age 10 years and had severe scoliosis, developed symptomatic hypercapnia at age 26 in 1977 with a vital capacity of 46% of predicted normal. He was placed on nocturnal mouthpiece IPPV, which he used without lipseal retention. By 1980 he required mouthpiece IPPV for increasing periods during daytime hours and used it 24 hours/day from 1981 to 1985, at which point vital capacity was 340 ml or 13% of predicted normal. Because he was not offered a lipseal retention system for nocturnal mouthpiece IPPV,[7] he had frequent sleep arousals and was convinced by his physicians to undergo elective tracheotomy during his first hospitalization in 1985.

However, with the tracheostomy he developed pneumonia. Because of malnutrition due to worsening dysphagia, a gastrostomy tube was placed; then a Hickman catheter was placed for hyperalimentation and long-term antibiotic therapy.

Once the patient was stable, he could not be discharged home because his wife, a survivor of poliomyelitis, could walk but had no upper extremity function and could not perform tracheal suctioning. Therefore, after a hospitalization of 6 months, the patient was forced to return to his parents' home. Because the tracheostomy tube cuff was never deflated, he could no longer verbalize. He received 24-hour oxygen therapy, and the Hickman catheter was not removed. In 1988, the family sent me a copy of his hospital records. His tracheostomy tube cuff was still inflated; he still received supplemental oxygen; he no longer had sufficient stamina to sit in a wheelchair and had not been placed in one since hospital discharge two and one-half years earlier; and he was extremely depressed because he could no longer live with his wife. I was told that the physicians had informed the family two and one-half years earlier that he was "being sent home to die and the oxygen will make him more comfortable." He died in October 1988 when he developed sepsis from the Hickman catheter.

This patient's depression and ultimate demise were the result of unnecessary tracheotomy, unnecessary long-term cuff inflation, an unnecessary central line, and failure to consider postdischarge tracheostomy management. With an optimal tracheostomy tube diameter and some residual vocal cord function, virtually no patient with primarily ventilation impairment requires cuff inflation unless pulmonary compliance is extremely poor.[11] Indeed, virtually no patient with NMD and sufficient bulbar musculature to speak should require a tracheostomy tube for ventilatory support or airway secretion management.[12]

Case 10: Inadequate Pressure-Assist Ventilation/Inappropriate Use of Pressure Rather Than Volume-Limited Ventilation/Failure to Extend Nocturnal Use of Noninvasive IPPV into Daytime Hours/Inappropriate Use of Oxygen/Unnecessary Emphasis On Tracheostomy

A cognitively intact patient with DMD underwent Harrington rod placement for scoliosis relief in 1989 at age 14 years. He remained stable until February of 1995 when a chest infection caused fatigue and cyanosis. $PaCO_2$ was 88 mmHg. He was treated with low-span PIP + PEEP (IPAP of 12 cmH_2O, EPAP of 6 cmH_2O) in a local emergency department with some improvement, then sent home using the same settings at night with supplemental oxygen. However, during the next month he had frequent nocturnal arousals with tachycardia, saying "breathe" to himself. He was readmitted, but because the hospital had no policy about PIP + PEEP, use of his ventilator was not permitted. On the first morning after admission he was found to be comatose with a $PaCO_2$ of 99 mmHg. The physicians advised his parents to "let him go," but they did not concur and he was placed on low-span PIP + PEEP. He developed severe anoxic encephalopathy. I advised discontinuation of oxygen therapy and use of high spans of IPAP at 18 cmH_2O and EPAP at 2 cmH_2O to normalize SpO_2 without supplemental oxygen therapy. This recommendation, however, was not followed.

Because he remained precariously underventilated, his parents were pressured to permit tracheotomy. At our urging against the procedure, his parents transferred him to our clinic. However, because the hospital believed that it was hazardous to discharge or transfer the patient using a BiPAP machine (Respironics, Inc., Murrysville, PA) and the ambulance "did not have oxygen," his parents had to sign him out against medical advice and bring him themselves. We were advised to admit him for tracheotomy.

In our outpatient clinic we converted the patient to nasal IPPV using the assist-control mode on a PLV-100 portable volume-limited ventilator (Respironics, Inc., Murrysville, PA). He and his family were instructed in the MAC protocol, which included discontinuation of oxygen therapy. SpO_2 became and remained normal, and the patient was sent home.

Despite requiring full-time noninvasive IPPV, he has had no subsequent respiratory complications and regained normal cognitive function over the next few years.

This case demonstrates failure to use PIP + PEEP at adequate spans, inappropriate use of a pressure- rather than volume-limited ventilator for a patient who required more than nocturnal aid and was capable of air-stacking, unnecessarily protracted hospitalization, failure to use expiratory muscle aids to eliminate airway secretions, hazardous use of oxygen therapy, needless emphasis on tracheostomy, and the paradigm paralysis of associating BiPAP machines with nasal-only, low-span PIP + PEEP for simple sleep-disordered breathing.

Case 11: Hazardous Oxygen Therapy/Overemphasis on Tracheostomy/ Increased Respiratory Muscle Endurance by Rest with IPPV

A floppy neonate was diagnosed clinically with probable SMA at 2 years of age in 1958. Despite never having had the ability to sit or walk and developing severe scoliosis, she achieved a Ph.D. and worked as a full-time leisure counselor from 1979 to 1991 until severe carbon dioxide retention caused symptoms that prevented continued employment. These symptoms included hypersomnolence with sleep episodes every 5–10 minutes, confusion, "black-outs," depression, headaches, nightmares, frequent nocturnal arousals and difficult morning arousals, and polycythemia (hematocrit = 55). She had been evaluated by physicians in three NMD clinics in Pennsylvania, had been prescribed continuous oxygen therapy that only exacerbated hypercapnia and hypersomnolence, and was advised that if she did undergo tracheotomy, she would die in a matter of weeks.

After reading an article about our approach she came to our clinic. She was extremely depressed. Vital capacity was 120 ml; she weighed 37 lb and had more than 120° of scoliosis. Baseline SpO_2 on room air was 70–78%. With 1 liter of oxygen, SpO_2 was greater than 94%, but end-tidal carbon dioxide increased to over 80 mmHg. As she fell asleep breathing room air, her oximeter read 37–44%; with oxygen therapy it read 70%.

Oxygen therapy was discontinued, and the patient was instructed in the use of respiratory muscle aids and oximetry feedback. She was immediately able to maintain normal SpO_2 when using mouthpiece IPPV on room air in the awake state. She also maintained normal SpO_2 when using nasal IPPV during sleep. All symptoms of hypercapnia cleared, and she returned to gainful employment in 1 month. Because compensatory metabolic alkalosis cleared and ventilatory drive normalized, she almost immediately became dependent on noninvasive IPPV with virtually no breathing tolerance. However, after 1–2 months, she developed up to 4 hours of breathing tolerance while maintaining normal SpO_2. Despite increased ventilatory ability, no change was observed in vital capacity. Over the past 10 years she has had no hospitalizations despite four chest infections, which she managed at home with continuous noninvasive IPPV and MAC. She continues full-time employment.

This case demonstrates the hazards of oxygen therapy, unnecessary insistence on tracheostomy, and the fact that breathing tolerance (inspiratory muscle endurance) initially can be entirely lost while ventilatory drive resets but subsequently may increase with the inspiratory muscle rest provided by the full-time use of noninvasive IPPV over time.

A 54-year-old high-school teacher with a history of Pott's disease at age 3 years, severe kyphoscoliosis, and a 5-year history of shortness of breath, hypersomnolence, fatigue, and headaches was hospitalized for ventilatory failure, informed that he would not survive for more than a few months without a tracheostomy tube, and sent home using continuous supplemental oxygen. With oxygen therapy, $PaCO_2$ increased to 74 mmHg and PaO_2 to 55 mmHg. Dyspnea eased, but hypersomnolence and other symptoms of hypercapnia worsened. The patient also complained that he frequently fell asleep while teaching classes. He had two additional hospitalizations for ventilatory failure over the next 4 months and continued to refuse to undergo tracheotomy, but he became quite depressed and thought that he was dying. His respiratory therapist referred him to our program.

Mean nocturnal SpO_2 on room air was 71%, and end-tidal carbon dioxide was 53 mmHg. With 4 L/min of oxygen via nasal cannula, SpO_2 was 89%; with nasal IPPV on room air, 91%; and with nasal IPPV with 2 L/min of oxygen, 95%. Supplemental oxygen use was discontinued to optimize nocturnal nasal IPPV (see Chapter 5).[1] Using oximetry for occasional feedback, the patient maintained SpO_2 greater than 94% during daytime hours by breathing more deeply and using mouthpiece IPPV for periods of time. He has continued to use nocturnal nasal IPPV with a custom-molded nasal interface (see Fig. 9 of Chapter 7) and has used mouthpiece IPPV during the day for 15 years. He continues to have no symptoms of alveolar hypoventilation.

Case 12: Overreliance on Tracheostomy/Benefits of Glossopharyngeal Breathing

A 43-year-old journalist with limb-girdle muscular dystrophy had been using IPPV via a tracheostomy with a vital capacity of 200 ml and no breathing tolerance for 5.5 years. During this time, as for other tracheostomy IPPV users, she could not be safely left alone to work and had had numerous febrile episodes that were treated with intravenous antibiotics. In July of 1992, the tracheostomy tube was removed and the site closed. The patient was converted to daytime mouthpiece and nighttime nasal IPPV (see Fig. 3 of Chapter 1). She also mastered GPB sufficiently for up to 8 hours of breathing tolerance. This strategy permitted her to work safely at home alone. With a maximal GPB single-breath capacity of 1200 ml, she also improved her ability to raise her voice and cough.

A 17-year-old girl had a complete C1–C2 cervical spine injury in January of 1993. Vital capacity was just under 200 ml with no breathing tolerance. The tracheostomy tube was removed and the site closed in May of 1993. She was converted to daytime mouthpiece IPPV and nocturnal nasal IPPV (Fig. 5), which she continues to use. She has achieved 20–30 minutes of breathing tolerance by GPB, but a partial leak of GPB-stacked gulps from the nose limits efficacy.

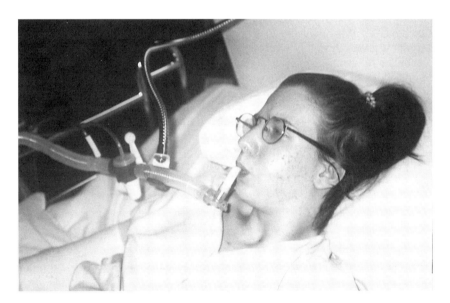

FIGURE 5. Seventeen-year-old girl with complete C2 tetraplegia, vital capacity under 200 ml, and no tolerance of ventilator-free breathing. She was decannulated and switched from tracheostomy to daytime mouthpiece IPPV and nocturnal nasal IPPV. She achieved breathing tolerance by glossopharyngeal breathing and has required noninvasive IPPV for 9 years with no respiratory complications.

Case 13: Unnecessary Endotracheal Intubation/Extubation and Conversion to 24-Hour Noninvasive IPPV

In 1990 an 18-year-old boy with DMD developed acute respiratory failure during an otherwise benign chest infection and was intubated in a local hospital. This episode occurred even though he had been previously instructed in how to use mouthpiece and nasal IPPV and air-stacked daily. While he was intubated, vital capacity decreased from an 800-ml baseline to 200 ml and he had no breathing tolerance. I was consulted at this point. Because the patient knew how to receive IPPV noninvasively, he was extubated and switched directly to continuous noninvasive IPPV and MAC. With aggressive MAC, vital capacity immediately increased to 400 ml, but he continued to have no breathing tolerance and airway secretions remained profuse for 5 days. At this point he weaned to nocturnal nasal IPPV and went home using MAC as needed. In 1996 he began to require daytime mouthpiece as well as nocturnal nasal IPPV. Thus far he has had five chest infections, which were managed at home with the oximetry feedback- respiratory aid protocol, and no further hospitalizations. During one such episode, nasal congestion rendered nasal IPPV ineffective, and he developed respiratory distress with a $PaCO_2$ of 55 mmHg. When given the choice between switching to lipseal IPPV or using nasal decongestants, he chose the decongestants and had no further elevations of end-tidal carbon dioxide or significant oxyhemoglobin desaturation. Hospitalization was avoided despite temperature elevations to 104°F and leukocytosis during at least three of the five infections. This patient also demonstrates postextubation ventilator weaning. He has now used noninvasive IPPV continuously for 6 years.

Case 14: Overreliance on Tracheal Suctioning

A 43-year-old man with C5 traumatic tetraplegia in a rehabilitation center had a vital capacity of 1900 ml and maintained normal alveolar ventilation and SpO_2 with unassisted breathing. His tracheostomy tube, however, had not yet been removed. While receiving physical therapy, he suddenly developed respiratory distress and oxyhemoglobin desaturation to 75–79%. Aggressive chest percussion, postural drainage, and tracheal suctioning were administered but failed to relieve his distress or improve SpO_2. An ambulance was called to transfer him to a local hospital for bronchoscopy. Before its arrival and after these efforts were continued for about 10 minutes, a Cough-Assist was ordered. He received MAC using MI-E through the tracheostomy tube with the cuff inflated. After only 1 cycle a large mucus plug was expelled. His dyspnea cleared, SpO_2 returned to normal, and the ambulance was canceled. Thus, MAC can be more effective than routine tracheal suctioning. Undoubtedly, the mucus emanated from the left airways, which were inaccessible to the suction catheter.[13]

Case 15: Noninvasive Nocturnal Blood Gas Monitoring/Need to Customize and Vary Interfaces/Oximetry Feedback/Improvement in Respiratory Muscle Endurance by Rest with IPPV

A patient with DMD had stopped walking at 30 months of age in 1972. Vital capacity plateaued at 1050 ml before 9 years of age. Spinal surgery was refused, and his spinal curve was 114° to the left (Cobb technique) in 1994. From January of 1985 to September of 1987 he was hospitalized five times for dyspnea, difficulties with managing airway secretions, and chest infections. His mother said that he had frequent "mucus attacks," which she described as episodes of profuse salivation, airway congestion, and uncontrolled drooling.

In October of 1987, he presented with a temperature of 104°F, complaints of chronic headaches, difficulty with swallowing, weight loss, vital capacity of 280 ml, and profuse mucopurulent airway secretions. Manually assisted coughing was not effective because of severe scoliosis. He received antibiotics and required intravenous fluids because of dehydration. $PaCO_2$ on admission was 57 mmHg. SpO_2 varied from 89% to 94% when the patient was awake with end-tidal carbon dioxide of 50–54 mmHg.

Trials of mouthpiece IPPV failed because oropharyngeal muscles were inadequate to grab the mouthpiece. He was taught and used nasal IPPV during the daytime with end-tidal carbon dioxide and pulse oximetry feedback. In this manner end-tidal carbon dioxide was maintained below 43 mmHg and SpO_2 above 94%. He napped using nasally delivered assist-control volumes of 560 ml (mask pressure of 23–25 cmH_2O) at a rate of 16 per minute. His expiratory volumes were 500 ml in the awake state with the mouth open or closed. During overnight sleep monitoring with nasal IPPV, end-tidal carbon dioxide varied from 40 to 47 mmHg, and SpO_2 averaged 95% with a low of 85% and few episodes of oxyhemoglobin desaturation. He was discharged home using nasal IPPV nocturnally.

The following week his mother stated that he felt stronger and was eating better. She also reported that the "mucus attacks" were less frequent and less severe but were not completely relieved until he began cardiac medications. He no longer required daytime ventilatory aid to maintain SpO_2 above 94%, except occasionally when he was tired. Repeat nocturnal sleep studies were performed with ventilator-delivered volumes of 1200 ml. The mean SpO_2 was 96–97%, and the maximal recorded end-tidal carbon dioxide was 40 cmH_2O. The low-pressure alarm, which was set at 14 cmH_2O, sounded often for a few seconds and about twice per night for longer periods. The alarms correlated with the dips in SpO_2, which at no time was lower than 82%. He now had excellent control of secretions, and swallowing improved. Vital capacity increased from 270 ml on October 27, 1987 to 330 ml on February 3, 1988. He gained weight and was able to sit in his wheelchair all day without fatigue.

This patient had four subsequent chest infections with fevers, elevated white blood cell counts, and profuse mucopurulent airway secretions during the first 15 months of using nocturnal nasal IPPV. Each infection was managed at home using the oximetry-MAC protocol and full-time noninvasive IPPV. On no occasion was supplemental oxygen administered. Sudden dips in SpO_2 that could not be corrected by taking large insufflation volumes were corrected by MAC. With only 1 L/sec of unassisted PCF, he required MAC about 4 times per hour during chest infections.

During a severe chest infection in August of 1988, SpO_2 ranged from 88% to 93% and PaO_2 from 62 to 70 mmHg; end-tidal carbon dioxide remained normal because he used nasal IPPV and frequent MAC around the clock. The patient apparently had diffuse microscopic atelectasis that could not be identified on chest radiographs. Desaturations as low as 70% were immediately corrected to a baseline of 91–93% after MAC. With continued aggressive MAC, baseline SpO_2 returned to normal over 4 days, and the patient weaned back to nocturnal-only nasal IPPV.

Except during chest infections, the patient used nasal IPPV only overnight and for short periods during the day until July of 1989 when his total sitting time was less than 2 hours per day. He complained of extreme fatigue, frequent "mucus attacks," dysphagia, and weight loss. Vital capacity was 250 ml. He then began to use nasal IPPV 24 hours/day. As a result, his symptoms once again cleared and he returned to sitting in his wheelchair 16 hours/day and to maintaining an active lifestyle that included frequent interstate travel with his family. Because of the need for 24-hour aid he alternated the use of four commercial CPAP and two custom-molded nasal interfaces. For 3 years he used only the interface for ventilator-assisted living[14] (IVAL; Fig. 6), which he alternated over 12-hour periods around the clock. IVAL sufficiently redistributed pressure around the nose to avert discomfort and skin irritation despite the requirement of increasingly higher pressures on the retention straps to avert insufflation leaks. Mask pressures gradually had increased to over 40 cmH_2O because of a chronic pneumothorax and severe scoliosis.

Nocturnal SpO_2 monitoring, which has been repeated every 12 months since August 1988, demonstrated mean SpO_2 at 95% or greater with a mean of 1.7 dips of 4% per hour and infrequent dips below 90%. Unassisted PCF were less than 50 L/min. With air-stacking of nasal insufflations, he generated PCF of 110 L/min; fully assisted PCF was only 110 L/min. PCF generated by MI-E was 555 L/min.[6]

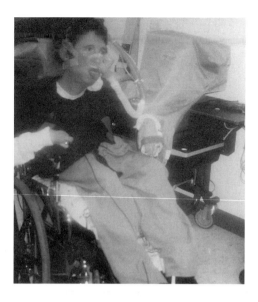

FIGURE 6. Twenty-five-year-old man with Duchenne muscular dystrophy and severe scoliosis. He required 24-hour nasal IPPV for over 5 years and used acrylic low-profile transparent nasal interfaces fabricated from plaster moulages.[14]

On May 3, 1995 the ventilator-delivered volumes were generating interface pressures averaging 52 cmH$_2$O; nocturnal mean SpO$_2$ had decreased to 92% (on room air); airway secretion production had increased; and the patient had become febrile with a white blood cell count of 16,000. He decompensated from a massive pneumothorax with complete collapse of the right lung. After chest tube placement the mild dyspnea was relieved, and ventilator pressures normalized with the same delivered volumes. Seven hours later, however, he developed repeated episodes of ventricular tachyarrhythmias and died. This patient had a severe cardiomyopathy. Correction of hemodynamic status led to acute cardiac decompensation.

This patient demonstrates the following principles:
1. The utility of oximetry feedback and sleep monitoring
2. The need for switching between various nasal interfaces for IPPV
3. Nasal IPPV can be used effectively 24 hours/day over the long term when the lips are too weak for effective mouthpiece IPPV, when scoliosis is too severe for use of an IAPV, and even when patients have no breathing tolerance, pulmonary compliance is poor, and ventilator-delivered volumes generate interface pressures exceeding 40 cmH$_2$O.
4. Breathing tolerance can increase with the respiratory muscle rest provided by noninvasive IPPV.
5. Use of respiratory muscle aids can be critical for avoiding pulmonary complications and hospitalizations.
6. Volume-limited ventilator gauge pressures should be monitored; when they increase, chest radiographs should be performed.
7. MAC can be effective even when manually assisted PCF cannot exceed 180 L/min.
8. "Mucus attacks," which probably are due in large part to heart failure, can be relieved by normalizing alveolar ventilation.

Case 16: Inability to Discharge a Conventionally Managed Patient to the Community and Benefits of Various Noninvasive Ventilation Approaches

A 31-year-old woman with a history of poliomyelitis at 4 years of age developed a chest infection and acute respiratory failure in April of 1987. She suffered a cardiopulmonary arrest on route to a local hospital. She was intubated and subsequently tracheostomized. Attempts at ventilator weaning failed, and, against her wishes, she was transferred to a chronic care facility despite the fact that she required only nocturnal ventilatory support.

Vital capacity was 1030 ml in the sitting position but only 630 ml in the supine position. She was not permitted to return home to her husband who had a "9 to 5" job because regulations prohibited tracheal suctioning by other than family members and licensed health care professionals, for whom no funds were available. She remained at the chronic care facility using nocturnal tracheostomy IPPV with an inflated cuff for 6 months. This technique caused severe tracheomalacia.

She was transferred to our rehabilitation unit for decannulation. On the first night the cuff was deflated, and the delivered ventilator volumes were increased to compensate for insufflation leakage through the upper airway. Deflation relieved the pressure on the trachea and permitted speech during use of tracheostomy IPPV. Then the tracheostomy tube was removed; a firm occlusive dressing was placed over the site; and the patient was placed on nocturnal nasal IPPV. She used this technique for 2 weeks until she complained of nasal bridge discomfort from the nasal interface. Once again an attempt at weaning failed when, after 10 days off assistance, severe fatigue and blood gas deterioration resulted in placement in an iron lung overnight for 2 weeks. She was converted to use of a Pulmowrap ventilator and discharged home. Since this device was too inconvenient to don, she eventually switched to a strapless oronasal interface (SONI) for IPPV. She continues to use nocturnal SONI IPPV and has not required rehospitalization.

A 49-year-old woman with congenital myopathy had a long history of fatigue, difficulties with concentration, dyspnea, and hypersomnolence. She developed pneumonia and was hospitalized and underwent tracheotomy in February of 1990. She was weaned from IPPV and breathed through an open tracheostomy tube. Unfortunately, she also was placed on continuous supplemental oxygen therapy but developed increasing hypercapnia ($PaCO_2$ of 55–93 mmHg) over a 3-week period. She could not tolerate plugging of the tube. Because of chronic hypercapnia and dyspnea she was returned to tracheostomy IPPV and continued to receive continuous oxygen therapy. Further attempts at ventilator weaning involved alternating use of diminishing rates and periods of SIMV with CPAP. Her arterial blood gases typically demonstrated normal pH, PaO_2 of 130–170 mmHg, $PaCO_2$ of 65–74 mmHg, and elevated bicarbonate levels. The patient lived in a communal Ashram; her caregivers were not relatives. Because no one could or would be permitted to take responsibility for tracheal suctioning, she could not be discharged.

After 5 months of unsuccessful ventilator weaning, she was transferred to our service for decannulation on July 27, 1990. Supplemental oxygen therapy, bronchodilators, and theophylline were discontinued on admission with no untoward effects. Oximetry feedback demonstrated that she could normalize SpO_2 and $PaCO_2$ by breathing more deeply for short periods before tiring. Decannulation was performed on admission, and she was ventilated by a chest-shell ventilator for 18 hours while the tracheostomy site closed (see Fig. 5 in Chapter 1). During overnight chest-shell use, mean SpO_2 was 89%; she had a maximal end-tidal carbon dioxide of 55 mmHg; and she was uncomfortable and vomited twice. With discontinuance of the chest-shell ventilator she could maintain normal SpO_2 by deep breathing supplemented by periods of mouthpiece IPPV. She was placed on nasal IPPV for nocturnal ventilatory aid. With nocturnal nasal IPPV, mean SpO_2 was 97% with a low of 89%. The airway secretions due to tracheostomy tube irritation were cleared by MAC for two days, after which no sputum remained. She was discharged to the Ashram on the fourth day after admission. Although at discharge breathing tolerance was less than 2 hours, the maintenance of normal alveolar ventilation around the clock with noninvasive IPPV kept her symptom-free. She returned to her active career as a professional writer and counselor and thus far has used noninvasive IPPV 16–20 hours/day for 10 years without further respiratory difficulties.

A 26-year-old man with DMD became wheelchair-dependent at age 12 years. He remained in good health until October of 1996 when a cold developed into pneumonia and respiratory failure. He was hospitalized for 7 days without requiring intubation. In

November another chest infection developed into pneumonia and respiratory failure, for which he was hospitalized for 4 days, again without requiring intubation. Then, one morning in December of 1996, he was found in hypercapnic coma. He was hospitalized for 32 days and intubated for 4 days and then underwent tracheotomy. He was discharged to a nursing home, where he remained for the next 7 months for tracheostomy care and continuous ventilator dependence that his parents felt they could not manage at home. However, because his parents wanted him to return home, they arranged for him to be transferred to our service in July of 1997 for decannulation and transition to noninvasive aids.

On admission supplemental oxygen was discontinued. Vital capacity was 650 ml, SpO_2 averaged 92%, and end-tidal carbon dioxide was 38 mmHg. Chest radiograph demonstrated gross atelectasis. The tracheostomy tube was changed to a fenestrated cuffed Shiley tube, and trials of mouthpiece and nasal IPPV were begun. He had no breathing tolerance and reported that he had had none since being intubated. At one point vital capacity was 250 ml and SpO_2 was 87%. After MAC vital capacity immediately returned to 650 ml and SpO_2 increased to the 92% baseline. MAC was used at least every 30 minutes for 24 hours while he was awake to reverse oxyhemoglobin desaturation. Within 24 hours after admission baseline SpO_2 had normalized to 97%. The fenestrated tracheostomy tube was then removed and nasal IPPV was begun with the PLV-100 portable volume-limited positive-pressure ventilator (Respironics, Inc., Murrysville, PA). After continuous nasal IPPV for 2 days, he was switched to daytime mouthpiece IPPV and required 2–3 mouthpiece IPPVs per minute. Over the next 4 days, he required assisted ventilation less and less frequently. The tracheostomy closed completely after 1 week, and SpO_2 continued to be normal. By the time of discharge home on day 8, vital capacity was 840 ml, assisted PCF was 200 L/m, and the patient required only nocturnal ventilatory assistance with a PLV-100, an oximeter, and a Cough-Assist for home use. He subsequently had one chest infection, which was managed at home with continuous noninvasive IPPV, expiratory aids, and oximetry feedback. Five years after discharge home, he remains without a tracheostomy tube and has had no further hospitalizations.

This patient had experienced no speech or swallowing difficulties and was also a good candidate for decannulation because assisted PCF was over 160 L/min. In addition, the patient and his care providers were cooperative in learning the respiratory aid/oximetry protocol. This case demonstrates that despite 7 months of continuous ventilator dependence with no breathing tolerance, decannulation and transition to noninvasive IPPV can result in weaning to nocturnal-only aid for the reasons noted in Chapter 5. Even patients with DMD who are generally not good candidates for GPB should be considered, under certain circumstances, for decannulation and transition to noninvasive alternatives. Decannulation and access to a variety of noninvasive inspiratory muscle aids and IPPV interfaces can facilitate discharge to the community.

Case 17: Intubation Avoided by Noninvasive IPPV

A 15-year-old boy with an odontoid fracture as the result of a diving accident in May of 1988 was hospitalized with C3 motor-complete tetraplegia. His ventilatory status deteriorated rapidly. Twenty-four hours after admission he had a vital capacity of 750 ml and complained of shortness of breath. Physical examination and chest radiographs demonstrated no lung pathology. Increasing dyspnea was managed with the use of a chest-shell ventilator (Fig. 7), which provided a tidal volume of 550 ml and normalized blood gases. Within 24 hours he had no breathing tolerance; vital capacity was less than 500 ml in the supine position; and unassisted tidal volumes were less than 200 ml.

The patient's neck was stabilized temporarily with a Philadelphia collar, and he was transferred to a trauma center. On June 2, 1988, 4 days after injury, the chest shell was removed so that halo traction with an anterior chest-wall jacket could be placed (Fig. 8). The patient was switched to mouthpiece IPPV. At this time vital capacity was 480 ml, and he

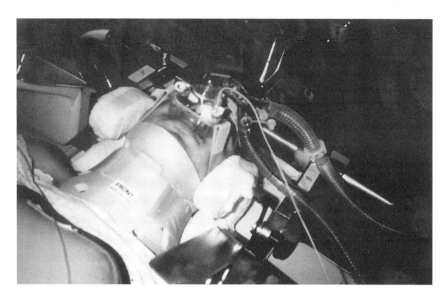

FIGURE 7. Fifteen-year-old boy with spinal cord injury. Ventilatory failure was relieved by chest-shell ventilator use. Because the chest shell had to be removed to accommodate a neck-stabilizing brace, he was trained in noninvasive IPPV.

continued to have no breathing tolerance. He mastered mouthpiece IPPV in less than 10 minutes. The assist-control mode at a volume of 890 ml maintained SpO_2 above 94%, $PaCO_2$ below 45 mmHg, and complete relief of dyspnea. Since he had no breathing tolerance and neither neck nor upper extremity movement, the mouthpiece had to be kept in his mouth. He switched from mouthpiece to nasal IPPV for sleep without changing ventilator settings.

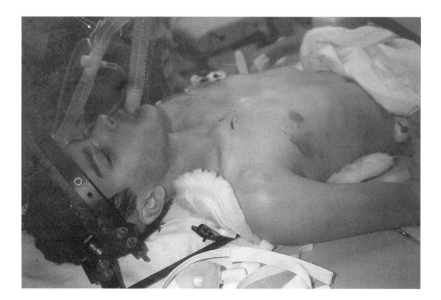

FIGURE 8. Same patient as in Figure 7. Once the chest shell was removed, a pressure ulcer became visible. He had no tactile sensation on his thorax. Here he is using mouthpiece IPPV as the four-poster brace is being placed.

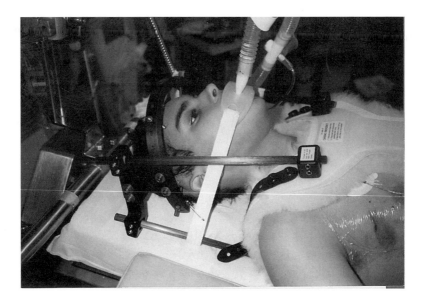

FIGURE 9. The same patient is pictured using mouthpiece IPPV with lipseal retention for nocturnal ventilatory support. A single cloth retention strap was attached around each posterior poster by Velcro to avoid straps that course above and below the ears.

He used noninvasive IPPV in this manner for 24 hours/day for 3 days. Nocturnal blood gas monitoring demonstrated no significant oxyhemoglobin desaturation. On June 6, 1988, at 1 AM he wanted to discontinue nasal IPPV because of nasal bridge irritation. Because no custom interface was available, he switched to lipseal IPPV (Fig. 9). Although lipseal retention was strongly recommended for mouthpiece IPPV, at 3 am he had the lipseal removed and continued mouthpiece IPPV without it. During sleep he maintained a firm oral grip on the mouthpiece and insufflation leakage-associated episodes of oxyhemoglobin desaturation were infrequent.

On June 7 vital capacity was 660 ml in the supine position (11% of predicted), and the patient had approximately 1 minute of breathing tolerance. He continued full-time mouthpiece IPPV from June 6 (vital capacity of 540 ml) through June 9 (vital capacity of 860 ml). On June 10, 1988 vital capacity was 940 ml, and the patient became free of daytime ventilatory support. On June 11, with a vital capacity of 1070 ml, he discontinued mouthpiece IPPV except for periodic air-stacking. He had no need for assisted coughing.

This patient would have been intubated or undergone tracheotomy if noninvasive techniques not been available. He also demonstrates the need for versatility in the use of noninvasive aids. Mouthpiece IPPV at times can be used even without a lipseal because patients with intact chemotaxic drive develop reflex muscle activity during sleep to periodically grab the mouthpiece more firmly and thus decrease insufflation air leakage and maintain adequate blood gases.[1] The appropriate methods of ventilatory support in patients with spinal cord injury should be determined largely as a function of the level of injury (see Table 2 of Chapter 8).

Case 18: Decannulation of Ventilator-Dependent Patients with Amyotrophic Lateral Sclerosis

When asked "What has it been like to be dependent upon a machine for your breathing?," without hesitation he responded, "It has been a friend. It has given me some extra years of life."[16]

Three patients with amyotrophic lateral sclerosis (ALS) were decannulated and converted to noninvasive IPPV. One had onset of nonbulbar disease at 37.5 years of age, was diagnosed at 37.9 years of age, and became wheelchair-dependent at 40.5 years of age in November of 1993. In June of 1993 he had developed symptoms of nocturnal hypoventilation and was placed on nocturnal low-span PIP + PEEP. He used PIP + PEEP for 1.5 years until diurnal dyspnea and chronic hypercapnia became severe. At this point he underwent elective tracheotomy and became continuously dependent on tracheostomy IPPV. However, because he wanted the tube removed, he was admitted to our intensive care unit, decannulated, converted to noninvasive IPPV, and discharged home in 4 days. He initially required noninvasive IPPV 18 hours/day, but over the next 3 months he became continuously dependent on daytime mouthpiece and nocturnal nasal IPPV. After tracheostomy closure vital capacity was 1400 ml (22% of expected normal) in the sitting position and 640 ml (9%) in the supine position. MIC was 2400 ml, unassisted PCF was 230 L/min, and assisted PCF was 380 L/min. By 1998 he had lost most bulbar muscle function and assisted PCF had become unmeasurable. Rather than undergo tracheotomy a second time, he died from aspiration pneumonia due to chronic saliva aspiration.

A second patient with onset at age 34 years became wheelchair-dependent and underwent tracheotomy for acute respiratory failure at age 36.3 years. Despite generalized weakness (with no further ventilator dependency), we removed his tracheostomy tube 3 months later. At that time vital capacity was 1600 ml (28% of expected normal) in the sitting position and 1200 ml (21%) in the supine position, PCF was 200 L/min, and assisted PCF was 230 L/min. He developed progressively severe hypercapnia (diurnal $PaCO_2$ of 66 mmHg) and chronic oxyhemoglobin desaturation. He used nocturnal nasal IPPV for 2 years, developed respiratory failure, underwent tracheotomy in a local hospital, and died 2 weeks later.

A third patient with onset at age 69 developed chronic dyspnea and was intubated and underwent tracheotomy for acute respiratory failure 2 months later at age 71.9 years. Four months later he was decannulated despite having no breathing tolerance and a vital capacity of 1260 ml (24% of expected normal) in the sitting position and 640 ml (12%) in the supine position with adequate assisted PCF. Five months after decannulation vital capacity was 800 ml in the sitting position and 400 ml in the supine position; the patient required continuous noninvasive IPPV; and maximal assisted PCF had decreased below 160 L/min. Tracheotomy was recommended, but he refused and died at home 2 months later of acute respiratory failure due to airway secretion aspiration.

Unlike patients with other NMDs, who, once decannulated, typically can use noninvasive IPPV and assisted coughing methods indefinitely, patients with ALS usually develop bulbar muscle dysfunction to the point of eventually requiring tracheotomy. Unfortunately, many of these patients with functional bulbar musculature and adequate assisted PCF too often undergo tracheotomy during an episode of respiratory failure triggered by an intercurrent chest infection. Such episodes usually can be managed by noninvasive IPPV and assisted coughing with oximetry feedback. Tracheostomy is warranted only when assisted PCF cannot exceed 160 L/min and either respiratory failure occurs or aspiration is so severe that baseline SpO_2 decreases below 95%.

Three additional patients with ALS failed extubation at other hospitals, refused tracheotomy, and were transferred to our service for extubation using our protocol, which involves the avoidance of supplemental oxygen, use of MAC, and extubation to full noninvasive ventilatory support. In one case, persistent pneumonia and failure to maintain extubation resulted in tracheotomy. The other two cases were successfully extubated to noninvasive IPPV. One of these two patients was averbal, had no residual bulbar muscle function, and no measurable assisted PCF. After extubation she had excessive insufflation leakage when using nasal or lipseal IPPV and could be maintained only with the use of IPPV via an oronasal interface. She required full-time oronasal IPPV for 4 months until she was weaned gradually to nocturnal-only IPPV. She died suddenly 9 months later.

Case 19: Unnecessary Resort to Endotracheal Intubation and Tracheostomy

A 62-year-old man with COPD, atherosclerotic heart and carotid artery disease, hypertension, peptic ulcers, and steroid-induced diabetes had a history of tachyarrhythmias and frequent hospitalizations and intubations for acute exacerbations of COPD, pneumonia, and respiratory failure. He signed a statement refusing further invasive interventions. During early April of 1992, with use of continuous oxygen therapy, baseline $PaCO_2$ was 48–61 mmHg. On April 30, 1992, he experienced severe dyspnea, tachypnea, disorientation, lethargy, and hypercapnia, which led to severe obtundation and agonal breathing. Because intubation was not an option, nasal IPPV was tried. However, because of rapid mouth breathing, obtundation, and depression of central chemotaxic centers by hypercapnia and oxygen therapy, he did not trigger the nasal IPPV and all delivered volumes leaked out of his mouth. Mouthpiece IPPV via a lipseal was then tried. With this essentially closed system of ventilatory support, carbon dioxide tensions decreased and the patient recovered consciousness. SpO_2 increased to 94–95% after 30 minutes of lipseal IPPV at delivered volumes of 800 ml, assist-control rate of 10, and FiO_2 of 30%. Because of improved chemotaxic responsiveness he was then switched to nasal IPPV, with which he fell asleep and maintained a mean SpO_2 of 91% with the above settings. When awake he required full-time mouthpiece IPPV and maintained normal SpO_2 and $PaCO_2$ of 40 mmHg with little supplemental oxygen. When he stopped using the ventilator for any period of time, he became dyspneic with or without supplemental oxygen. He, therefore, had become dependent on 24-hour noninvasive IPPV. He weaned downward to 6 hours of daytime noninvasive IPPV but suffered another episode of acute respiratory failure and hospitalization with reinstitution of 24-hour noninvasive IPPV. He continued continuous noninvasive IPPV for 2 years before dying suddenly. This patient used a rolling walker with a ventilator tray for daytime mouthpiece IPPV (see Fig. 2).

Another patient in our service with severe lung disease and a history of 24 episodes of respiratory failure, who was managed by endotracheal intubation, refused further invasive interventions. He, too, was resuscitated from hypercapnic coma by lipseal IPPV and maintained by 24-hour noninvasive IPPV for 14 months before dying suddenly.

Another study of one obtunded patient and four comatose patients who were severely hypercapnic (4 with COPD, 1 with morbid obesity) and treated by IPPV via oronasal interface reported successful recovery of consciousness in all five patients. Three were discharged home and two died, one from septic shock and the other after refusing to continue noninvasive IPPV.[15]

Case 20: Death Due to Unnecessary Tracheostomy after Coronary Artery Bypass

An otherwise healthy 51-year-old lawyer underwent apparently uneventful coronary artery bypass surgery. On the third day after surgery he developed ventilatory failure, for which he underwent tracheotomy. He required nocturnal-only tracheostomy IPPV. Three months after discharge a tracheoesophageal fistula was diagnosed and surgically closed. The fistula repair broke down because the trachea had been destroyed by infection to the level of the carina. A muscle flap and tracheal prosthesis were implanted. At 11 months after surgery he suddenly bled to death as tracheal cartilage eroded through the aortic arch. The patient had been unable to return to work because of inability to speak effectively due to tracheal obstruction. He died because he underwent tracheotomy rather than received nocturnal-only nasal IPPV.

Dios, que es proveedor de todas las cosas, no nos faltará. No les falta a los mosquitos del aire, ni a los gusanillos de la tierra, ni a los renacuajos del agua. Es tan piadoso que hace salir su sol sobre los buenos y los malos, y llueve sobre los injustos y justos.

(God, who provides all things, does not fail us. He does not fail the mosquitoes of the air, nor the worms of the earth, nor the tadpoles of the water. In his mercy he makes the sun rise on the good and the bad and makes the unjust suffer along with the just.)

Miguel de Cervantes, *Don Quijote de La Mancha*

REFERENCES

1. Bach JR, Robert D, Leger P, Langevin B: Sleep fragmentation in kyphoscoliotic individuals with alveolar hypoventilation treated by nasal IPPV. Chest 107:1552–1558, 1995.
2. Kirshblum SC, Bach JR: Walker modification for ventilator assisted individuals. Am J Phys Med Rehabil 71:304–306, 1992.
3. Rochester DF, Braun NMT: Determinants of maximal inspiratory pressure in chronic obstructive pulmonary disease. Am Rev Respir Dis 132:42–47, 1985.
4. Richard I, Giraud M, Perrouin-Verbe B, et al: Laryngotracheal stenosis after intubation or tracheostomy in patients with neurological disease. Arch Phys Med Rehabil 77:493–496, 1996.
5. Bach JR: Amyotrophic lateral sclerosis: Predictors for prolongation of life by noninvasive respiratory aids. Arch Phys Med Rehabil 76:828–832, 1995.
6. Bach JR: Mechanical insufflation-exsufflation: Comparison of peak expiratory flows with manually assisted and unassisted coughing techniques. Chest 104:1553–1562, 1993.
7. Bach JR, Alba AS, Saporito LR: Intermittent positive pressure ventilation via the mouth as an alternative to tracheostomy for 257 ventilator users. Chest 103:174–182, 1993.
8. Bach JR, Alba AS, Bodofsky E, et al: Glossopharyngeal breathing and non-invasive aids in the management of post-polio respiratory insufficiency. Birth Defects 23:99–113, 1987.
9. Bach JR, O'Connor K: Electrophrenic ventilation: A different perspective. J Am Parapleg Soc 14:9–17, 1991.
10. Scala R, Archinucci I, Naldi M, et al: Noninvasive nasal ventilation in a case of hypercapnic coma [in Italian]. Minerva Anestesiol 63:245–248, 1997.
11. Bach JR, Alba AS: Tracheostomy ventilation: A study of efficacy with deflated cuffs and cuffless tubes. Chest 97:679–683, 1990.
12. Bach JR, Ishikawa Y, Kim H: Prevention of pulmonary morbidity for patients with Duchenne muscular dystrophy. Chest 112:1024–1028, 1997.
13. Fishburn MJ, Marino RJ, Ditunno JF: Atelectasis and pneumonia in acute spinal cord injury. Arch Phys Med Rehabil 71:197–200, 1990.
14. McDermott I, Bach JR, Parker C, Sortor S: Custom-fabricated interfaces for intermittent positive pressure ventilation. Int J Prosthod 2:224–233, 1989.
15. Severa E, Sancho J, Catala A, et al: Noninvasive ventilation in patients with severe hypercapnic respiratory failure and altered consciousness who refused ICU treatment. Eighth Journées Internationales de Ventilation à Domicile, abstract 85, March 7, 2001, Hopital de la Croix-Rousse, Lyon, France.
16. Sivak ED, Gipson WT, Hanson MR: Long-term management of respiratory failure in amyotrophic lateral sclerosis. Ann Neurol 12:18–23, 1982.

—— Glossary

Air-stacking—Insufflations are stacked in the lungs to maximally expand them. This is done by taking a deep breath then adding consecutive volumes of air delivered through a mouthpiece or nasal interface and holding them with a closed glottis until no more air can be held and the lungs and chest wall are fully expanded.

Alveolar ventilation—The passage of air into and out of the small air sacs (alveoli) of the lungs' respiratory exchange membrane by the intermittent action of the diaphragm and other inspiratory muscles.

Alveolus—The microscopic air sacs of the lung from which oxygen diffuses into the blood and carbon dioxide diffuses out of the blood. Plural: *alveoli*.

Apnea—Absence of breathing for an abnormally long period of time.

Atelectasis—Areas of collapse of lung air sacs (alveoli) due to underventilation or accumulation of airway secretions.

Atrophy—Muscle wasting (thinning) due to loss of function of the nerve that innervates the muscle.

Autosomal dominant—Disorders in which only one abnormal gene must be inherited from either parent and that respective parent is also affected.

Autosomal recessive—Disorders that can affect either sex in which abnormal genes must be inherited on the chromosomes from both the mother and the father. Both parents therefore are carriers.

Autosome—*See* Chromosome.

Breathing tolerance—Said to be limited when acute respiratory distress and blood gas derangements occur within minutes or seconds of discontinuing ventilator use.

Bulbar muscles—Muscles located in the head and neck that permit speech, swallowing, and coughing. This include the oropharyngeal (mouth and throat) muscles.

Cannula—Tubing entering the nose or mouth to deliver air or supplemental oxygen.

Carbon dioxide (CO_2)—The gas in the blood that reflects the ability of the inspiratory muscles to ventilate the lungs. Blood carbon dioxide levels increase (hypercapnia) when the lungs are under (hypo-) ventilated and decrease (hypocapnia) when the lungs are over (hyper-) ventilated.

Cardiomyopathy—Weakness of the heart muscle caused by muscle pathology affecting the heart.

Chromosome—A long string of connected genes. Every cell has 48 chromosomes, 46 autosomes, and 2 sex chromosomes, either 2 X chromosomes for females or an X and a Y chromosome for males.

CO_2—Carbon dioxide.

Compliance (pulmonary compliance)—Essentially, the elasticity of the lungs that decreases when one cannot take or does not receive deep breaths, leading to loss of lung tissue and lung stiffening.

Congenital—Medical conditions with which one is born.

Contracture—Rigid shortening (tightness) of muscles and other soft tissues caused by muscle weakness at any joint; the side with the weaker muscles is stretched and the joint has decreased range of motion.

Cor pulmonale—Failure of the right side of the heart due to decreased blood oxygen levels (hypoxia) and increased blood carbon dioxide levels (hypercapnia) from lung underventilation.

Corticosteroids—Anti-inflammatory steroid medications that have been helpful in treating Duchenne muscular dystrophy, multiple sclerosis, myasthenia gravis, and polymyositis. Unfortunately, these medications also cause weight gain; adversely affect the immune system, bone development, metabolism, and protein synthesis; can alter mood; and cause intestinal disturbances, excessive hair growth, and cataracts.

Continuous positive airway pressure (CPAP)—Continuous pressure applied through a mask covering the nose, mouth, or nose and mouth that acts as a splint to keep the otherwise obstructed upper airway open and acts to expand the lungs but does not directly help one breathe. This is not a method of ventilatory or inspiratory muscle assistance.

CPAP—*See* Continuous positive airway pressure.

CPAP masks—Nasal interfaces for the delivery of CPAP or nasal ventilation for ventilatory assistance.

Dorsiflexion—Upward rotation or extension of the ankle.

Dysarthria—Difficulty speaking.

Dysphagia—Difficulty swallowing.

Dyspnea—Shortness of breath.

End-tidal carbon dioxide—The concentration of carbon dioxide in the exhaled air. It serves as an estimate of blood carbon dioxide levels.

End-tidal carbon dioxide levels—The concentration or partial pressure of carbon dioxide in the last bit of air that one exhales that closely reflects the partial pressure of carbon dioxide in the arterial blood.

Electrodiagnosis—A study of nerve conduction velocities and muscle membrane stability that can be helpful in differentiating muscular from neurologic conditions and diagnosing myasthenia gravis.

Fasciculations—Muscle twitching.

Gastroesophageal reflux—Foods regurgitated back up into the esophagus that cause choking or increased airway secretions.

Gastrostomy tube—A tube placed into the stomach for direct delivery of food for people who cannot take food safely by mouth.

Glossopharyngeal breathing (GPB)—The "gulping" of air into the lungs to permit ventilator-free breathing or to provide maximal insufflations (deep lung volumes) without need for a ventilator or other air delivery system.

Glottis—The opening between the vocal cords at the upper orifice of the larynx; the mouth of the windpipe.

Hypercapnia—Increased blood carbon dioxide levels due to inability of the breathing muscles to adequately ventilate the lungs.

Hypoxia—Decreased blood oxygen levels due to increased blood carbon dioxide levels, mucus plugging of the airways, or lung disease such as pneumonia.

Inspiratory capacity (predicted)—The volume of air that one should be able to inhale as a function of age, sex, and height. For example, most adult males have predicted inspiratory capacities of over 3000 ml.

Insufflation—Providing greater volumes of air than one can breathe in with one's own inspiratory muscles.

Insufflation leakage—Air delivered from a ventilator that leaks out of the nose or mouth rather than entering the lungs.

Insufflation-exsufflation—A technique whereby a device is used to provide a deep volume of air to the lungs (insufflation) immediately followed by a forced expiration (exsufflation) to expel airway secretions.

Intermittent positive-pressure breathing (IPPB)—The delivery of deep insufflations to more fully expand the lungs.

Intermittent positive-pressure ventilation (IPPV)—A form of inspiratory muscle aid or ventilatory assistance provided by delivering air to the lungs via the mouth, nose, mouth-and-nose, or indwelling tracheostomy tube.

Intubation—Passage of a tube via the nose (nasotracheal tube) or via the mouth (orotracheal tube), through the throat and larynx (translaryngeally), and into the trachea for ventilatory assistance and airway suctioning.

IPPB—*See* Intermittent positive-pressure breathing.

IPPV—*See* Intermittent positive-pressure ventilation.

Mechanically assisted coughing (MAC)—A combination of mechanical insufflation-exsufflation and manually assisted coughing with an exsufflation timed abdominal thrust.

Mask leakage—Air leakage from a ventilator-delivered volume caused by a loosely fitting or leaky interface.

Maximum insufflation capacity—The maximum volume of air that can be mechanically delivered to the patient's lungs and held by the patient in the lungs.

Mechanical insufflation-exsufflation—A mechanical method to create 10 liters per second of expiratory flow to clear airway secretions (*see* Insufflation-exsufflation).

Narcosis—Coma or death resulting from high levels of carbon dioxide in the blood, most often due to an inability to adequately ventilate the lungs to eliminate the carbon dioxide that the body continuously produces.

Nasogastric tube—A feeding tube passed through the nose and esophagus and into the stomach.

Negative pressure body ventilators—Body ventilators that work by creating negative pressure around the chest and abdomen to cause air to enter the nose and mouth to ventilate the lungs.

Neuropathy—Any general anatomic, biochemical, or electrical disorder of nerves.

O_2—Oxygen.

Oximeter—A device that can continuously measure the oxyhemoglobin saturation of the blood.

Oxygen—A gas needed by the body's metabolic processes. Oxygen blood levels are decreased by underventilation (hypercapnia), by airway mucus plugging, and by lung disease.

Oxyhemoglobin saturation—Oxyhemoglobin is the main oxygen-carrying protein in the blood, and normally it is 95% or more saturated with oxygen.

Pectus excavatum—Failure of the normal development of the chest and rib cage due to an inability to take deep breaths during childhood. The breast bone has a caved in appearance.

Peak cough flows—The maximum flows that can be generated while coughing with or without assistance.

PEEP—*See* Positive end-expiratory pressure.

Positive end-expiratory pressure (PEEP)—Pressure given at the end of a mechanically assisted breath.

Respirator—*See* Ventilator.

Respiratory failure—Acute decompensation in pulmonary function due to intrinsic lung or chronic obstructive pulmonary disease (COPD) with deterioration in arterial blood gases to pH levels of 7.25 or less. Hypoxia cannot be resolved simply by ventilator use or assisted coughing.

Respiratory insufficiency—Hypoxia in the presence of normal or low blood carbon dioxide levels. The hypoxia cannot be reversed by normalizing lung ventilation, normalizing carbon dioxide levels, or using assisted coughing to clear bronchial mucus plugs.

Spinal muscular atrophy—An inherited disease of peripheral nerves (anterior horn cells in the spinal cord) that has been separated arbitrarily into types 1 through 5 based on perceived onset of weakness.

Spirometer—A device used for measuring volumes of air such as with vital capacity measurements.

Stenosis—Narrowing of a passage. For example, the narrowing of the trachea caused by complications of translaryngeal intubation or an indwelling tracheostomy tube.

Suctioning—The passage of a catheter into the airways to aspirate out airway secretions and other debris.

Tidal volume—The volume of air one inhales during one normal breath. Measured in milliliters.

Trachea—The wind pipe.

Tracheostomy—A surgical hole (stoma) that creates a passage through the neck to the windpipe (trachea) for placement of a tube (tracheostomy tube) through which ventilatory support and airway suctioning can be done.

Ventilator—A device that intermittently provides negative or positive pressure to assist or substitute for the inspiratory muscle function needed for breathing (sometimes called a "respirator").

Ventilation—*See* Alveolar ventilation.

Ventilatory assistance—Ventilator use by patients with periods of 12 or more hours of breathing tolerance.

Ventilatory failure—The inability to sustain one's respiration without ventilator use.

Ventilatory insufficiency—The presence of hypercapnia not caused by intrinsic lung disease or irreversible upper airway collapse.

Ventilatory support—Ventilator use by patients with no significant breathing tolerance.

Vital capacity—The maximum volume of air that one can inhale then blow through a device (spirometer). Measured in milliliters.

X-linked—An inherited trait or disease that generally affects only boys.

Index

Page numbers in **boldface type** indicate complete chapters.